Cardiothoracic Surgery

Editor

DANIEL G. CUADRADO

SURGICAL CLINICS
OF NORTH AMERICA

www.surgical.theclinics.com

Consulting Editor
RONALD F. MARTIN

June 2022 • Volume 102 • Number 3

ELSEVIER

1600 John F. Kennedy Boulevard • Suite 1800 • Philadelphia, Pennsylvania, 19103-2899

http://www.surgical.theclinics.com

SURGICAL CLINICS OF NORTH AMERICA Volume 102, Number 3
June 2022 ISSN 0039–6109, ISBN-13: 978-0-323-91965-4

Editor: John Vassallo, j.vassallo@elsevier.com
Developmental Editor: Arlene Campos

Surgical Clinics of North America (ISSN 0039–6109) is published bimonthly by Elsevier Inc., 360 Park Avenue South, New York, NY 10010-1710. Months of publication are February, April, June, August, October, and December. Business and Editorial Offices: 1600 John F. Kennedy Blvd., Suite 1800, Philadelphia, PA 19103-2899. Periodicals postage paid at New York, NY and additional mailing offices. Subscription prices are $456.00 per year for US individuals, $1240.00 per year for US institutions, $100.00 per year for US & Canadian students and residents, $547.00 per year for Canadian individuals, $1283.00 per year for Canadian institutions, $552.00 for international individuals, $1283.00 per year for international institutions and $250.00 per year for foreign students/residents. To receive student/resident rate, orders must be accompanied by name of affiliated institution, date of term, and the *signature* of program/residency coordinator on institution letterhead. Orders will be billed at individual rate until proof of status is received. Foreign air speed delivery is included in all *Clinics* subscription prices. All prices are subject to change without notice. POSTMASTER: Send address changes to *Surgical Clinics*, Elsevier Health Sciences Division, Subscription Customer Service, 3251 Riverport Lane, Maryland Heights, MO 63043. **Customer Service (orders, claims, online, change of address): Telephone: 1-800-654-2452 (U.S. and Canada); 314-447-8871 (outside U.S. and Canada). Fax: 314-447-8029. E-mail: journalscustomerservice-usa@elsevier.com (for print support); journalsonlinesupport-usa@elsevier.com (for online support).**

Reprints. For copies of 100 or more, of articles in this publication, please contact the Commercial Reprints Department, Elsevier Inc., 360 Park Avenue South, New York, New York 10010-1710. Tel. 212-633-3874, Fax: 212-633-3820, E-mail: reprints@elsevier.com.

Surgical Clinics of North America is also published in Spanish by McGraw-Hill Interamericana Editores S.A., P.O. Box 5-237 06500 Mexico D.F. Mexico; and in Portuguese by Interlivros Edicoes Ltda., Rua Comandante Coelho 1085, CEP 21250, Rio de Janeiro, Brazil; and in Greek by Paschalidis Medical Publications, Athens Greece.

Surgical Clinics of North America is covered in *MEDLINE/PubMed (Index Medicus)*, *EMBASE/Excerpta Medica*, *Current Contents/Clinical Medicine*, *Current Contents/Life Sciences*, *Science Citation Index*, and *ISI/BIOMED*.

Contributors

CONSULTING EDITOR

RONALD F. MARTIN, MD, FACS
Colonel (Retired), United States Army Reserve, Department of General Surgery, Pullman
Regional Hospital and Clinic Network, Pullman, Washington

EDITOR

DANIEL G. CUADRADO, MD, FACS, FCCP
Chief, Cardiothoracic Surgery, Madigan Army Medical Center, Joint Base
Lewis-McChord, Washington

AUTHORS

JARED L. ANTEVIL, MD
Cardiothoracic Surgeon, Division of Cardiothoracic Surgery, Veterans Affairs Medical
Center, Washington, DC

SAMEER K. AVASARALA, MD
Division of Pulmonary, Critical Care and Sleep Medicine, University Hospitals – Case
Western Reserve University School of Medicine, Cleveland, Ohio

JUSTIN D. BLASBERG, MD, MPH
Associate Professor, Division of Thoracic Surgery, Yale School of Medicine, New Haven,
Connecticut

RAPHAEL BUENO, MD
Chief, Division of Thoracic and Cardiac Surgery, Brigham and Women's Hospital, Boston,
Massachusetts

MIA DEBARROS, MD
Thoracic Surgeon, Thoracic Surgery, Madigan Army Medical Center, Tacoma,
Washington

ANDREW P. DHANASOPON, MD
Assistant Professor, Division of Thoracic Surgery, Yale School of Medicine, New Haven,
Connecticut

DAVID M. DUDZINSKI, MD
Director, Cardiac Intensive Care Unit, Assistant Professor of Medicine, Department of
Cardiology, Heart Center Intensive Care Unit, Massachusetts General Hospital, Boston,
Massachusetts

JOHN P. DUGGAN, MD
Resident in General Surgery, Department of Surgery, Walter Reed National Military
Medical Center, Bethesda, Maryland

ANDREW FRANCIS, MD
General Surgery Department, Madigan Army Medical Center, Tacoma, Washington

CAROLINE M. GODFREY, MD
Postdoctoral Fellow, Department of Thoracic Surgery, Vanderbilt University Medical Center, Nashville, Tennessee

ERIC L. GROGAN, MD, MPH
Associate Professor, Section of Thoracic Surgery, Tennessee Valley VA Healthcare System; Associate Professor, Department of Thoracic Surgery, Vanderbilt University Medical Center, Nashville, Tennessee

STEVEN J. HOFF, MD, FACS, FHRS
Orlando Health Heart and Vascular Institute, Orlando, Florida

JEFFERY CHAD JOHNSON, MD
Department of Surgery, Division of Cardiothoracic Surgery, Naval Medical Readiness and Training Center Portsmouth, Portsmouth, Virginia

BAHIRATHAN KRISHNADASAN, MD, FACS
Medical Director, Cardiothoracic Surgery, Chief of Surgery, St. Joseph Medical Center, Tacoma, Washington

JOHN KUCKELMAN, DO
Thoracic Surgery Resident, Division of Thoracic and Cardiac Surgery, Brigham and Women's Hospital, Boston, Massachusetts

ERIC S. LAMBRIGHT, MD
Associate Professor, Department of Thoracic Surgery, Vanderbilt University Medical Center, Nashville, Tennessee

HANNAH N. MARMOR, MD
Postdoctoral Fellow, Department of Thoracic Surgery, Vanderbilt University Medical Center, Nashville, Tennessee

VINCENT J. MASE JR., MD
Assistant Professor, Division of Thoracic Surgery, Yale School of Medicine, New Haven, Connecticut

AUNDREA L. OLIVER, MD, FACS
Assistant Professor, Department of Cardiovascular Sciences, Brody School of Medicine, East Carolina University, East Carolina Heart Institute, Greenville, North California

ASISHANA A. OSHO, MD, MPH
Cardiac Surgeon, Division of Cardiac Surgery, Massachusetts General Hospital, Boston, Massachusetts

ALEX S. PETERS, MD
Resident in General Surgery, Department of Surgery, Walter Reed National Military Medical Center, Bethesda, Maryland

BEAU PREY, MD
General Surgery Department, Madigan Army Medical Center, Tacoma, Washington

OTIS B. RICKMAN, DO, FCCP
Director of Interventional Pulmonology, Associate Professor, Department of Internal Medicine and Thoracic Surgery, Vanderbilt University Medical Center, Nashville, Tennessee

RAFAEL SANTANA-DAVILA, MD
Associate Professor of Medicine, Fred Hutch Cancer Center, University of Washington, Seattle, Washington

ERIC FRANCIS SULAVA, MD
Department of Emergency Medicine, Naval Medical Readiness and Training Center Portsmouth, Portsmouth, Virginia

GREGORY D. TRACHIOTIS, MD
Professor of Surgery and Biomedical Engineering, George Washington University; Department of Surgery, George Washington University Hospital; Cardiothoracic Surgeon and Chief, Division of Cardiology, Cardiothoracic Surgery and Heart Center, Washington DC Veterans Affairs Medical Center; Washington, DC

JAMES WILLIAMS, MD
General Surgery Department, Madigan Army Medical Center, Tacoma, Washington

RAFAEL SANTIAGA-DAVILA, MD
Associate Professor of Medicine, Fred Hutch Cancer Center, University of Washington, Seattle, Washington

ERIC FRANCIS SULAVA, MD
Department of Emergency Medicine, Navy Medical Readiness and Training Center, Portsmouth, Portsmouth, Virginia

GREGORY D. TRACHIOTIS, MD
Professor of Surgery and Biomedical Engineering, George Washington University, Department of Surgery, George Washington University Hospital, Cardiothoracic Surgeon and Chief, Division of Cardiology, Cardiothoracic Surgery and Heart Center, Washington DC Veterans Affairs Medical Center, Washington DC

JAMES WILLIAMS, MD
General Surgery Department, Madigan Army Medical Center, Tacoma, Washington

Contents

Foreword: Cardiothoracic Surgery   **xiii**

Ronald F. Martin

Preface: Cardiothoracic Surgery: Present and Future   **xv**

Daniel G. Cuadrado

Lung Cancer: Epidemiology and Screening   **335**

Aundrea L. Oliver

> Lung cancer remains the leading cause of cancer mortality in the United States and Worldwide. Incidence and mortality have been on the decline in the United States, while worldwide cases continue to increase. Risk factor modification and screening are critical to improving survival in patients with lung cancer. Identifying at-risk populations for access to care and screening programs will improve overall outcomes. Understanding environmental and carcinogenic sources are integral to public health policy and education. Innovations in population health and translational research will be essential in the future to improve lung cancer survival.

Extended Resections for Lung Cancer   **345**

John Kuckelman, Mia Debarros, and Raphael Bueno

> This article briefly reviews the literature supporting the practice of extended pulmonary resection followed by a comprehensive description of the indications, workup, and technique commonly used for patients requiring extended pulmonary resections for advance lung cancers. The article also provides up-to-date advances in the field that have aided in the safe and effective practice of extended pulmonary resections.

Evaluation and Interventional Management of Cardiac Dysrhythmias   **365**

Steven J. Hoff

> This article focuses on the guideline-directed evaluation and management of cardiac dysrhythmias, particularly as they are important to the practice of a noncardiac surgeon. The focus is on atrial fibrillation (AF) as the most common arrhythmia encountered by surgeons. The authors discuss the importance of AF as a risk factor for perioperative morbidity and mortality. They pay particular attention to topics such as postoperative AF and options for its acute treatment and perioperative anticoagulation management. They discuss nonpharmacologic left atrial appendage management and nonpharmacologic AF management, including catheter-based therapy, surgical-based therapy, and hybrid therapies.

Endobronchial Therapies for Diagnosis, Staging, and Treatment of Lung Cancer   393

Sameer K. Avasarala and Otis B. Rickman

Lung cancer is the leading cause of cancer-related death worldwide and within the United States. Although evidence-based screening has been shown to reduce cancer-related mortality, the late-stage presentation remains common. Bronchoscopy has been proven to be an essential tool in the diagnosis and management of lung cancer. Basic and advanced diagnostic bronchoscopic techniques offer a minimally invasive modality for diagnosing and staging patients with lung cancer. In patients with malignant endotracheobronchial disease, therapeutic bronchoscopy (flexible or rigid) is a safe procedure that palliates symptoms such as dyspnea and hemoptysis. In this article, we review the various endobronchial tools and strategies essential for the management of lung cancer.

Surgical Management of Pneumothorax and Pleural Space Disease   413

Andrew P. Dhanasopon, Justin D. Blasberg, and Vincent J. Mase Jr.

Pleural space diseases constitute a wide range of benign and malignant conditions, including pneumothorax, pleural effusion and empyema, chylothorax, pleural-based tumors, and mesothelioma. The focus of this article is the surgical management of the 2 most common pleural disorders seen in modern thoracic surgery practice: spontaneous pneumothorax and empyema.

Interventional Therapies for Acute Pulmonary Embolism   429

Asishana A. Osho and David M. Dudzinski

Pulmonary embolism (PE) is the third leading cause of cardiovascular mortality in the United States. Unfortunately, significant gaps exist in outcome data around many interventional therapies, a fact that is reflected in the low strength of management recommendations found in consensus major society guidelines. In addition to careful risk stratification, therapeutic anticoagulation generally should be an early part of PE management in all cases. For patients presenting with acute high-risk PE or intermediate-risk PE with higher risk features, consideration should be given to systemic thrombolysis after careful evaluation for potential bleeding complications. In patients with contraindications to systemic thrombolysis, failure of this therapy, or significant ongoing cardiopulmonary distress, consideration should be given to interventional therapies like catheter-directed lysis, catheter-directed embolectomy, surgical embolectomy, and mechanical circulatory support. Until more robust comparative outcome data are put forward, pulmonary embolism response teams (PERT) should be considered for multi-disciplinary patient evaluation and management.

Management of Coronary Artery Disease   449

Eric Francis Sulava and Jeffery Chad Johnson

This article reviews the surgical management of coronary artery disease (CAD). The authors cover the background, presentation, diagnosis, heart team evaluation, and development of treatment strategies tailored to individual patients with significant CAD. Special attention is given to conduit selection and configuration as well as alternative revascularization approaches that differ from traditional coronary artery bypass grafting.

Evaluation and Treatment of Massive Hemoptysis 465

Beau Prey, Andrew Francis, James Williams, and Bahirathan Krishnadasan

> Massive hemoptysis is appropriately defined as life-threatening hemoptysis that causes airway obstruction, respiratory failure, and/or hypotension. Patients with this condition die from asphyxiation, not hemorrhagic shock. Any patient who presents with life-threatening hemoptysis requires immediate treatment to secure the airway and stabilize hemodynamics. Early activation and coordinated response from a multidisciplinary team is critical. Once the airway is secure and appropriate resuscitation is initiated, priorities are to localize the source of the bleeding and gain hemorrhage control. Nonsurgical control of hemorrhage is superior to surgery in the acute situation.

Minimally Invasive and Sublobar Resections for Lung Cancer 483

Caroline M. Godfrey, Hannah N. Marmor, Eric S. Lambright, and Eric L. Grogan

> Current guidelines for non–small cell lung cancer (NSCLC) recommend segmentectomy over lobectomy for patients with poor pulmonary reserve or for peripheral nodules less than or equal to 2 cm with adenocarcinoma in situ histology, greater than 50% ground-glass opacity on computed tomography, or radiologic doubling time greater than or equal to 400 days. However, emerging data suggest oncologic equivalence of segmentectomy to lobectomy for less than or equal to 2 cm, peripheral stage IA NSCLC regardless of histologic type or radiographic findings.

Chemo and Immuno-Therapeutic Options for Non-small Cell Lung Cancer Lung Cancer 493

Rafael Santana-Davila

> Over the last decade, the use of immune checkpoint inhibitors (ICI) has dramatically changed the treatment paradigm and outcome of patients with non-small cell lung cancer (NSCLC) across all stages of the disease. In this review, we provide a concise history of the use of ICIs in the treatment of NSCLC and review discuss the data behind the different indications.

Epidemiology of Coronary Artery Disease 499

John P. Duggan, Alex S. Peters, Gregory D. Trachiotis, and Jared L. Antevil

> Although the mortality of coronary artery disease (CAD) has declined over recent decades, CAD remains the leading cause of death in the United States (US) and presents a significant economic burden. Epidemiologic studies have identified numerous risk factors for CAD. Some risk factors–including smoking, hypertension, dyslipidemia, and physical inactivity–are decreasing within the US population while others, including advanced age, diabetes, and obesity are increasing. The most significant historic advances in CAD therapy were the development of coronary artery bypass grafting (CABG), percutaneous coronary intervention (PCI), and lipid-lowering medications. Contemporary management of CAD includes primary and secondary prevention via medical management and revascularization when appropriate based on best available evidence. Despite the increasing prevalence of CAD nationwide, there has been a steady decline

in the number of CABGs and PCIs performed in the US for the past decade. Patients with CABG are becoming older and with more comorbid conditions, although mortality associated with CABG has remained steady.

Epidemiology of Valvular Heart Disease   517

Alex S. Peters, John P. Duggan, Gregory D. Trachiotis, and Jared L. Antevil

Acquired diseases of the aortic and mitral valves are the most common cause of morbidity and mortality among Valvular heart diseases. Aortic stenosis (AS) is increasing in incidence in the United States (4,43 US), driven largely by an aging demographic. Aortic valve replacement is the only effective treatment of AS and has a dramatic mortality benefit. Mitral valve regurgitation (MR) is the most common form of valvular heart disease (VHD) in the US, whereby MR is most often the result of mitral valve pro-lapse; rheumatic heart disease (RHD) is a more common etiology of MR in underdeveloped countries. interventions for MR in the US are increasing.

SURGICAL CLINICS
OF NORTH AMERICA

FORTHCOMING ISSUES

AUGUST 2022
A Surgeon's Guide to Sarcomas and Other Soft Tissue Tumors
John M. Kane III, *Editor*

OCTOBER 2022
Pediatric Surgery
John D. Horton, *Editor*

DECEMBER 2022
Management of Benign Breast Disease
Melisa Kaptanian, *Editor*

RECENT ISSUES

APRIL 2022
Head and Neck Surgery
Brian J. Mitchell and Kyle Tubbs, *Editors*

FEBRUARY 2022
Surgical Critical Care
Brett H. Waibel, *Editor*

DECEMBER 2021
Controversies in General Surgery
Sean J. Langenfeld, *Editor*

SERIES OF RELATED INTEREST

Advances in Surgery
https://www.advancessurgery.com/
Surgical Oncology Clinics
https://www.surgonc.theclinics.com/
Thoracic Surgery Clinics
http://www.thoracic.theclinics.com/

Foreword

Cardiothoracic Surgery

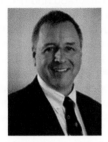

Ronald F. Martin, MD, FACS
Consulting Editor

When I was a very junior resident, one of my staff surgical mentors told me that if I ever had a profoundly sick patient and wasn't sure what to do, just treat them as I would a postoperative cardiac patient. That was some of the best advice I ever received. My very first rotation as a surgical intern was on the cardiothoracic service. To be sure, the idea of covering a large volume of patients in the ICU, many of whom had vast arrays of tubes and monitoring devices with which I had only passing familiarity, was daunting to say the least. However, in those days where "on-boarding" largely consisted of a quick push into the deep end of the pool, it was a fantastic chance to learn at an accelerated rate. At first one realized that all the gadgets and devices made a great deal of sense once you learned the basics. After becoming comfortable, sometimes perhaps too comfortable, with the large-volume data analytics, one then had to learn when the numbers did not tell the whole story, and going back to good clinical skills and pattern recognition was essential. Still, getting a handle on those basic functions and how to assess them in real time was excellent training for taking care of every other kind of patient who might be struggling.

In previous issues of our series that we have presented on critically ill patients, I have written that there are three basic concepts that drive our ability to keep profoundly ill people alive: air goes in and out, blood goes around and around, and oxygen is good. As overly simplified as that is, it remains fundamentally true at most levels. As with many parts of life, the basics of this paradigm can be learned in short periods of time, but even a lifetime will only let you approach mastery.

When Dr Cuadrado and I first discussed this issue of the *Surgical Clinics*, we wanted to assure that we covered topics that could be useful to all manner of surgeons as well as nonsurgeons in the care of complicated patients. The goal was to provide a concise resource for understanding the evaluation of cardiopulmonary performance under more routine conditions as well as updating people on interventional capabilities for either cardiac or pulmonary dysfunction as stand-alone problems or in the setting of

Surg Clin N Am 102 (2022) xiii–xiv
https://doi.org/10.1016/j.suc.2022.03.003
0039-6109/22/© 2022 Published by Elsevier Inc.

other clinical maladies. By necessity, there is considerable overlap in the topics covered here or covered in issues we have created on surgical critical care or emergency care of other types. However, since our goal at the *Surgical Clinics* series is to put clinical content in context, it is vital to look at these topics through the varied lenses of all of our colleagues.

This issue on cardiothoracic surgery that is compiled by Dr Cuadrado and his colleagues is an exceptional collection of articles that address the essential components of cardiac and pulmonary function as well as give us a broad overview of treating the dysfunction that may arise in those organs. We are indebted to them as a group, and I am indebted to them personally. Many of our contributors to this issue are not only members of our surgical community but also members of our military community. I have had the opportunity to work alongside many of them personally in varying capacities. They are extraordinary people who give selflessly to care for our service members and their families. We should all be grateful for their personal sacrifices as well as the sacrifices endured by their families.

No matter what kind of physician, surgeon, or caregiver one is, each patient we care for needs the core elements of cardiopulmonary function to be viable. That vital core cardiopulmonary component can and will falter, frequently at the worst time and frequently without much warning. Having an excellent grounding in these systems as a baseline will be quite comforting in times of unexpected trouble. As I stated earlier, one can learn the basics quickly, but mastery takes time—lots of time. Beginning clinicians tend to first look at the monitors; more seasoned clinicians tend to look first at the patient. I would submit the latter approach is adopted by those who have honed their ability to recognize more complex patterns. That experience comes from developing a good foundation of understanding followed by long-term correlations between the numeric data stream and clinical observations. We hope that this issue of the *Surgical Clinics* helps our readers in their quest of mastery.

Ronald F. Martin, MD, FACS
Colonel (retired), United States Army
Department of General Surgery
Pullman Surgical Associates
Pullman Regional Hospital and Clinic Network
825 SE Bishop Boulevard, Suite 130
Pullman, WA 99163, USA

E-mail address:
rfmcescna@gmail.com

Preface

Cardiothoracic Surgery: Present and Future

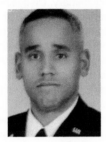

Daniel G. Cuadrado MD, FACS, FCCP
Editor

Interventional treatments to manage diseases of the chest have existed since the time of Hippocrates. An understanding of the role of tracheal intubation and thoracotomy for the treatment of empyema thoracis dates back to antiquity.[1] Francisco Romero performed the first pericardial window in 1801 to relieve a symptomatic pericardial effusion.[2] Following John Gibbon's repair of an atrial septal defect using cardiopulmonary bypass in 1953, the world entered a new era of cardiac surgery.[3] The pace of innovations in the discipline of cardiothoracic surgery rivals that seen in any field of medicine.

Furthermore, diseases of the chest present a significant burden to US and global health. Based on data from the American Cancer Society, over 250,000 cases of lung cancer were diagnosed in 2021 in the United States. Lung cancer remains the leading cause of cancer death irrespective of gender.[4] Heart disease remains the leading cause of death across gender, racial, and ethnic groups, accounting for 1 in every 4 deaths in the United States.[5] Significant disparities exist among certain groups, which are discussed in the following articles.

Along with significant innovations in the field of cardiothoracic surgery, there has been a paradigm shift in the surgical training pathway. Accreditation Council for Graduate Medical Education general surgery training no longer requires experience in cardiac surgery. The minimum requirement in thoracic surgical caseload for a

Surg Clin N Am 102 (2022) xv–xvii
https://doi.org/10.1016/j.suc.2022.03.002
0039-6109/22/© 2022 Published by Elsevier Inc.

surgical.theclinics.com

general surgical resident is 20 cases, 5 of which must be performed via thoracotomy. Over the past 10 years, there has been a 30% decrease in the number of traditional cardiothoracic residency programs with a shift to integrated (I-6) programs.[6] In total, over 97% of training slots are filled, which is a significant increase from 68% in 2008.[6] These I-6 programs have shifted the decision to pursue cardiothoracic surgery to earlier in medical training.

Simultaneously, as the pace of innovation increases, the management of cardiothoracic disease has become increasingly complex and multidisciplinary. Discussions on the management of coronary artery disease, valvular heart disease, and thoracic oncology now frequently fall to the Heart Team or Tumor Board. Surgeons in-training now choose from either the cardiothoracic or general thoracic training pathways. Although initial certification is accomplished via a common examination, subsequent maintenance of certification allows for differentiation based on a predominantly cardiac or thoracic practice. As the respective fields continue to advance at unprecedented rates, further divergence into two distinct fields may eventually be required.

As with the changing nature of cardiothoracic surgical training, the tools of the trade are ever evolving. The skills of open and thoracoscopic surgery are now further complemented by endovascular, endobronchial, and robotic technologies and techniques. Full-spectrum cardiac and thoracic surgical care now requires this understanding and a partnership with our colleagues in cardiology, pulmonology, and interventional radiology. As medicine continues to develop a deeper understanding of the biology of cancer, surgeons must now keep pace with the ever-changing role of chemotherapy, radiation therapy, and immunotherapy. As leaders on multidisciplinary teams, surgeons must be aware of the full spectrum of treatment options available for the care of our patients.

The future of cardiothoracic surgery has never been brighter. The following articles covers a broad spectrum of the disease processes encountered by cardiothoracic surgeons. Although not all-encompassing, the authors present an expert perspective on the burden of disease, management, and advanced interventional techniques. Both benign and malignant diseases of the thorax affect patients throughout the health care system, and a familiarity with their treatment is important for all surgical disciplines. In this unprecedented time of health care upheaval from the COVID-19 pandemic, I would like to commend the authors on their resiliency and perseverance.

Daniel G. Cuadrado, MD, FACS, FCCP
COL, US Army
Department of Surgery
9040 Jackson Avenue
Madigan Army Medical Center
Joint Base Lewis-McChord, WA 98431, USA

E-mail address:
daniel.cuadrado2.mil@mail.mil

REFERENCES

1. Tsoucalas G, Sgantzos M. Hippocrates (ca 460-375 bc), introducing thoracotomy combined with a tracheal intubation for the parapneumonic pleural effusions and empyema thoracis. Surg Innov 2016;23(6):642–3.
2. Aris AMD. Francisco Romero, the first heart surgeon. Ann Thorac Surg 1997;64(3): 870–1.
3. Cohn LH. Fifty years of open-heart surgery. Circulation 2003;107(17):2168–70.

4. Siegel RL, Miller KD, Fuchs HE, et al. Cancer statistics, 2021. CA Cancer J Clin 2021;71(1):7–33.
5. Virani SS, Alonso A, Aparicio HJ, et al. Heart disease and stroke statistics—2021 update: a report from the American Heart Association. Circulation 2021;143(8): e254–743.
6. Bui J, Bennett WC, Long J, et al. Recent trends in cardiothoracic surgery training: data from the National Resident Matching Program. J Surg Educ 2021;78(2): 672–8.

Lung Cancer
Epidemiology and Screening

Aundrea L. Oliver, MD

KEYWORDS

• Lung cancer • Epidemiology • Disparities • Screening

KEY POINTS

- Lung cancer remains the leading cause of cancer mortality in the United States and worldwide
- Despite improvement in incidence and mortality, significant disparities in outcomes remain prevalent
- Tobacco smoke is the primary cause of lung cancer, followed by radon and other environmental factors
- Lung cancer screening has a clear mortality benefit and further work is required to improve participation by eligible individuals

INTRODUCTION

Despite a consistent decline in incidence and mortality for more than a decade, lung cancer continues to rank as the leading cause of cancer mortality.[1,2] In incidence it is second only to prostate and breast for men and women respectively. In stark contrast it accounts for over 20% of the cancer deaths annually, more than the burden of prostate, breast, and colon cancers combined. This mortality has two main drivers, late stage at initial diagnosis and poor overall survival. There have been major strides in lung cancer therapeutics and awareness; however, the burden of lung cancer remains significant in the United States and worldwide.

Epidemiology

In 2021, it is estimated that there will be 235,760 new lung cancer diagnoses and 131,880 lung cancer deaths in the United States.[2] The rate of new cases has declined by an average of 2% per year since 2000, arriving at approximately 53.1 per 100,000 persons in 2018. The death rate has decreased even more dramatically at an average of 4% per year over the same interval with a current estimated death rate of 36.7 per 100,000 persons. **Fig. 1**

Department of Cardiovascular Sciences, Brody School of Medicine, East Carolina University, East Carolina Heart Institute, 115 Heart Drive Mailstop 651, Greenville, NC 27834, USA
E-mail address: oliverau15@ecu.edu

Surg Clin N Am 102 (2022) 335–344
https://doi.org/10.1016/j.suc.2021.12.001
0039-6109/22/© 2021 Elsevier Inc. All rights reserved.

surgical.theclinics.com

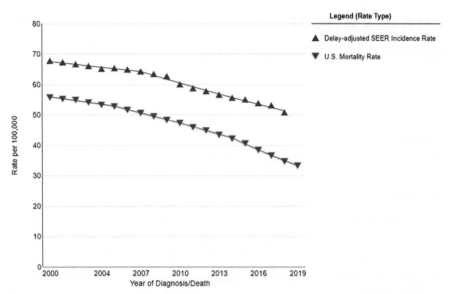

Fig. 1. Lung and bronchus stage distribution of SEER Incidence cases, 2009 to 2018 By Race/Ethnicity, Both Sexes, All Ages. (*Created by* https://seer.cancer.gov/explorer on Fri Oct 15, 2021)

The lifetime risk of lung cancer for the average individual in the United States is 6.1% or approximately 1 in 16 people. In 2018 it was estimated that over 500,000 individuals were living with lung cancer, the majority (55%) of which were women. Although men are more likely to have lung cancer, the incidence of lung cancer is decreasing more slowly among women in comparison to men. It is the leading cause of death for women aged 40 to 80 and men 60 to 80 years of age.[1] Lung cancer remains diagnosed at a relatively late stage, with most of the new diagnoses presenting with advanced disease. This directly affects survival with a steep drop in survival between the local and regional burden of disease. **Figs. 2** and **3**

Globally, lung cancer incidence is on the rise and given patterns of tobacco use throughout the world we expect this trend to continue. The most recently reported global data from 2018 indicates that lung cancer was the most commonly diagnosed cancer with 2,093,900 new cases, and likewise the most common cause of cancer death at 1,761,000 deaths globally. Of distribution throughout the world, lung cancer is the leading cancer diagnosis in most of the Asian continent and Eastern Europe for men, and the leading cause of cancer death for men in the same region. Women in those regions are more likely to be diagnosed with breast cancer, but more likely to die of lung cancer in most of Europe, and Eastern Asian continent.[3]

Disparities

A great deal of focus has shifted in recent years to broadening our view of social determinants of health beyond census-based descriptors of race or socioeconomic status. Historically, qualitative data have been limited to race and binary gender. The medical community has come to understand forces which dictate and influence health and access are far more complex than previously understood. However, these historical categories can prove a starting point to look at disease among population groups over decades. Within these constructs, we find that the rate of new

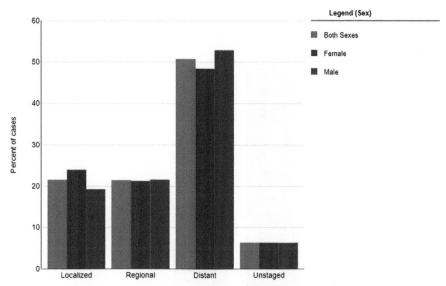

Fig. 2. Lung and bronchus stage distribution of SEER Incidence cases, 2009 to 2018 By Sex, All Races (includes Hispanic), All Ages. (*Created by* https://seer.cancer.gov/explorer on Fri Oct 15, 2021)

cases is highest among black men, followed by white men and Asian/pacific islander men. There is a shift in the death rate, while black men are most likely to die of lung cancer followed by white men, Native American men and women are more likely to die than Asian men or women despite the lower incidence of disease among Native Americans.[2] **Figs. 4** and **5**

It has been established that social determinants of health such as education, employment status and safety, food security, housing and hygiene, social inclusion, structural conflict, and environmental health, are better predictors of health access and outcomes than income or race alone. Factors such as education level, insurance status, along with income, and at times geographic location can have greater impact on stage at diagnosis, treatment, and survival over race alone. These disparities were found to persist when applied to communities outside the United States.[4] This supports the need for a more detailed understanding of how societal factors can have as much impact as the biology of disease. We have learned in our mechanistic understanding of cancer that our shift toward biologically tailored treatment has had an impact on survival. Likewise, our ability to contextualize disease and therapy within the complex social constructs our patients' experience will break down unnecessary barriers to care and improve health outcomes for all patients. There are emerging data investigating barriers to care for transgender communities with cancer. A recent study retrospectively reviewed access to care, stage at diagnosis, and mortality for transgender patients compared with cisgender controls. For lung cancer, they found transgender patients were more likely to present with advanced disease and had slightly increased rates of mortality, although not statistically significant.[5] Visibility of marginal groups is key in identifying potentially vulnerable cancer populations. More research is required to capture previously under-identified groups such as homeless or displaced individuals, severely mentally ill, and incarcerated persons. In one Seattle hospital, 17% of patients treated for nonsmall cell lung cancer were homeless. Homeless patients experienced a longer delay from radiographic finding to biopsy (248 days compared with 116), missed

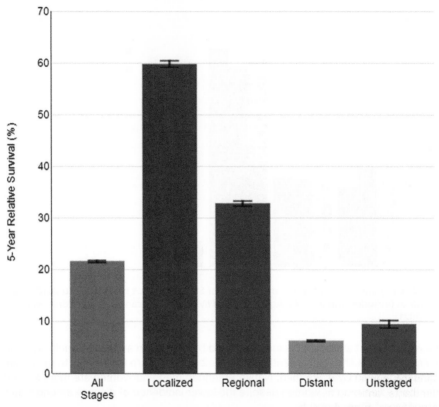

Fig. 3. Lung and bronchus SEER 5-year relative survival rates, 2011 to 2017 by stage at diagnosis, both sexes, all races (includes Hispanic), all ages. (*Created by* https://seer.cancer.gov/explorer on Fri Oct 15, 2021)

more appointments, and worse median survival (0.58 years vs 1.30 years) when compared with housed patients.[6] Patients with schizophrenia were more likely to present with earlier stage disease, however 50% less likely to receive stage-appropriate therapy.[7] Lung cancer accounted for 8% of deaths in state prisons, and the population of incarcerated individuals over 55 continues to grow disproportionately.[8] Understanding the complexity of medical care for our most vulnerable populations can only help us to work better within existing limitations, and hopefully translate into models of care that uphold the humanity and health of all individuals.

RISK FACTORS

There are several risk factors for developing lung cancer that are well established. Most of the sporadic lung cancers are attributed to tobacco cigarettes both via primary and second-hand exposure.[4] Current data from 2019 indicate that the rate of smoking has declined from approximately 20% in 2005% to 14% in 2019. The rates of smoking are highest among non-Hispanic Native American, three times the rate of Asian Americans. Individuals with GED or limited high school education were as much as twice as likely to smoke in comparison to persons with an associate degree. Individuals who live in households with annual income less than $35,000 were twice as likely to smoke compared with those in households with income >$75,000.[9]

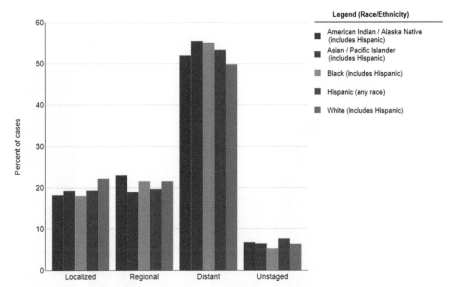

Fig. 4. Lung and bronchus stage distribution of SEER incidence cases, 2009 to 2018 by race/ethnicity, both sexes, all ages. (*Created by* https://seer.cancer.gov/explorer on Fri Oct 15, 2021)

The progressive legalization of marijuana has made its widespread use more visible. Cannabis derivatives have long been used as adjuncts to cancer therapy as appetite stimulants, antiemetics, and anxiolytics. What is less well understood are the long-term effects of smoking marijuana in comparison to tobacco products as it relates to lung cancer risk. The International Lung Cancer Consortium reviewed 6 case-controlled studies from the US, UK, Canada, and New Zealand. Their analysis indicated inconclusive association between cannabis smoking and lung cancer.[10] It is known that the combustion of cannabis produces similar toxins to tobacco smoke, with an similar airway inflammatory response. There is not, however, the data to indicate that it results in similar oncogenic transformation as seen with other carcinogenic exposures.[11] The lack of standardization of production and variable regulation limits the ability to study broadly its effects as it relates to lung cancer. The ability to better quantify exposure via the various delivery systems, potency of active metabolites and carcinogens, and define frequency or intensity of use is required for meaningful data to be obtained. Furthermore, overlap with tobacco smoking that can confound observed effect as it relates to lung health.[9]

Environmental risk factors include asbestos and radon, which exhibit synergistic carcinogenesis when combined with cigarette smoking. Radon is considered the second most common cause of lung cancer after cigarette smoking alone, accounting for up to 15% of lung cancer cases.[4,12] Although originally identified in miners, it has also been found to have an increased risk for the general population.[8] Radon is a naturally occurring gas that emits alpha particles in its process of radioactive decay.[13] The initial association between radon and lung cancer was noted in miner communities and reported in the 1990s.[14] The pooled study by Lubin and colleagues was able to identify a clear risk of 40% of lung cancer deaths in miners attributable to radon exposure. They used their model to extrapolate to the residential population resulting in an estimate of 2% to 10% of lung cancer deaths attributed to radon exposure. A more recent, meta-

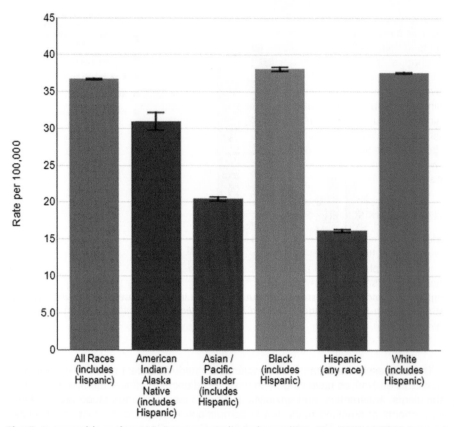

Fig. 5. Lung and bronchus U.S. 5-year age-adjusted morality rates, 2015 to 2019 by race/ethnicity, both sexes, all ages. (*Created by* https://seer.cancer.gov/explorer on Fri Oct 15, 2021)

analysis of several North American residential studies supported the link between radon exposure and lung cancer.[11] There is a need for large-scale systematic research to better define the association seen in earlier case-control studies performed over the last 30 years.

Asbestos is a well-established risk factor for lung cancer and is synergistic with tobacco cigarette exposure. Klebe and colleagues provided a thorough review of the historical and current literature around asbestos-related lung cancer. In short, the authors reiterated that all asbestos fiber types have been associated with lung cancer, there is no anatomic or histologic pattern associated with asbestos-related lung cancer, and a near-linear dose–response relationship exists.[15] Asbestos use has been in decline in most countries worldwide since the 1980s and 1990s; however, there are still countries who have yet to curtail its use despite the overwhelming body of evidence that exists for its health risk. The United States reached its peak in 1970 and had a steep drop off after regulation. Most of the current asbestos production and use remains in the Russian Federation, China, and India.[16]

Finally, e-cigarettes or electronic nicotine delivery systems (ENDS) have exploded in use with a predominance in the late adolescent and young adult population. These noncombustible delivery systems still require heat, and furthermore, have a myriad of chemical additives that independently can affect the function of the respiratory system. In a review by Gotts and colleagues, they defined the immediate respiratory effects of ENDS use on the airway cilia function, immune cell function, and alveolar gas exchange. This was further supported by a flurry of cases of respiratory insufficiency in 2019, hypothesized to be related to glycerol-based additives or oil-based preservatives in various ENDS. Their review went on to describe acute airway inflammation, similar to tobacco cigarette-induced injury, and changes in spirometry mimicking airway obstruction. Their review detailed several mechanistic and regulatory concerns as well as called for robust systematic research to evaluate risk over time. In short, to date, there is no clear evidence linking ENDS to lung cancer, but there is overlap between certain documented acute changes seen in tobacco cigarette use that may have similar long-term effects.[17]

LUNG CANCER SCREENING

Most of lung cancers are diagnosed at the advanced stage, which directly affects survival despite the current advances in therapy. The key to lowering mortality from lung cancer is 2-fold, minimizing risk by identifying modifiable risk factors and early detection through screening. In 2011, the National Lung Screening Trial (NLST) reported its initial results of screening high-risk adults for lung cancer. This trial evaluated adults 55 to 74 with a minimum of 30 pack-year smoking history, and if former smokers had quit within 15 years of enrollment in the study. It randomized participants to either low-dose CT or chest radiography for their screening modality. Participants were screened annually for 3 years and in this trial, a 20% decrease in lung cancer mortality was seen with low-dose CT chest in comparison to the chest radiograph arm.[18] The extended follow-up in this study supported their original results, and there were no changes in the number needed to screen to have the mortality benefit seen in the initial study.[19]

This study revolutionized our perspective regarding the ability to establish a reasonable screening model for lung cancer. The NELSON trial in Europe found similar results screening current or former smokers ages 50 to 74. This trial randomized participants to low-dose CT versus no screening. This study also included a growth-rate assessment for indeterminate results. The limitations of this study were the small sample size of women in the study, as well as the variable screening interval (1, 2, 2.5 years). The strength of the trial was the initial longer follow-up time of 10 years. This study reported a 24% reduction in lung cancer mortality in men and a 33% reduction in women in comparison to the control group at 10 years. This was also associated with lower stage at diagnosis and increased eligibility for surgical resection.[20]

These data are compelling for low-dose screening, and in 2014, the U.S. Preventative Services Task Force recommended screening for asymptomatic adults 55 to 80 years of age based on the initial NLST criteria. They included that after 15 years of abstinence from smoking or if health problems limiting life expectancy arise that screening should be discontinued.[21] These recommendations were updated and expanded in 2021 to include the NELSON trial findings. Low-dose CT screening is recommended for persons aged 50 to 80 with a 20 pack-year smoking history who are current smokers or have quit within 15 yrs. The USPFT concluded in this statement that annual screening with low-dose CT had a moderate net benefit for high-risk individuals.[22] In addition, they did not recommend chest radiography, sputum cytology, or biomarker studies as screening alternatives.

Expansion of these criteria has an impact beyond simply a larger potential cohort of eligible persons. This change has allowed for the inclusion of high-risk groups that would more likely fall outside the initial criteria. This includes women, younger current smokers, and under-represented minority groups with higher incidence of lung cancer. However, there is criticism that despite this inclusion the disparities remain. Transgender persons who qualify for lung cancer screening are far less likely to undergo screening compared with cisgender controls (2.3% vs 17.2%).[23] Landy and colleagues have proposed using prediction models to reduce disparity. They found that despite larger rates of inclusion of minority populations, the disparate outcomes persisted, indicating that additional criteria for inclusion in screening are needed. In particular, they indicate that the additional calculation of individual life-years gained would better identify true risk and prove to provide a more robust correction for disparities.[24]

Despite this large and longitudinal body of evidence supporting annual screening for high-risk patients with low-dose CT, adoption of these protocols has been slow to gain traction in the United States. In 2015, data from the National Health Interview Survey indicated that only 3.9% of eligible individuals had undergone lung cancer screening with low-dose CT. In 2017, 10 states participating in the behavioral risk factor surveillance system survey elected to include a module on lung cancer screening. Of the survey participants who met the criteria for lung cancer screening, only 14.4% had undergone screening low-dose CT.[25] In 2018, this increased to 19.2%, although the data were only collected from 8 states in this study.[26]

Innovation has always been a hallmark of cancer therapy and research. Currently, liquid biopsy or circulating biomarkers have gained visibility as potential diagnostic or prognostic tools. Among these potential targets, research continues to understand the role of circulating microRNA (miRNA), circulating tumor cells (CTC), circulating tumor DNA (ctDNA), and noncoding RNAs (ncRNA). The challenges with these modalities are the variable presence, stability, and signature based on the malignancy. There is currently no consistent biologic target for all nonsmall cell lung cancers, and likely any liquid biopsy would require a panel to maximize sensitivity. Most current studies are designed to augment radiographic screening, and potentially increase the specificity of low-dose screening CT.[27]

SUMMARY

Lung cancer has remained the most lethal cancer in the United States and worldwide. The incidence and mortality declined in the United States over the last 2 decades; however, the burden of disease remains significant. Accurate understanding of social determinants of health will be critical in identifying risk and barriers to screening and treatment of all populations. Worldwide lung cancer rates continue to rise in Asia, whereby the largest concentration of the world population resides. This parallels current tobacco cigarette use in that region. Interestingly, this region along with Eastern Europe also continues to produce and consume asbestos which has synergistic carcinogenic potential with tobacco smoking. Radon remains a ubiquitous environmental risk for smokers and nonsmokers alike in developing lung cancer. There is a need for ongoing research to understand the relationship between cannabis smoking, ENDS, and lung cancer due to the exponential increase in the consumption of both in recent decades. Finally, after smoking cessation, screening is currently our most powerful tool to decrease mortality from lung cancer. Increasing participation in low-dose CT screening programs among all eligible individuals is critical in improving survival and mitigating disparities in lung cancer outcomes among all people. Understanding the complex biology of disease within various populations, and how to identify high-risk individuals for screening is still an area of ongoing research. The frontier of liquid biopsy is a potential area of noninvasive diagnosis and monitoring in lung cancer. Using shed tumor proteins to help increase the precision of radiographic screening is promising for diagnosis. Liquid biopsy has far-reaching implications for accelerating treatment planning, avoiding unnecessary invasive procedures, and potentially providing better indicators of true prognosis. Ultimately if we can reach our most vulnerable populations with effective lung cancer screening programs, we will offer all patients their best chance at survival and possibly cure.

CLINICS CARE POINTS

- Lung cancer screening criteria has expanded to include: patients age 50-80, >20pkyr smoking history or current smoker, former smoker having quit within 15yrs.
- Clinicians need to understand how social determinants of health affect access to screening and therefore outcomes in lung cancer.
- Clinicians should remain vigilant to ensure our most vulnerable patients not only have access to lung cancer screening, but recieve stage appropriate standard of care.

DISCLOSURE

The author has nothing to disclose.

REFERENCES

1. Siegel RL, Miller KD, Fuchs HE, et al. Cancer Statistics, 2021. CA Cancer J Clin 2021;71(1):7–33 [Erratum appears in CA Cancer J Clin 202171(4):359].
2. Howlader N, Noone AM, Krapcho M, et al, editors. SEER Cancer Statistics Review, 1975-2018. Bethesda (MD): National Cancer Institute; 2021. Available at: https://seer.cancer.gov/csr/1975_2018/.
3. Ferlay J, Colombet M, Soerjomataram I, et al. Estimating the global cancer incidence and mortality in 2018: GLOBOCAN sources and methods. Int J Cancer 2019;144(8):1941–53.
4. Alberg AJ, Brock MV, Ford JG, et al. Epidemiology of lung cancer: Diagnosis and management of lung cancer, 3rd ed: American College of Chest Physicians evidence-based clinical practice guidelines. Chest 2013;143(5 Suppl):e1S–29S.
5. Jackson SS, Han X, Mao Z, et al. Cancer Stage, Treatment, and Survival Among Transgender Patients in the United States. J Natl Cancer Inst 2021;113(9): 1221–7.
6. Concannon KF, Thayer JH, Wu QV, et al. Outcomes among homeless patients with non-small-cell lung cancer: a county hospital experience. JCO Oncol Pract 2020;16(9):e1004–14.
7. Bergamo C, Sigel K, Mhango G, et al. Inequalities in lung cancer care of elderly patients with schizophrenia: an observational cohort study. Psychosom Med 2014;76(3):215–20.
8. Aziz H, Ackah RL, Whitson A, et al. Cancer care in the incarcerated population: barriers to quality care and opportunities for improvement. JAMA Surg 2021; 156(10):964–73.
9. Cornelius ME, Wang TW, Jamal A, et al. Tobacco Product Use Among Adults – United States, 2019. Morbidity Mortality Weekly Rep 2020;69(46):1736–42. Available at: https://www.cdc.gov/tobacco/data_statistics/fact_sheets/adult_data/cig_smoking/#nation. Accessed November 19, 2020.
10. Zhang LR, Morgenstern H, Greenland S, et al, Cannabis and Respiratory Disease Research Group of New Zealand, Brhane Y, Liu G, Hung RJ. Cannabis smoking

and lung cancer risk: pooled analysis in the International Lung Cancer Consortium. Int J Cancer 2015;136(4):894–903.

11. Jett J, Stone E, Warren G, et al. Cannabis Use, Lung Cancer, and Related Issues. J Thorac Oncol 2018;13(4):480–7.

12. Choi H, Mazzone P. Radon and lung cancer: assessing and mitigating the risk. Cleve Clin J Med 2014;81(9):567–75.

13. Krewski D, Lubin JH, Zielinski JM, et al. A combined analysis of North American case-control studies of residential radon and lung cancer. J Toxicol Environ Health A 2006;69(7):533–97.

14. Lubin JH, Boice JD Jr, Edling C, et al. Lung cancer in radon-exposed miners and estimation of risk from indoor exposure. J Natl Cancer Inst 1995;87(11):817–27.

15. Klebe S, Leigh J, Henderson DW, et al. Asbestos, smoking and lung cancer: an update. Int J Environ Res Public Health 2019;17(1):258.

16. Allen LP, Baez J, Stern MEC, et al. Trends and the economic effect of asbestos bans and decline in asbestos consumption and production worldwide. Int J Environ Res Public Health 2018;15(3):531.

17. Gotts JE, Jordt SE, McConnell R, et al. What are the respiratory effects of e-cigarettes? BMJ 2019;366:l5275 [Erratum appears in BMJ 2019;367:l5980].

18. National Lung Screening Trial Research Team, Aberle DR, Adams AM, Berg CD, et al. Reduced lung-cancer mortality with low-dose computed tomographic screening. N Engl J Med 2011;365(5):395–409.

19. National Lung Screening Trial Research Team. Lung cancer incidence and mortality with extended follow-up in the national lung screening trial. J Thorac Oncol 2019;14(10):1732–42.

20. de Koning HJ, van der Aalst CM, de Jong PA, et al. Reduced lung-cancer mortality with volume ct screening in a randomized trial. N Engl J Med 2020;382(6):503–13.

21. Moyer VA, U.S. Preventive Services Task Force. Screening for lung cancer: U.S. preventive services task force recommendation statement. Ann Intern Med 2014;160(5):330–8.

22. US Preventive Services Task Force, Krist AH, Davidson KW, Mangione CM, et al. Screening for lung cancer: US preventive services task force recommendation statement. JAMA 2021;325(10):962–70.

23. Stowell JT, Parikh Y, Tilson K, et al. Lung cancer screening eligibility and utilization among transgender patients: an analysis of the 2017-2018 United States Behavioral Risk Factor Surveillance System Survey. Nicotine Tob Res 2020;22(12):2164–9.

24. Landy R, Young CD, Skarzynski M, et al. Using Prediction-Models to Reduce Persistent Racial/Ethnic Disparities in Draft 2020 USPSTF Lung-Cancer Screening Guidelines. J Natl Cancer Inst 2021;djaa211. https://doi.org/10.1093/jnci/djaa211.

25. Zahnd WE, Eberth JM. Lung cancer screening utilization: a behavioral risk factor surveillance system analysis. Am J Prev Med 2019;57(2):250–5.

26. Narayan AK, Gupta Y, Little BP, et al. Lung cancer screening eligibility and use with low-dose computed tomography: Results from the 2018 Behavioral Risk Factor Surveillance System cross-sectional survey. Cancer 2021;127(5):748–56.

27. Kan CFK, Unis GD, Li LZ, et al. Circulating Biomarkers for Early Stage Non-Small Cell Lung Carcinoma Detection: Supplementation to Low-Dose Computed Tomography. Front Oncol 2021;11:555331.

Extended Resections for Lung Cancer

John Kuckelman, DO[a],*, Mia Debarros, MD[b], Raphael Bueno, MD[c]

KEYWORDS

- Extended resections • Lung cancer • Pulmonary reconstruction • Lobectomy
- Pneumonectomy

KEY POINTS

- Extended pulmonary resections for advanced lung cancers are feasible and safe and provide acceptable oncologic benefit in appropriately selected patients.
- Every effort should be made to preserve lung parenchyma favoring airway reconstructions over pneumonectomy when appropriate.
- Advances in mechanical circulation may allow for the safe resection of previously unresectable locally advanced disease.
- Extended pulmonary resection can be done via minimally invasive approaches as the field continues to improve and progress.

INTRODUCTION

Locally advanced lung cancer represents a diverse group encompassing several different patient populations as defined by the American Joint Committee on Cancer (AJCC, **Box 1**).[1] Stage IIIA represents a heterogeneous group making it a unique subset within lung cancer subjected to much research and debate. Stage IIIA includes the following clinical realities:

1. T1 to T2 tumors with mediastinal lymph node involvement.
2. T3 and T4 tumors without mediastinal lymph node involvement.
3. Involvement of chest wall, pericardium, phrenic nerve, or separate tumors in the same lobe without mediastinal lymph node involvement
4. Direct tumor invasion of the mediastinum, heart, esophagus, great vessels, diaphragm, recurrent laryngeal nerve, carina, trachea, spine, or tumor nodules in different ipsilateral lobes.

[a] Thoracic Surgery, Brigham and Women's Hospital, 25 Francis Street, Boston, MA 02215, USA;
[b] Thoracic Surgery, Madigan Army Medical Center, 9040A Jackson Avenue, Joint Base Lewis-McChord, WA 98431, USA; [c] Division of Thoracic and Cardiac Surgery, Brigham and Women's Hospital, 25 Francis Street, Boston, MA 02215, USA
* Corresponding author.
E-mail address: jkuckelman@partners.org

Surg Clin N Am 102 (2022) 345–363
https://doi.org/10.1016/j.suc.2022.02.003
0039-6109/22/Published by Elsevier Inc.

surgical.theclinics.com

Box 1
Lung cancer staging groups, American Joint Committee on Cancer, eighth edition[1]

IIIA: T1N2M0
T2N2M0
T3N1
T4N0
T4N1

IIIB: T1N3M0
T2N3M0
T3N2M0
T4N2M0

IIIC: T3N3M0
T4N3M0

T1 = tumors less than 3 cm.

T2 = 3 to 4 cm, or visceral pleura/main bronchus involvement or atelectasis to hilum.

T3 = 5 to 7 cm or chest wall, pericardium, or phrenic nerve involvement or separate tumors in the same lobe.

T4 = Tumors greater than 7 cm or mediastinal, diaphragm, heart, great vessels, or esophageal invasion or multiple tumor nodules in ipsilateral lung.

Within stage IIIA, upfront surgical resection is recommended for patients with T3N1 disease followed by appropriate adjuvant therapy. Occasionally, mediastinal lymph node (N2) involvement consisting of "unexpected," intranodal/extracapsular, single, or multistation and limited or bulky lymph nodes is discovered at an index operation for T1 or T2 tumors. Although grouped as stage IIIA, these patients have varied treatment approaches.

Studies from the early 1990s laid the groundwork for improved treatment in patients with N2 involvement by demonstrating that induction chemotherapy followed by surgery showed improved clinical outcomes compared with chemotherapy or surgery only.[2–4] Based on these landmark trials, several randomized controlled trials sought to determine the best multimodality treatment of these patients. The EORTC 08941 trial analyzed patients with stage IIIA N2 cancer given induction chemotherapy and randomized to either surgical resection or definitive radiation therapy. The surgical group demonstrated improved local control, but this failed to translate into improved progression-free or overall survival between groups. However, a subgroup analysis found improved 5-year survival of 27% in the surgical cohort achieving R0 resection and lobectomy.[5] The Intergroup 0139 trial randomized patients with stage IIIA N2 cancer to induction chemoradiation followed by surgical resection or further concurrent chemoradiation. The surgical cohort had significantly improved progression-free survival. The trial confirmed prior findings of improved survival in complete pathologic responders and lobectomy compared with matched definitive chemoradiation (33.6 months vs 22 months). Given the poor outcomes initially seen after pneumonectomy for patients with N2 disease, there was some debate regarding the benefit of surgical resection when pneumonectomy was required. The initially high mortality of pneumonectomy reported in the 0139 study has not been redemonstrated in subsequent analysis and thus is an acceptable resection for fit individuals with resectable disease[6–9]; this may be in part because the study included low-volume centers as well as resections done by surgeons whose majority practice did not include thoracic surgery.

Several nonrandomized studies have found that for highly selected patients with good performance status, long-term survival is possible even with larger tumors that invade mediastinal organs, with reported 5-year survival rates of 9% to 48%. The current recommendations include induction chemoradiation therapy followed by surgical resection if no tumor progression on restaging and adjuvant chemotherapy and immunotherapy. The morbidity and mortality and long-term survival seems to be directly associated with the invaded structure. Several single-center retrospective studies report postoperative organ-specific mortality rates, the highest being left atrial resection (up to 50%) and the lowest being aorta or esophagus (14%). The 5-year survivals range from 44% to 22% depending on the structure involved. All studies confirm that N0 status and achieving an R0 resection confers improved overall survival.[10]

DISCUSSION

It is crucial to have a fluid knowledge of the incisions at the thoracic surgeon's disposal because each provides its own unique advantages for a wide variety of operations and approaches. It is not uncommon for the preoperative planning for extended resections to first focus on the most appropriate incision; this is particularly true for tumors involving mediastinal and apical structures. An apt quote from Robert Gross summarizes it nicely: "If an operation is difficult, you are not doing it properly." **Table 1** reviews incisions for extended pulmonary resections. Importantly, excellent pain control is necessary postoperatively to maintain chest wall mechanics and thus positive progression in recovery. A multimodality approach to include epidural anesthesia or rib nerve blocks with long-acting injectable anesthesia in conjunction with scheduled antiinflammatory medications is typically required. Gabapentin should be added when patients describe pain related to potential intercostal nerve irritation. These measures will help limit the need of opioid medications. In addition, early mobilization is key to successful recovery, aiding tremendously with respiratory mechanics.

SPECIFIC RESECTIONS
Sleeve Lobectomy

Sleeve resection (SL) is indicated when tumor originates or extends to the main bronchus or in rare instances, carinal invasion (carinal sleeve discussed separately). The most common malignant histology and reason for SL is carcinoid or mucoepidermoid carcinoma. Centrally invasive non–small cell carcinoma (NSCLC) tumors are also amenable to resection provided an R0 resection is feasible. Even when resecting advanced neoplasms, lung preservation, whenever possible, should be the preference.

Since it was first described in the 1940s, there have been multiple studies evaluating the safety and feasibility of sleeve lobectomy for centrally located lung cancer. This culminated in the early 2000s with Deslauriers and colleagues[11] reviewing 1230 patients undergoing sleeve lobectomy or pneumonectomy for central tumors. Operative mortality was low for both groups (1.3% vs 5.3% in pneumonectomy group, $P < .05$) with a 5-year survival of 52% in the sleeve group compared with 31% in the pneumonectomy group. In 2010, a propensity-matched study of patients undergoing sleeve lobectomy and pneumonectomy confirmed the safety and feasibility of sleeve lobectomy with similar findings (mortality of 1.0% vs 8.6%, $P < .05$ and 5-year survival of 58.4% in sleeve group vs 32.1% in pneumonectomies). Recurrence was also similar between the 2 groups (30.5% with sleeve vs 38.1%, $P = .180$). The investigators noted that lymph node status was the most important factor in long-term survival.[12]

Table 1
Commonly used incision for extended pulmonary resections

Incision	Technique	Advantages	Disadvantages
Posterolateral thoracotomy	Position: lateral decubitus position ± flexed bed Landmarks: Tip of the scapula and nipple Incisions: Begins 3 cm posterior to the scapula and ends at the anterior axillary line, latissimus dorsi typically divided and serratus anterior (deep and anterior to Lat) preserved. Scapula raised and ribs counted. Sixth rib is identified and intercostals divided on the superior border of the rib extended to transverse vertebral process posteriorly and anteriorly to sternum as needed. Rib can be shingled or removed if additional exposure needed	Superb visualization of the hilum, pulmonary artery as it branches in the fissure, diaphragm, as well as the apex. It is the standard incision for anatomic pneumonectomy as well as anatomic lobectomies	Morbid incision, unilateral
Anterior thoracotomy	Position: lateral decubitus position ± flexed bed Landmarks: fourth rib posterior to the lateral border of the pectoralis major Incisions: Progresses along the course of the rib to the midaxillary line. Less common to shingle or remove a rib in this space because the intercostal space tends to larger	Excellent access to the apices, localized to the upper and middle lobes as well as the mediastinum. Generally better tolerated than posterolateral thoracotomy	Limited access to posterior hilum, lower lobes, and diaphragm

Bilateral thoracosternotomy (Clamshell)	Position: supine, extended with shoulder roll, arms out Landmarks: pectoralis major, posterior axillary line Incisions: made in the shape of a 'W' under bilateral pectoralis, across the sternum at the fifth rib terminating at the posterior axilla. Internal mammary located, clipped, and divided, sternum divided with a bone saw or Libschki knife and the anterior mediastinum is dissected from the posterior sternum. Rib spreaders are placed lateral and posterior on both sides.	Excellent visualization of the entire thorax bilaterally. Best incision for neoplasms that have resectable extension across the mediastinum or bilateral oligometastatic disease	Rarely needed for lung cancer. Most morbid incision. Somewhat limited access to posterior mediastinum
Sternotomy	Position: Supine, shoulder roll, arms tucked Landmarks: Sternal notch, sternal border, xyphoid process Incision: Confirm midline of sternum, create partial tunnel under sternal plate superiorly and inferiorly. Division with sternal saw followed by periosteal and marrow-directed hemostasis	Helpful for invasive cancers invading mediastinal or cardiac structures. Ease of initiation of cardiopulmonary bypass. Easy access to intrapericardial structures including proximal or main pulmonary artery	Limited views of posterior hilum and left lower lobe hilar structures
Sternothoracotomy (Fig. 1)	Position: Supine, shoulder roll, arms tucked Landmarks: Sternal notch, sternal border, fifth rib Incision: Divide soft tissue to level desired for thoracotomy (intercostal spaces 2–5). Enter intercostal space just lateral to mammary and carry toward sternum, identifying and controlling mammary vessels. Partial sternotomy with right angle connection followed by anterolateral thoracotomy. Rultract retractor placement	Benefits of sternotomy with added access to apices and hilar structures. Better inferior access than sternotomy alone. Ease of lung manipulation Well tolerated	Limited posterior exposure. Somewhat limited inferior exposure

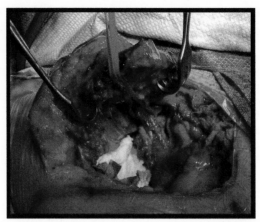

Fig. 1. Example of sternothoractomy in the second intercostal space using the Rultract retractor. This incision was used in this case for apical tumor that invaded the anterior mediastinum including the superior vena cava.

There are several different techniques used in tracheobronchial resections, all of which fall loosely under the terms "sleeve resection" or "bronchoplasty." A bronchoplasty is defined as "removal of lung at the bronchial orifice without removal of the main bronchus" and completed by simple primary defect closure. Standard SL refers to "circumferential resection of a bronchial section with reconstruction." Extended sleeve resection (ESL) is a "bronchoplastic procedure with resection of more than one lobe" usually an additional wedge or segmentectomy. The different types are classified A to E (**Box 2**).[13] A double SL refers to lobectomy and resection of pulmonary artery segment with reconstruction of both structures.

All patients should undergo the standard preoperative workup to include full pulmonary function testing and chest computed tomographic (CT) and PET imaging. The imaging defines the extent of disease and aids in preoperative planning. Doppler echocardiography is helpful to evaluate right ventricular function and pulmonary hypertension, which make extended and carinal resections prohibitive. Ventilation perfusion scans assist in determination of preoperative and postoperative lung function and support patient fitness for pneumonectomy. Preoperative bronchoscopy is often

---

Box 2
Okada/Berthet/Bolukbas classification of extended sleeve lobectomy[15,16,24]

A. Resection of the upper and middle lobes with or without superior segment (6) and anastomosis between the right main and lower lobe bronchus/basilar segmental bronchus.

B. Resection of the upper lobe and superior segment of the lower lobe and anastomosis between the left main and basal segment bronchi.

C. Resection of the lingular segment and lower lobe and anastomosis between the left main and upper division bronchi.

D. Resection of the middle and lower lobe and anastomosis between the right main and superior bronchi.

E. En bloc resection of the middle lobe and superior segment with anastomosis between bronchus intermedius and basilar segmental bronchus

essential to obtain tissue diagnosis and to determine the exact location and length of proposed bronchial resection. Mediastinal staging is aggressively pursued beginning with PET-CT imaging but requires confirmatory invasive staging. Cervical mediastinoscopy may be performed at the time of proposed SL providing the added benefit of tracheal mobilization. Conversely, mediastinoscopy is preferably performed earlier than 2 weeks before the operation to prevent anastomotic tension related to adhesion formation. Confirmed N2 disease requires induction chemotherapy with or without concurrent radiation followed by restaging. Recent radiation (within 3 months) warrants consideration of an anastomotic buttress. Neoadjuvant immunotherapy has been shown to be safe in small series reports with no differences in technical difficulty or postoperative complications compared with patients treated without immunotherapy.[14] Careful patient selection is paramount, particularly in the case of extended and carinal resections. All patients must be evaluated for cardiopulmonary fitness for pneumonectomy because this is the "fallback" procedure in the event the tumor is deemed not amenable or in the event of failure of SL.

Technique
When contemplating an SL, the surgeon must consider the principles of bronchoplastic surgery: complete resection of the lesion, construction of a tension-free anastomosis, and alternative options if R0 resection or tension-free anastomosis is not possible. For an SL, single lung isolation is required with a double lumen tube with the bronchial side opposite of the intended resection side. The typical incision is a posterior lateral thoracotomy with muscle-sparing techniques if possible. If an intercostal muscle flap is intended, then it requires harvest at this time.

A right-sided upper lobe standard SL is the most common and technically simple SL performed. Right middle lobe sleeves may be difficult due to the middle lobe orifice in relation to the superior and basilar segmental orifices of the lower lobe. In many cases, it is preferable to perform a superior segmentectomy to prevent stenosis of the segment after reconstruction. Right lower lobe SLs can present a size mismatch between the bronchus intermedius and the middle lobe bronchus. Left-sided resections are more technically demanding because of difficult exposure. In all resections, the creation of tension-free anastomosis requires complete lung mobilization and standard release maneuvers. Lung mobilization includes division of anterior and posterior hilar pleural reflections and the pulmonary ligament to the level of the inferior pulmonary vein. The intralobar fissures are opened, and the blood supply is separated from the lung remaining behind. A complete lymphadenectomy is performed. The subcarinal space is cleared to expose the pericardium and carina. The esophagus is mobilized away from the airway. On the right, the main bronchus and bronchus intermedius are mobilized away from the pulmonary artery and distal trachea taking care to avoid disrupting the lateral blood supply. Intraoperative bronchoscopy is used to confirm the extent of proximal and distal macroscopic disease, and the airway is sharply divided in a transverse fashion. The resected portion is sent for frozen analysis to confirm adequate margins before reconstruction.

Upon confirmation of negative margins, the cut ends of the bronchi are reapproximated, and tension is assessed. Additional mobilization can be accomplished with full hilar release by opening the pericardium anteriorly at the level of the superior pulmonary vein and extending the incision posteriorly in a C-loop to the inferior pulmonary vein. Stay sutures are placed at both membranous-cartilaginous junctions to ensure proper alignment and decrease tension during reconstruction. A 4-0 Vicryl suture is typically used, but material and size depend on the surgeon preference and type of anastomosis performed. A permanent suture such as prolene should be considered for immunosuppressed patients. There are several techniques available for anastomosis construction. The continuous suture technique is best suited for size-matched bronchi. The suture is started at one membranous-cartilaginous junction and used to reapproximate the membranous portion. A second suture is used to close the cartilaginous portion. All knots are extraluminal. The interrupted technique is equally suited for size-matched and mismatched bronchi. Suture organization is paramount, and confusion is eliminated using alternating dyed and undyed sutures. The anastomosis is completed with full-thickness bites beginning at the membranous portion and moving anteriorly. The extraluminal knots are tied posterior to anterior. Finally, a hybrid technique uses continuous running suture on the membranous portion and interrupted sutures in the cartilaginous portion. For extreme size mismatch, particularly those present in ESL, several techniques assist with reconstruction:

1. Telescope anastomosis: smaller distal bronchus is inserted into the larger bronchus (**Fig. 2**)
2. Proximal bronchial stump membranous plication
3. Oblique resection of the distal bronchus[15]

Once reconstruction is complete, an air leak test up to 25 to 30 cm H_2O is mandatory. No air leak is acceptable. Bronchial anastomotic dehiscence is reported to be 5% to 8% and can result in pulmonary artery erosion with lethal hemorrhage. To prevent this devastating complication, buttressing the anastomosis is recommended.[13] Common buttress materials include intercostal muscle, pericardium, pleura, thymic fat pads, or omentum. SL interrupts the natural lymphatic drainage so postoperative fluid management is paramount to prevent edema in the reconstructed lobe (**Fig. 3**).

Double SLs involve the resection and reconstruction of the pulmonary artery. Reconstruction of the pulmonary vein is not recommended due to propensity for thrombosis and life-threatening thromboembolism. The most common reason is tumor or metastatic disease invading the main pulmonary artery or disease preventing ligation of segmental or lobar arteries. Resection and reconstruction may also be required to prevent kinking of the artery after bronchial reconstruction due to length differences. Resection is either circumferential (SL) or noncircumferential (arterioplasty). Proximal and distal control of the pulmonary artery is obtained, and low-

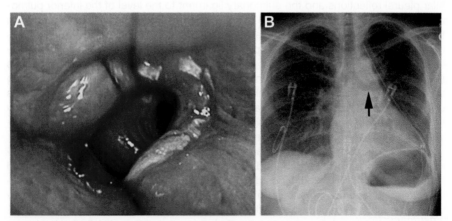

Fig. 2. Left lower lobe resection with upper lobe reconstruction. (*A*) Endobronchial view of the anastomosis. (*B*) Postoperative chest radiograph with arrow designating patient anastomosis.

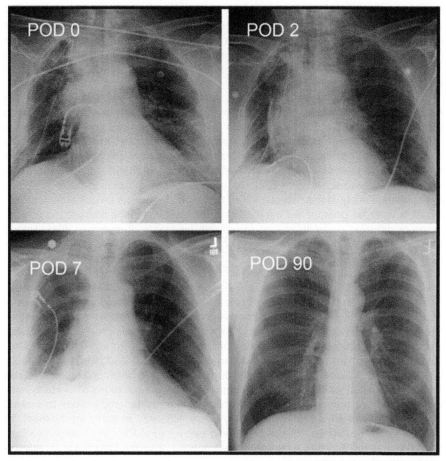

Fig. 3. Example of pulmonary edema seen over first week post opeartively of the right lower lobe after a right upper lobe sleeve resection.

dose heparin (2000–3000 IU) is administered before clamping proximal and distal to the planned resection. The affected area is removed, and reconstruction is predicated on how much lumen has been resected. A 5-0 permanent monofilament suture is used. A simple, primary repair (arterioplasty) is sufficient if the arterial narrowing does not compromise outflow by 10% to 20%. If the narrowing exceeds 20% then patch angioplasty is recommended with native azygous, pericardium or bovine pericardium, all being equally acceptable. A greater than 50% resection necessitates SL. For shorter segments (<2.5 cm) an end-to-end anastomosis is acceptable provided it is tension free, whereas longer segments require an interposition conduit. In a double SL, the vascular sleeve is performed first. Intra-anastomotic tissue buttressing prevents formation of a bronchovascular fistula. Postoperatively, therapeutic anticoagulation is not required, and low-dose aspirin is favored by some centers.[16]

Pneumonectomy, Sleeve Pneumonectomy, and Extrapleural Pneumonectomy

Most pneumonectomies are performed for oncologic curative intent. Removal of the entire lung on one side is reserved for tumors involving the main stem bronchus or carina (requiring sleeve pneumonectomy), and those with extensive involvement across a major fissure. Rarely are pneumonectomies indicated for the intrapulmonary metastasis. Generally, extrapulmonary pneumonectomy is reserved for resectable mesothelioma and thymoma with extensive hilar involvement precluding decortication alone and in patients whose tumor has created an inflammatory response leading to complete pleural symphysis.

Inherently, these patients tend to have at least stage IIIA disease and thus often receive neoadjuvant chemoradiation or definitive chemoradiation. Multiple studies in the first decade of the 2000s called into question the utility of pneumonectomy in the age of definitive chemoradiation with increasing efficacy given the high morbidity and mortality.[6,17] Since these landmark randomized trials there have been multiple studies showing the safety of pneumonectomy following chemoradiation with many showing increased survival for patients receiving a combination of the 2, justifying the continued utility of this resection.[18–21] Distant metastasis is an absolute contraindication, whereas postoperative forced expiratory volume in the first second of expiration or diffusing capacity of lung for carbon monoxide of less than 40%, limited fitness determined by maximum oxygen consumption or 6-minute walk test, poor cardiac function, severe pulmonary hypertension, or evidence of decreased right heart function are all relative contraindications.[22]

Historically the quoted perioperative mortality ranges up to 20% for pneumonectomy, thus preoperative workup and patient selection are critical to the success of this operation.[17,23] However, outcomes reported by high-volume centers such as those shown by White and colleagues,[21] show considerably improved mortality less than 10% at 90 days. A thorough review of the preoperative workup for pneumonectomy has been reviewed for patients undergoing SL. Right-sided procedures, preoperative cardiac disease, and current smoking status tend to be among the highest risk factors associated with mortality.[23–25] Although often safer in terms of mortality, left-sided pneumonectomies are fraught with dissection-related morbidities to include negotiation of a short left main pulmonary artery, left heart or aortic involvement, as well as recurrent laryngeal nerve or phrenic nerve injury. Overall preoperative lung function does not seem to affect mortality because often the lung to be resected is not functional preoperatively.[25]

Technique

The procedure is performed through a posterior lateral thoracotomy. For both sides, the pleura is opened circumferentially at the level of the hilum. Evaluation of the ability to limit the resection with a sleeve reconstruction should be made in every case. Complete hilar lymph node dissection allows for a complete oncologic resection as well as detailed evaluation of the bronchial resection margin. After the main vascular and bronchus is dissected, vascular TA staplers are useful for completed control and division the pulmonary veins and pulmonary trunk with a thicker stapler (4.8 mm, green loaded) for the bronchus or parenchyma. Test clamping and monitoring the patient's hemodynamic tolerance is a crucial step before the division of the hilar vasculature. Bronchoscopic guidance can be used to ensure bronchial division is flush with the carina and uninvolved with tumor. On the left, additional length of the main PA may be obtained by division of the ligamentum arteriosum using meticulous dissection to avoid the RLN. Intrapericardial dissection with dissection off the pericardium will also afford the surgeon additional length. On the right division of the azygous vein will aid in obtaining control of the main pulmonary artery as will dissection of the PA medially off the superior vena cava (SVC) intrapericardially. Reconstruction of the surrounding structures may be needed and is discussed separately.

Circumstances that may require extrapleural dissection include instances of pleural symphysis (complete fusion of the visceral and parietal pleura) from chronic inflammation or tumor involvement limited to the pleura. If this is expected, an extralateral plane can be developed at the time of thoracotomy using blunt dissection to free the pleura and lung from the chest wall before placing retraction; this can be done around the entire lung or limited to only areas necessary to facilitate dissection.

Carinal resection and sleeve pneumonectomy are more commonly performed on the right side. Unique to this operation is careful and thoughtout ventilation management in coordination with our anesthesia colleagues. There are multiple techniques used to include jet ventilation, cross-field sterile endobronchial ventilation, intermittent apneic ventilation, and even venovenous extracorporeal membrane oxygenation (ECMO).[26] Performing the tracheal division and tracheobronchial anastomosis in general follows the same principles discussed for SL. Most extended SLs (right and left sided) are approached through right-sided thoracotomy.[27–29] Banki and Wood[30] provide a detailed step by step review of a left carinal pneumonectomy in their 2007 article for operative techniques.

Pancoast Tumors

Tumors in the apex of the lung with extension into the thoracic inlet are known as Pancoast or superior sulcus tumors; have the potential to involve the first and second ribs and associated vertebral bodies, the brachial plexus, the sympathetic chain, as well as the subclavian vessels; and thus require dedicated attention. Pancoast tumors are by definition at least T3 tumors and make up to 5% of all NSCLC. Pathopneumonic findings on physical examination include Horner syndrome (ptosis, miosis, and anhidrosis from the ipsilateral stellate ganglion), arm pain in the ulnar distribution, hoarseness from RLN involvement, and thenar/hypothenar muscle wasting. Induction chemoradiation followed by surgical resection is the NCCN recommended gold standard for these patients due to the improved survival findings of the Southwest Oncology Group and Japanese Clinical Oncology phase 2 prospective trials.[31,32] Unique but necessary to the preoperative workup for these tumors is an MRI of the neck and chest to determine what structures are involved. Long-term outcomes originally were largely affected by the presence of T4 tumors and N2 disease; however, since the implementation of neoadjuvant therapy, R0 resection and complete pathologic response seem to be the most important factors effecting long-term survival.[6,32–35] Complete pathologic response may be seen in up to 18% of patients; however, guidelines recommend that R0 surgical resection remains the standard for all patients. Absolute and relative contraindications to resection are listed in **Table 2**.

Technique

Various incisions have been described as approaches for Pancoast tumor resection with each providing their own unique advantages and access to potentially involved

Table 2
Absolute and relative contraindications for Pancoast tumor resection

Absolute Contraindications	Relative Contraindications
• Poor functional status	• Inability to tolerate neoadjuvant chemoradiation
• Brachial trunk involvement	• Oligometastatic disease
• C8 nerve root involvement	• Poor response to induction therapy
• Multisite metastasis	• Extensive vascular disease precluding reconstruction
• Persistent N2/N3 disease	(extension into carotid/vertebral/subclavian is not absolute contraindication)

structures. Oftentimes the choice of incision is determined based on a combined consideration for tumor location, involved thoracic inlet structures, and surgeon preference. Up to the first 5 ribs may need to be resected, and this requires division of the anterior, middle, and posterior scalene from their respective attachments to the first and second ribs before entrance into the chest, which will be below the lowest rib to be resected. Typically, if only the posterior portion of the first 3 ribs is needed for R0 resection then reconstruction of the chest wall is not necessary because the scapula will provide adequate coverage. Anterior rib removal or greater than 3 ribs posteriorly requires chest wall reconstruction to avoid flail chest, lung herniation, or entrapment of the tip of the scapula. A multidisciplinary surgical approach should be taken if vascular reconstruction, neurolysis, or vertebral stabilization will be required to accomplish R0 resection. Resection of the T1 nerve root is acceptable for complete resection and will result in ipsilateral arm weakness; however, extension to the C8 nerve root will result in complete paralysis of the upper extremity and usually precludes resection.

Chest Wall Involvement

Chest wall invasion outside of superior sulcus tumors is rare and accounts for approximately 5% to 10% of all NSCLC tumors and is classified as T3 tumor according to eighth edition of AJCC.[36] The NCCN guideline recommends upfront resection for chest wall involvement outside of superior sulcus tumors. Standard oncologic staging and determination of preoperative fitness remains necessary. Patients with N2 disease represent stage IIIB disease and should be referred for definitive chemoradiation except in very select cases. Uniquely, chest and/or spine MRI with respiratory gating is helpful for preoperative assessment for the depth of parietal pleural invasion, involvement of the diaphragm, or vertebral encroachment or involvement.[37] Thoracic spine involvement should be addressed with spinal surgeon assistance. Anticipated large defects requiring extensive soft tissue coverage will benefit from preoperative plastic surgery consultation.

Technique

Tumor location determines the surgical approach with posterior lateral thoracotomy remaining the most common approach. The entry is typically tailored to the tumor level. Tumors anterior to the midaxillary line or involving the sternum are approached by anterolateral thoracotomy.[36] Entry must be away from chest wall involvement. Video-assisted thoracoscopy (VATS) can aid in the determination of appropriate level of entry. Exploration to ensure metastatic disease is undertaken, and chest wall resection is usually completed before lung resection. En bloc resection is recommended over extrapleural dissection if there is parietal pleural violation. Resection margin of 1 cm in all directions is considered adequate. Traditionally, margins of one rib above and below with 3 to 4 cm lateral margins were advocated.[37] The routine use of intraoperative frozen margin analysis is impractical because bone requires decalcification.

Principles of chest wall reconstruction include protection of the heart and mediastinal structures, prevention of flail chest, preservation of ventilation mechanics, judicious use of prosthetic material, and coverage of all prosthetic material with viable tissue.[36] Defects less than 3 cm or larger defects covered by the scapula do not require reconstruction. Defects just below the scapular tip in the fifth or sixth intercostal space should be closed to avoid scapular entrapment and chronic pain. Most defects are reconstructed using 2-mm-thick Gore-Tex mesh (Gore, Newark, DE, USA). Rigid prosthesis such as methyl methacrylate is difficult to use and can often be avoided except for defects involving the anterolateral chest or sternum where it is needed to preserve pulmonary mechanics and protection of the heart. For larger defects, skeletal reconstruction can be achieved using a variety of materials such as titanium plates and rods, costal and scapular autographs, cryopreserved iliac crest or ribs, or polylactic acid bars.[38–41] Prosthetic material requires coverage with viable soft tissue. The assistance of plastic surgery in preoperative planning for this purpose cannot be understated. Once the defect is closed drains are placed under the flap in addition to standard chest tubes to prevent seroma formation and kept in place until output is less than 25 to 30 mL/day.[42] Postoperative care is centered on aggressive pulmonary toilet and pain control to prevent respiratory complications. The reconstructed site is monitored closely for signs of infection and treated aggressively, although infected synthetic prostheses such as prolene, Marlex, or polytetrafluoroethylene mesh usually must be explanted and replaced with temporizing biological materials.

Extended Resections with Mechanical Circulatory Support

Circulatory bypass may be necessary to facilitate or make extended pulmonary resections possible for T4 tumors invading the heart, vena cava, aorta, subclavian arteries, innominate artery, and/or proximal pulmonary arteries. The intraoperative use of full cardiopulmonary bypass (CPB) or ECMO adds considerable complexity to what is likely an already complex resection and should be reserved for instances when it is absolutely necessary for R0 resection. Although bypass support provides the advantages of decompressing the heart to allow for safe dissection and reconstruction of tumors invading mediastinal structures such as the atrium or main pulmonary artery, it also carries significant inherent disadvantages. These disadvantages include the need for anticoagulation, access to cannulation sites, longer operative times, as well as increased risk of postoperative arrhythmias, pulmonary complications, and the largely theoretic risk of hematogenous spread.[43,44] A recent meta-analysis of studies performed from 2000 to 2016 found that most cases requiring bypass involved a single location, most commonly the left atrium (72%) or the great vessels (63%), with R0 resection being possible in more than 75% of patients.[44] Reported survival for patients undergoing these extended resections is not significantly different for patients with the same T stage who do not need bypass for resection and is approximately 40% at 5 years and 26% at 10 years.[45] However, intraoperative and in-hospital mortality is higher. One study looking at planned compared with unplanned CPB found the in-hospital mortalities were 22% and 57%, respectively.[46]

Technical considerations

Anticipated CPB-aided resection requires meticulous preoperative planning with special consideration to patient positioning and cannulation strategy. These decisions will be largely guided by tumor location, which structures are anticipated to need resection, and surgeon preference. Femoral artery and vein access for peripheral cannulation should be obtained and prepped into the field; cardiac anesthesiology and a perfusionist should be available when CPB is even potentially needed based on preoperative evaluation. Standard to all bypass procedures, cannulation strategies should consider which structures will need to be isolated as well as appropriate aortic root and pulmonary artery venting if appropriate. In general, we suggest prioritizing positioning and incision for dissection with cannulation strategies designed to accommodate the desired patient position. Nearly any position will accommodate arterial cannulation of femoral, axillary ascending, and descending aorta with venous drainage being easily accomplished in the SVC/inferior vena cava/right atrium for resection on the right (**Fig. 4**) and limited to the femoral vein and pulmonary artery

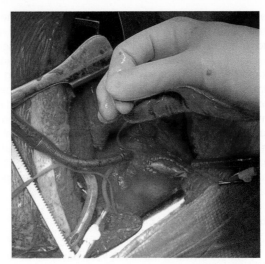

Fig. 4. Venovenous bypass (SVC-innominate and right atrium cannulas) through a right posterolateral thoracotomy with SVC pair using bovine pericardium (repair is denoted by the *arrow*).

for operations performed on the left side. Aortic cross-clamping and cardiac arrest is rarely needed except in cases were a concomitant cardiac operation (valve replacement or coronary bypass) is being performed.[46] Completion of as much dissection of structures as possible with meticulous hemostasis before initiation of bypass may aid with bleeding related to anticoagulation as well as limiting time on CPB. Prior to closure, hemostasis should be excellent and postoperatively patients are monitored closely for bleeding and pulmonary complications.

If no major vessel or heart chamber will need to be entered but mechanical circulation is needed to make resection feasible then the use of venovenous or venoarterial ECMO affords many advantages over CPB. ECMO can be used with minimal (3–5000 IU of heparin) or even no anticoagulation if necessary.[47,48] In addition, ECMO use results in less hemodilution, less blood-air interface, less postoperative coagulopathy, and less of an inflammatory response when compared with CPB.[49,50] Perhaps the best example of how ECMO can aid an operation is in the case of a sleeve pneumonectomy, doing away with awkward or cumbersome cross-field ventilation.[51]

Superior vena cava involvement

SVC involvement represents a small subset of patients with stage IIIA disease but deserves specific attention here. Involvement is either by direct tumor invasion (T4) or metastatic lymph node invasion or compression (N2). It should be noted that not all patients with SVC involvement have SVC syndrome; however, all patients are thoroughly evaluated for the syndrome and managed appropriately; incomplete resection should be avoided. Venography and or MRI may aid in determining the exact location of obstruction, presence of collaterals, patency of distal veins, and sites for proximal graft anastomosis.[52]

If the tumor involvement is not extensive (<50% and not involving the innominate vein), the use of venovenous bypass may be avoided and a side-biting Satinsky clamp can be used to excise and repair the SVC (see **Fig. 4**). Tumor invasion more than 50% requires SVC cross-clamping, excision, and reconstruction. Reconstruction is usually completed with a synthetic prosthesis, Gore-tex ringed PTFE being the most common (**Fig. 5**), but other materials such as cryopreserved arterial allograft, spiral saphenous vein, and bovine pericardial or fixed glutaraldehyde autologous pericardium tubes are also described as possible conduits.[40,53,54] Interposition reconstruction uses ringed PTFE to prevent kinking; however, Dartevelle and colleagues[55] recommend straight PTFE instead of ringed in isolated truncal reconstruction. If complete SVC resection is required, intravascular volume and vasoactive agents are used to maintain preload. Intravenous heparin (50–100 U/kg) is administered before clamping. The clamp should not be placed near the cavoatrial junction to avoid postoperative sinoatrial node dysfunction. Cross-clamp times of less than 60 minutes are well-tolerated, particularly for patients with extensive venous collaterals. Clamp time can be reduced by performing the distal anastomosis before clamping. If cross-clamp times are expected to exceed 60 minutes, innominate vein reconstruction is required or the proximal clamping will need to be below the azygous vein; then caval shunting (internal or external) or full CPB can be used to maintain adequate hemodynamics and prevent cerebral edema. Postoperatively, oral anticoagulation is maintained for 3 to 6 months.[56] Patency rates with PTFE grafts are reported at 10% to 24%, most occurring within the first month postoperatively.[57] The presence of extensive venous collaterals is considered a risk factor due to the competitive flow.[56]

Minimally Invasive Extended Resections

Because thoracic surgeons and their operative teams have become more comfortable with minimally invasive techniques for both thoracic and cardiac operations, there has been an increase in their utilization for extended resections. A full review of these

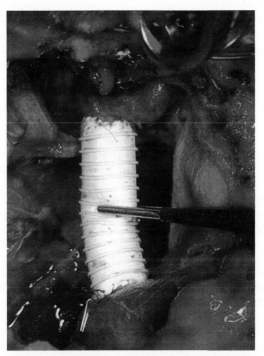

Fig. 5. SVC reconstruction using PTFE. Superiorly the subclavian-jugular junction can be seen, whereas inferiorly the innominate can be seen entering a remaining cuff of SVC.

techniques is beyond the scope of this discussion; however, it should be noted that these approaches have been noted to be safe and oncologically sound. As the technology continues to improve, as it has with robotic thoracic surgery, it is reasonable to assume that the utilization of minimally invasive extended pulmonary resection techniques will continue to grow. For example, chest wall resections can even be done via VATS or robotic means using a Gigli saw. However, this frontier may only be successfully embarked upon by individuals with a thorough understanding of traditional techniques and the ability to rapidly convert to an open resection as needed.

SUMMARY

Multiple advances in surgical technique, anesthesia, perfusion, medical oncology, and critical care over the past few decades have allowed thoracic surgeons to push the boundaries of R0 resection for advanced lung cancers. Many of these advanced operations can be done by teams in experienced centers with acceptable morbidity and mortality and improved mid- and long-term survival when compared with palliative chemoradiation.

CLINICS CARE POINTS

- Advanced lung cancer includes a diverse group of patients requiring multimodality therapeutic approaches that often require extended resections.
- Parenchymal-sparing techniques provide complete oncologic resection with similar survival and are preferred whenever possible.
- Tumors involving the thoracic inlet, mediastinal structures, or the chest wall require unique approaches and techniques.
- The advent of mechanical circulatory support has broadened the scope of what can be deemed.

DISCLOSURE

The authors have nothing to disclose.

REFERENCES

1. Detterbeck FC. The eighth edition TNM stage classification for lung cancer: what does it mean on main street? J Thorac Cardiovasc Surg 2018;155(1): 356–9.
2. Martini N, Kris MG, Flehinger BJ, et al. Preoperative chemotherapy for stage IIIa (N2) lung cancer: the Sloan-Kettering experience with 136 patients. Ann Thorac Surg 1993;55(6):1365–73 [discussion: 1373-1374].
3. Rosell R, Gómez-Codina J, Camps C, et al. A randomized trial comparing preoperative chemotherapy plus surgery with surgery alone in patients with non-small-cell lung cancer. N Engl J Med 1994;330(3):153–8.
4. Roth JA, Atkinson EN, Fossella F, et al. Long-term follow-up of patients enrolled in a randomized trial comparing perioperative chemotherapy and surgery with surgery alone in resectable stage IIIA non-small-cell lung cancer. Lung Cancer Amst Neth 1998;21(1):1–6.
5. van Meerbeeck JP, Kramer GWPM, Van Schil PEY, et al. Randomized controlled trial of resection versus radiotherapy after induction chemotherapy in stage IIIA-N2 non-small-cell lung cancer. J Natl Cancer Inst 2007;99(6):442–50.

6. Albain KS, Swann RS, Rusch VW, et al. Radiotherapy plus chemotherapy with or without surgical resection for stage III non-small-cell lung cancer: a phase III randomised controlled trial. Lancet Lond Engl 2009;374(9687):379–86.

7. Bograd AJ, Vallières E. Surgery as a component of multimodality care for known stage IIIA-N2 non-small cell lung cancer. Semin Respir Crit Care Med 2020;41(3): 346–53.

8. Gillaspie EA, Wigle DA. Management of stage IIIA (N2) non-small cell lung cancer. Thorac Surg Clin 2016;26(3):271–85.

9. Eberhardt WEE, Pöttgen C, Gauler TC, et al. Phase III study of surgery versus definitive concurrent chemoradiotherapy boost in patients with resectable stage IIIA(N2) and selected IIIB non-small-cell lung cancer after induction chemotherapy and concurrent chemoradiotherapy (ESPATUE). J Clin Oncol 2015; 33(35):4194–201.

10. Reardon ES, Schrump DS. Extended resections of non-small cell lung cancers invading the aorta, pulmonary artery, left atrium, or esophagus: can they be justified? Thorac Surg Clin 2014;24(4):457–64.

11. Deslauriers J, Grégoire J, Jacques LF, et al. Sleeve lobectomy versus pneumonectomy for lung cancer: a comparative analysis of survival and sites or recurrences. Ann Thorac Surg 2004;77(4):1152–6 [discussion: 1156].

12. Park JS, Yang HC, Kim HK, et al. Sleeve lobectomy as an alternative procedure to pneumonectomy for non-small cell lung cancer. J Thorac Oncol 2010;5(4): 517–20.

13. Okada M, Tsubota N, Yoshimura M, et al. Extended sleeve lobectomy for lung cancer: the avoidance of pneumonectomy. J Thorac Cardiovasc Surg 1999; 118(4):710–3 [discussion: 713-714].

14. Chen Y, Zhang L, Yan B, et al. Feasibility of sleeve lobectomy after neo-adjuvant chemo-immunotherapy in non-small cell lung cancer. Transl Lung Cancer Res 2020;9(3):761–7.

15. Bölükbas S, Baldes N, Bergmann T, et al. Standard and extended sleeve resections of the tracheobronchial tree. J Thorac Dis 2020;12(10):6163–72.

16. Raja S, Mason DP, Murthy SC. Sleeve resection/bronchoplasty for lung cancer. In: Sugarbaker DJ, Bueno R, Colson YL, et al, editors. Adult chest surgery. 2nd edition. McGraw-Hill Education; 2015. Available at: accesssurgery.mhmedical.com/content.aspx?aid=1105842464. Accessed November 30, 2021.

17. Shapiro M, Swanson SJ, Wright CD, et al. Predictors of major morbidity and mortality after pneumonectomy utilizing the Society for Thoracic Surgeons General Thoracic Surgery Database. Ann Thorac Surg 2010;90(3):927–34 [discussion: 934-935].

18. Couñago F, Rodriguez de Dios N, Montemuiño S, et al. Neoadjuvant treatment followed by surgery versus definitive chemoradiation in stage IIIA-N2 non-small-cell lung cancer: A multi-institutional study by the oncologic group for the study of lung cancer (Spanish Radiation Oncology Society). Lung Cancer Amst Neth 2018;118:119–27.

19. Refai M, Brunelli A, Rocco G, et al. Does induction treatment increase the risk of morbidity and mortality after pneumonectomy? A multicentre case-matched analysis. Eur J Cardiothorac Surg 2010;37(3):535–9.

20. Alifano M, Boudaya MS, Salvi M, et al. Pneumonectomy after chemotherapy: morbidity, mortality, and long-term outcome. Ann Thorac Surg 2008;85(6): 1866–72 [discussion: 1872-1873].

21. White A, Kucukak S, Bueno R, et al. Pneumonectomy is safe and effective for non-small cell lung cancer following induction therapy. J Thorac Dis 2017; 9(11):4447–53.
22. Brunelli A, Kim AW, Berger KI, et al. Physiologic evaluation of the patient with lung cancer being considered for resectional surgery: Diagnosis and management of lung cancer, 3rd ed: American College of Chest Physicians evidence-based clinical practice guidelines. Chest 2013;143(5 Suppl):e166S–90S.
23. Kim AW, Boffa DJ, Wang Z, et al. An analysis, systematic review, and meta-analysis of the perioperative mortality after neoadjuvant therapy and pneumonectomy for non-small cell lung cancer. J Thorac Cardiovasc Surg 2012;143(1):55–63.
24. Stolz A, Pafko P, Harustiak T, et al. Risk factor analysis for early mortality and morbidity following pneumonectomy for non-small cell lung cancer. Bratisl Lek Listy 2011;112(4):165–9.
25. Bernard A, Deschamps C, Allen MS, et al. Pneumonectomy for malignant disease: factors affecting early morbidity and mortality. J Thorac Cardiovasc Surg 2001;121(6):1076–82.
26. Schleicher A, Groeben H. Anesthetic considerations for tracheobronchial surgery. J Thorac Dis 2020;12(10):6138–42.
27. Costantino CL, Geller AD, Wright CD, et al. Carinal surgery: a single-institution experience spanning 2 decades. J Thorac Cardiovasc Surg 2019;157(5):2073–83.e1.
28. Costantino CL, Wright CD. Extended Pulmonary Resection by Sleeve Lobectomy and Carinal Pneumonectomy: Selection and Technique. Thorac Surg Clin 2021; 31(3):273–81.
29. Weder W, Inci I. Carinal resection and sleeve pneumonectomy. J Thorac Dis 2016;8(Suppl 11):S882–8.
30. Banki F, Wood DE. Techniques of performing left carinal pneumonectomy. Oper Tech Thorac Cardiovasc Surg 2007;12(3):194–209.
31. Rusch VW, Giroux DJ, Kraut MJ, et al. Induction chemoradiation and surgical resection for superior sulcus non-small-cell lung carcinomas: long-term results of Southwest Oncology Group Trial 9416 (Intergroup Trial 0160). J Clin Oncol 2007;25(3):313–8.
32. Kunitoh H, Kato H, Tsuboi M, et al. Phase II trial of preoperative chemoradiotherapy followed by surgical resection in patients with superior sulcus non-small-cell lung cancers: report of Japan Clinical Oncology Group trial 9806. J Clin Oncol Off J Am Soc Clin Oncol 2008;26(4):644–9.
33. Rusch VW, Parekh KR, Leon L, et al. Factors determining outcome after surgical resection of T3 and T4 lung cancers of the superior sulcus. J Thorac Cardiovasc Surg 2000;119(6):1147–53.
34. Hagan MP, Choi NC, Mathisen DJ, et al. Superior sulcus lung tumors: impact of local control on survival. J Thorac Cardiovasc Surg 1999;117(6):1086–94.
35. Marulli G, Battistella L, Perissinotto E, et al. Results of surgical resection after induction chemoradiation for Pancoast tumours. Interact Cardiovasc Thorac Surg 2015;20(6):805–11 [discussion: 811-812].
36. Loi M, Mazzella A, Desideri I, et al. Chest wall resection and reconstruction for lung cancer: surgical techniques and example of integrated multimodality approach. J Thorac Dis 2020;12(1):22–30.
37. Lanuti M. Surgical management of lung cancer involving the chest wall. Thorac Surg Clin 2017;27(2):195–9.
38. Boerma LM, Bemelman M, van Dalen T. Chest wall reconstruction after resection of a chest wall sarcoma by osteosynthesis with the titanium MatrixRIB (Synthes) system. J Thorac Cardiovasc Surg 2013;146(4):e37–40.

39. Miller DL, Force SD, Pickens A, et al. Chest wall reconstruction using biomaterials. Ann Thorac Surg 2013;95(3):1050–6.
40. Garcia A, Flores RM. Surgical management of tumors invading the superior vena cava. Ann Thorac Surg 2008;85(6):2144–6.
41. Rocco G. Anterior chest wall resection and reconstruction. Oper Tech Thorac Cardiovasc Surg 2013;18(1):32–41.
42. Bennett DT, Weyant MJ. Extended chest wall resection and reconstruction in the setting of lung cancer. Thorac Surg Clin 2014;24(4):383–90.
43. Dartevelle PG, Mitilian D, Fadel E. Extended surgery for T4 lung cancer: a 30 years' experience. Gen Thorac Cardiovasc Surg 2017;65(6):321–8.
44. Yuan SM. Extended pneumonectomy for advanced lung cancer with cardiovascular structural invasions. Turk Gogus Kalp Dama Cerrahisi Derg 2018;26(2):336–42.
45. Langer NB, Mercier O, Fabre D, et al. Outcomes after resection of T4 non-small cell lung cancer using cardiopulmonary bypass. Ann Thorac Surg 2016;102(3):902–10.
46. de Biasi AR, Nasar A, Lee PC, et al. National analysis of short-term outcomes after pulmonary resections on cardiopulmonary bypass. Ann Thorac Surg 2015;100(6):2064–71.
47. Raman J, Alimohamed M, Dobrilovic N, et al. A comparison of low and standard anti-coagulation regimens in extracorporeal membrane oxygenation. J Heart Lung Transplant 2019;38(4):433–9.
48. Pabst D, Boone JB, Soleimani B, et al. Heparin-induced thrombocytopenia in patients on extracorporeal membrane oxygenation and the role of a heparin-bonded circuit. Perfusion 2019;34(7):584–9.
49. Bermudez CA, Shiose A, Esper SA, et al. Outcomes of intraoperative venoarterial extracorporeal membrane oxygenation versus cardiopulmonary bypass during lung transplantation. Ann Thorac Surg 2014;98(6):1936–43.
50. Parikh AN, Merritt TC, Carvajal HG, et al. A comparison of cardiopulmonary bypass versus extracorporeal membrane oxygenation: Does intraoperative circulatory support strategy affect outcomes in pediatric lung transplantation? Clin Transplant 2021;35(6). https://doi.org/10.1111/ctr.14289.
51. Spaggiari L, Sedda G, Petrella F, et al. Preliminary Results of Extracorporeal Membrane Oxygenation Assisted Tracheal Sleeve Pneumonectomy for Cancer. Thorac Cardiovasc Surg 2021;69(03):240–5.
52. Al-Ayoubi AM, Flores RM. Surgery for lung cancer invading the mediastinum. J Thorac Dis 2016;8(Suppl 11):S889–94.
53. D'Andrilli A, Venuta F, Rendina EA. Surgical approaches for invasive tumors of the anterior mediastinum. Thorac Surg Clin 2010;20(2):265–84.
54. Spaggiari L, Veronesi G, D'Aiuto M, et al. Superior vena cava reconstruction using heterologous pericardial tube after extended resection for lung cancer. Eur J Cardiothorac 2004;26(3):649–51.
55. Dartevelle P, Chapelier A, Navajas M, et al. Replacement of the superior vena cava with polytetrafluoroethylene grafts combined with resection of mediastinal-pulmonary malignant tumors. Report of thirteen cases. J Thorac Cardiovasc Surg 1987;94(3):361–6.
56. Lee DSD, Flores RM. Superior vena caval resection in lung cancer. Thorac Surg Clin 2014;24(4):441–7.
57. Lanuti M, De Delva PE, Gaissert HA, et al. Review of superior vena cava resection in the management of benign disease and pulmonary or mediastinal malignancies. Ann Thorac Surg 2009;88(2):392–7.

Evaluation and Interventional Management of Cardiac Dysrhythmias

Steven J. Hoff, MD, FHRS

KEYWORDS

- Atrial fibrillation • Ablation • Postoperative atrial fibrillation
- Perioperative cardiac implantable electronic device management

KEY POINTS

- Postoperative atrial fibrillation has unique mechanisms of initiation and provides special challenges for treatment.
- Concomitant surgical ablation for atrial fibrillation can be performed without additional morbidity and mortality.
- Nonpharmacologic left atrial appendage management offers an alternative to standard anticoagulation for stroke risk reduction.
- Hybrid therapies for stand-alone ablation of atrial fibrillation are safe and effective.

EVALUATION AND MANAGEMENT OF ATRIAL FIBRILLATION
Introduction

Definitions and prevalence

Atrial fibrillation (AF) is defined as a supraventricular tachycardia characterized by irregular RR intervals with the absence of distinct P waves and irregular and ineffective atrial contraction.[1–8] AF is the most common sustained arrhythmia encountered in clinical practice and affects approximately 33 million people worldwide.[9] It is currently estimated that the prevalence of AF in adults is between 2% and 4%[10] and expected to increase given increased longevity and better diagnosis. In 2010, the prevalence of AF in the United States was estimated to be between 2.7 and 6.1 million. This is expected to increase to about 5.6 million to 12 million in 2050.[2] The incidence of AF increases with age.[11] Other identified risk factors for AF include hypertension, valvular heart disease, obesity, sleep apnea, diabetes, coronary disease, hyperthyroidism, excessive alcohol use, drug use, and heart failure/cardiomyopathy.[11,12]

Orlando Health Heart and Vascular Institute, 1222 South Orange Avenue, Orlando, FL 32806, USA
E-mail address: steve.hoff@orlandohealth.com

Surg Clin N Am 102 (2022) 365–391
https://doi.org/10.1016/j.suc.2022.01.003
surgical.theclinics.com

Abbreviations	
AF	Atrial Fibrillation
MI	Myocardial Infarction
INR	Internatyional Normalized Ratio
DOAC	Direct Oral Anticoagulant
NOAC	Novel Anticoagulant
AHA	American Heart Association
ACC	American College of Cardiology
HRS	Heart Rhythm Society
CAB	Coronary Artery Bypass
PVI	Pulmonary Vein Isolation
AV	Atrioventricular
LAA	Left Atrial Appendage
CIED	Cardiovascualr Implantable Electric Device
EMI	Electromechanical Inhibition
ICD	Internal Cardiac Defibrillator
	RRRelative Risk

AF tends to be a progressive disease. More than half of individuals who experience an initial episode of AF will eventually develop recurrent AF, typically within the first 2 years of follow-up.

Pathogenesis of AF can be described as mechanisms for the initiation of AF and for its maintenance. If the patient has the former without the latter, they typically developed paroxysmal AF. It is generally agreed upon that mechanisms for initiation are results of focal electrical triggers, which in humans originate more than 90% of the time from atrial myocytes in the pulmonary veins. This was first described by Haissaguerre and colleagues[13] in 1996. As AF continues, ion channel remodeling alters electrophysiologic substrate perpetuating macro-reentrant circuits and increases the activity of these triggers.[6] This downward pathophysiologic spiral gives rise to the clinical concept that "AF begets AF."[14] This will be important in later discussions of rhythm versus rate control. The mechanisms of maintenance of AF are more complicated and multifactorial and include abnormal substrate within the atrial myocardium, such as atrial fibrosis, or atrial stretch, such as is seen in valvular heart disease. It is complicated by other physiologic factors, including electrolyte disturbances, inflammation, and autonomic influences. Some of these have been implicated in the development of postoperative AF.

AF is independently associated with significantly increased morbidity and mortality, including a fivefold increased risk for stroke, twofold increased risk for dementia, threefold increased risk for heart failure, and a twofold increased risk for myocardial infarction (MI). The mortality of patients with AF is approximately double that of patients in sinus rhythm and linked to the severity of underlying heart disease and associated comorbidities.[15]

AF can be classified as paroxysmal or persistent (**Table 1**). Paroxysmal AF is defined as AF that terminates spontaneously or with intervention within 7 days of onset and may reoccur with a variable frequency. Persistent AF is defined as continuous AF that is sustained for greater than 7 days, including episodes that are terminated by pharmacologic or electrical cardioversion after 7 days or more. Longstanding persistent AF is defined as continuous AF of greater than 12 months' duration. Permanent AF is used to describe AF in a patient whereby no further attempts to restore/maintain sinus rhythm are being sought. Terms, such as lone AF, chronic AF, and valvular/nonvalvular AF, tend to be confusing, and most Societies discourage their use.[1,2]

Table 1 Definitions of atrial fibrillation: a simplified scheme	
Term	**Definition**
Paroxysmal AF	• AF that terminates spontaneously or with intervention within 7 d of onset • Episodes may recur with variable frequency
Persistent AF	• Continuous AF that is sustained >7 d
Long-standing persistent AF	• Continuous AF >12 mo in duration
Permanent AF	• When the patient and clinician make a joint decision to stop further attempts to restore and/or maintain sinus rhythm
Nonvalvular AF	• AF in the absence of rheumatic mitral stenosis, mechanical or bioprosthetic heart valve, or mitral valve repair

MEDICAL THERAPY FOR ATRIAL FIBRILLATION

A detailed discourse regarding medical therapy and drugs for AF is beyond the scope of this article. Detailed discussion can be found in recently published guidelines.[2,3,5] This discussion focuses on several topics of utility to the surgeon, including acute rate control, controversies regarding rhythm versus rate control, anticoagulation for stroke prevention, and postoperative AF.

Antiarrhythmic Therapy

Current available antiarrhythmics can be separated into 4 classes based on their mode of action. They include the following:

- Class I, sodium channel blockers: Their usage has become less commonly related to adverse long-term effects. Procainamide (1A) and lidocaine (1B) are used intravenously for acute ventricular arrhythmias. Flecainide (1C) and propafenone (1C) are generally considered safe only in the absence of structural heart disease.
- Class II, beta-blocker: These drugs are particularly effective in an hyperadrenergic state, such as chronic heart failure and ischemic arrhythmias, as well as for reentrant tachyarrhythmias.
- Class III, potassium channel blocker: Amiodarone is effective for both ventricular and supraventricular arrhythmias but potentially toxic even in low doses. Sotalol and dofetilide can lead to torsades de pointes in the face of baseline prolonged QTc and therefore must be carefully loaded in a hospital setting.
- Class IV, calcium channel blocker: Verapamil and diltiazem are used to reduce the ventricular rate in acute or chronic AF. Adenosine can be effectively used to terminate acute supraventricular tachycardias.

Acute Rate Control of Atrial Fibrillation

Rapid control of accelerated ventricular response to AF can be controlled in the inpatient setting using intravenous diltiazem or esmolol. It is managed in the outpatient setting typically with a class II or class IV agent. It should be noted that in either setting, the use of digoxin intravenously or orally is reserved for patients with uncontrolled ventricular response to AF where other agents have failed and only in the face of reduced ventricular function. Its current use is controversial, and it has been associated with an increased risk of all-cause mortality.[16,17] Recent guidelines have relaxed recommendations for heart rate target in the rate control strategy based on data that suggest a lenient rate control strategy (goal resting heart rate <110 bpm) is as effective as a strict rate energy control previously recommended (goal resting heart rate <80 bpm) but has far fewer side effects leading to seeking medical attention.[18]

Rhythm Control Strategy for Atrial Fibrillation

Pharmacologic cardioversion can often be achieved with intravenous ibutilide or oral sotalol. Amiodarone has been used for pharmacologic cardioversion but because of its long half-life has a much slower onset of action even if loaded intravenously. Given pathophysiologic mechanisms of AF generation resulting from substrate modification supporting the theory of "AF begets AF," a rhythm control strategy could be supported. Symptomatic benefit could be explained by improved hemodynamics with atrial contraction and augmentation of left ventricular filling.

Several older trials have investigated rate versus rhythm control and failed to identify differences between strategies in terms of overall survival, overall cardiovascular death, worsening heart failure, or stroke. They have documented significant improvement in symptoms and quality of life with rhythm restoration.[19–21] A more recent observational study suggested an increased rate of all-cause death at 1 year with a rate control strategy.[22] Accordingly, recent guidelines currently recommend antiarrhythmic therapy and a rhythm control strategy only for symptom amelioration and improvement in quality of life.[5]

POSTOPERATIVE ATRIAL FIBRILLATION

Postoperative AF, defined as new-onset AF in the immediate postoperative period, occurs with a peak incidence between postoperative day 2 and 4.[23] Mechanisms for the initiation of AF in the postoperative period are thought to be different from those generally associated with AF. They include pericardial inflammation, particularly after cardiac surgery, acute atrial stretch associated with volume expansion and fluid shifts after surgery, and hyperadrenergic states related to postoperative pain. It occurs in 20% to 50% of patients after cardiac surgery,[24–26] in 10% to 30% after noncardiac thoracic surgery,[27] and in 5% to 10% of patients after vascular or large colorectal procedures.[28] Postoperative AF has been shown to be a risk factor for stroke, MI, and death compared with patients who do not develop AF in the postoperative setting.[29,30] It has also been associated with hemodynamic instability, prolonged hospital stays, infections, renal complications, bleeding, increased in-hospital deaths, and increased health care costs.[31,32] The development of AF in the postoperative setting has been associated with a four- to fivefold increase in the risk of recurrent AF over the ensuing 5 years.[33,34]

Several agents have been tested to prevent or reduce the incidence of postoperative AF. Preoperative beta-blocker therapy has been the most frequently studied in its use in cardiac and noncardiac surgery and is associated with a reduced incidence of postoperative AF,[35–38] but not major adverse events, such as death, stroke, or acute kidney injury.[39] Amiodarone, with or without beta-blockers, has also shown some promise in reducing postoperative AF.[40,41] Other agents, such as statins, magnesium, sotalol, colchicine, and steroids, have been used with varying results. Colchicine is currently being reevaluated in a randomized controlled trial.[42]

The acute treatment of AF has been previously discussed. Effective intravenous agents for acute rate control include Lopressor and Cardizem. Amiodarone has been used effectively as rhythm control, but its pharmacokinetics are suboptimal owing to a long half-life and slow onset of action. It generally requires central venous access for intravenous loading to prevent cellulitis. Oral sotalol has been used effectively for acute rhythm control. Chronic rate control is generally accomplished with oral beta-blocker, calcium channel blockers, and amiodarone.

Prevention of thromboembolism in the postoperative setting often requires individualized therapy. In enlargement analysis, patients with postoperative AF had a 62% higher risk of early stroke compared with those without postoperative AF in patients who have been in AF for more than 48 hours postoperatively, and anticoagulation is indicated but must be individualized regarding the risk of bleeding complications.[29] Unfractionated heparin can be used under strict protocols to prevent supratherapeutic levels. Its short half-life and reversibility are advantageous in the situation. Long-term anticoagulation options include warfarin and non-vitamin K dependent oral anticoagulants (NOACs) as discussed later.

A treatment algorithm for the management of postoperative AF can be found in **Fig. 1**.

ANTICOAGULATION FOR STROKE PREVENTION IN ATRIAL FIBRILLATION

The most devastating complication related to AF is ischemic stroke related to thromboembolism. Stroke-related AF is associated with a higher stroke severity, more permanent disability, and greater short-term and long-term mortality.[43–45] Multiple clinical trials have shown anticoagulation lowers stroke risk owing to AF.[46–48] Pharmacologic and nonpharmacologic strategies for stroke risk reduction in AF are discussed.

Stratification Schemes for Thromboembolism Risk and Bleeding Risk

Several risk-stratification schemes have been developed to help predict the risk of ischemic stroke and other systemic thromboembolisms that may benefit from anticoagulation therapy. These indexes initially relied on age and cardiovascular factors to help predict stroke risk. Developed in 2001, the CHADS2 index was the first risk-stratification scheme to gain wide acceptance.[49] It used commonly known associated risk factors to help predict stroke owing to AF and categorize them as low, moderate, and high risk based on a weighted scoring system. A newer CHA2DS2-VASc scoring system has been shown to be more reliable at identifying truly low-risk patients that will not benefit from anticoagulation (**Table 2**).[50] A low-risk score is defined as a CHA2DS2-VASc score of 0 or 1, identifying a group of patients that are sufficiently low risk from thromboembolic complications and who do not benefit from anticoagulation therapy. A CHA2DS2-VASc 2 score of 2 or greater indicates a higher risk whereby anticoagulation should be considered. It should be emphasized that these risk-stratification schemes have been validated in the overall population, not in postoperative patients. It is used in most major guidelines as the recommended stroke risk-stratification tool.[2,5] In addition, cardiac imaging may provide additional information regarding patients with increased stroke risk. Echocardiographic determination of increased left atrial dimensions, the presence of spontaneous echo contrast, and left atrial appendage flow peak velocity less than 20 cm/s as well as left atrial appendage non–chicken wing morphology assessed by cardiac CT or MRI have been associated with increased stroke risk in patients with AF.[51–53]

Oral anticoagulation is associated with increased risk of bleeding particularly in the postoperative setting. His estimated up to 44% of patients with AF have 1 or more absolute or relative complications for long-term oral anticoagulation therapy. Therefore, an assessment of bleeding risk seems particularly pertinent in the postoperative setting. The risk of bleeding should be weighed against the potential benefit of stroke prevention for individual patients. Several risk models have been posed to predict

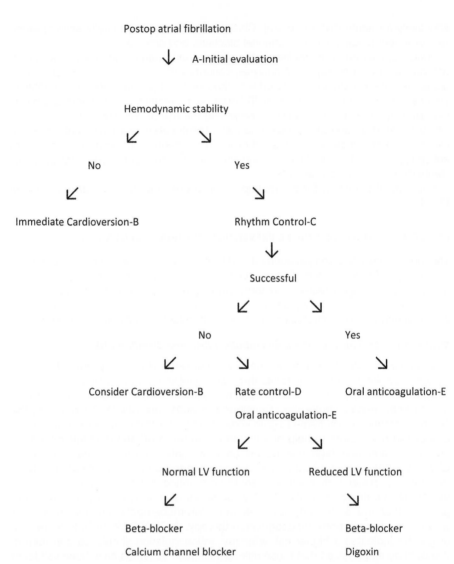

Fig. 1. Algorithm for treatment of postoperative AF. (*A*) Check potassium/magnesium levels and replete if necessary; check baseline EKG. (*B*) Periprocedural anticoagulation recommended. (*C*) Normal left ventricular (LV) function; load amiodarone intravenously if central access—sotalol if QTc < 450 and normal renal function; load amiodarone orally; reduced left ventricular function; load amiodarone IV or orally. (*D*) Target heart rate less than 110 bpm (*E*) if anticoagulation deemed safe: Eliquis 2.5 mg twice daily, consider warfarin. postop, postoperatively.

bleeding risk with antithrombotic therapy. Only the HAS-BLED score has been validated in the AF population (**Table 3**).[54] HAS-BLED has not been validated in the postoperative setting. Furthermore, bleeding risk in the postoperative setting should be individualized and include aggressive efforts at reduction of potentially reversible bleeding risk factor, such as uncontrolled hypertension concomitant use of antiplatelet therapy, anemia, and renal or hepatic insufficiency.

Table 2
CHADS2-VASC score

Letter	Clinical Characteristics	Points
C	Congestive heart failure, LV dysfunction	1
H	Hypertension	1
A2	Age ≥75 y	2
D	Diabetes	1
S2	Stroke, transient ischemic attack	2
V	Vascular (MI, peripheral vascualr disease, aortic disease)	1
A	Age 65–74 y	1
S	Sex (female gender)	1
	Maximum points	9

Anticoagulation Strategies in Atrial Fibrillation

Until 2000, study showed warfarin was better than placebo or aspirin for the prevention of AF-related strokes and was the standard of care in patients at high risk for stroke from AF[55] despite attempts at adherence to the target international normalized ratio (INR) range of 2.0 to 3.0, patient compliance, need for regular monitoring, and significant interactions with medications and food, and led to an increased risk of bleeding complications. Warfarin or aspirin therapy was generally recommended for patients at intermediate risk of stroke.

Beginning in 2009, four direct oral anticoagulants (DOACs) have been compared with warfarin therapy for stroke prevention and nonvalvular AF.[56–59] These trials demonstrated that the DOAC studied was noninferior to Coumadin for the prevention of stroke and thromboembolism. The Aristotle trial showed apixaban was superior in preventing stroke and thromboembolism compared with warfarin. In addition, these trials showed that apixaban and edoxaban had a significantly lower risk of major bleeding compared with warfarin. These results, reflected in the 2019 American Heart Association (AHA)/American College of Cardiology (ACC)/Heart Rhythm Society (HRS) focused update on the management of patients with AF, have led to a shift away from warfarin and have made apixaban first-line therapy for stroke prevention and nonvalvular AF owing to its superiority over warfarin in the prevention of stroke and thromboembolism with a lower overall rate of bleeding.[5]

Table 3
HAS-BLED score

Letter	Clinical Characteristics	Points
H	Hypertension	1
A	Abnormal liver/renal function	1 or 2
S	Stroke	1
B	Bleeding	1
L	Labile INR	1
E	Elderly (age >65)	1
D	Drug or alcohol use	1 or 2
	Maximum points	9

Interruption/Bridging of Oral Anticoagulation

In patients taking warfarin as stroke prophylaxis for AF, the Bridge Trial in 2015 demonstrated noninferiority for the prevention of arterial thromboembolism and a decreased risk of major bleeding in patients whose Coumadin was stopped before surgery without bridging.[60] This finding was confirmed by recent meta-analysis.[61]

Recommendations for patients undergoing planned invasive procedures taking DOACs were recently addressed in a 2018 consensus statement.[62] It was recommended not to interrupt oral adequate anticoagulation for most minor surgical procedures and those procedures whereby bleeding could easily be controlled. These procedures can be performed 12 to 24 hours after the last DOAC dose, with a DOAC restart 6 hours later. For invasive procedures with low bleeding risk, such as cardiac device implantation, it was recommended to take the last dose of DOAC 24 hours before the procedure in patients with normal kidney function. In the case of invasive procedures carrying a high risk for major bleeding, it remained recommended to take the last DOAC dose 48 hours or longer before surgery. Preoperative bridging with low-molecular-weight heparin was not recommended in DOAC-treated patients. Postoperatively, when postoperative bleeding has been controlled, DOACs can generally be resumed at 6 to 8 hours after the end of the procedure. For surgical procedures whereby bleeding risk may outweigh the risk of a fibrillated embolism, restarting DOACs 48 to 72 hours postoperatively should be considered.

Reversal of Oral Anticoagulation

It is well accepted that the traditional use of Coumadin has definitive reversal options with the administration of vitamin K orally or intravenously, prothrombin complex concentrate, or fresh frozen plasma. Rapid reversal in the patient with a mechanical heart valve should be done with caution. For instance, fresh frozen plasma is preferred. Reversal agents for DOAC have recently been approved.[5,63,64] Andexanet alfa can be used in the reversal of apixaban and Rivaroxaban. It is extremely expensive and unpredictably reliable. Apixaban and Rivaroxaban are not dialyzable, whereas dabigatran is dialyzable.

NONPHARMACOLOGIC INTERVENTIONS: LEFT ATRIAL APPENDAGE MANAGEMENT

Left atrial appendage is a site of thrombus formation and subsequent thromboembolism in greater than 90% of patients with nonvalvular AF who have a stroke.[65] This is related to its complex and highly variable anatomy.[66,67] The left atrial appendage is divided into 3 anatomic regions, the ostium or orifice, the neck, and the lobar region. The endocardium of the left atrial appendage contains pectinate muscles, particularly in the lobar region. A CT-based classification of left atrial appendage morphology has divided this into 4 types: the chicken wing (48%), the cactus (30%), the windsock (19%), and the cauliflower (3%).[68] The chicken wing has a dominant central lobe with a sharp bend in the proximal or midsection that can fall back on itself. The cactus has a dominant central lobe with secondary lobes extending above or below it. The windsock has one main lobe and other smaller lobes arising from it. The cauliflower is shorter in length and more complex. A recent study showed patients with chicken wing morphology had the lowest risk of cardioembolic events (4%), and the cauliflower morphology had the highest prevalence of embolic events (18%).[52] A subsequent study suggested a chicken wing morphology with greater than 90° bend had a similar risk of stroke as non–chicken wing appendages.[69] These morphologic differences become important in thrombus formation as well as in nonpharmacologic efforts to exclude the left atrial appendage from the circulation, therefore reducing thromboembolic risk.

In addition to a role in stroke prophylaxis, left atrial appendage ligation may have other benefits. As an important source of atrial natriuretic peptide, it could have a role in neurohormonal modulation.[70] It may also have a role in arrhythmia management. Dibiase and colleagues[71] concluded that abherent firings from the left atrial appendage occurred in 27% of patients with 1 implant repeat catheter ablation for AF and at 8.7% it was the only source of AF. Other recent studies have suggested that the addition of left atrial appendage ligation that leads to appendage necrosis is associated with improved success rates after AF ablation.[72,73]

Anticoagulation with vitamin K antagonists or NOACs is the gold standard for stroke prevention but is contraindicated in some patients. Interventional left atrial appendage occlusion devices are a valid alternative to anticoagulation; however, their use is limited by a high rate of periprocedural complications and the unknown long-term clinical implications of residual peridevice flow. Studies on surgical left atrial appendage have resulted in heterogeneous outcomes owing to failure to achieve occlusion.[74] Epicardial devices for left atrial appendage occlusion offer a safe and durable treatment with robust clinical data, but randomized control trials are lacking.

Clinically Available Devices

Endocardial: Watchman
Currently, the only Food and Drug Administration (FDA) -approved device for endovascular left atrial appendage closure is the Watchman device (Boston Scientific, Marlborough, MA)). It consists of a nitinol frame and polyethylene membrane that covers the surface facing the left atrium. In the protect-AF trial, which led to FDA approval, the rate of successful device implantation, defined as a peridevice leak of less than 5 mm, was 88%.[75] Long-term follow-up from the PROTECT-AF trial as well as the PREVAIL trial showed the Watchman device was comparable to warfarin for the prevention of stroke, with reductions in major bleeding, hemorrhagic stroke, and mortality.[76] A second generation of the device is in clinical trials.

Epicardial: AtriClip
First introduced in 2007, the Atriclip device (Atricure, Inc, Cincinnati, OH) has been used in more than 100,000 patients for left atrial appendage occlusion. Early studies showed excellent results with 100% appendage occlusion with an excellent safety and durability profile.[77,78] In long-term follow-up, a relative stroke risk reduction of 87.5% was observed in patients who had oral anticoagulation discontinued with an observed rate of ischemic stroke of 0.5 per 100 patient-years, compared with the rate expected in the group of patients with similar CHA2DS2-VASc scores of 4 events per 100 patient-years.[79] Expected data from the third left atrial appendage occlusion during cardiac surgery (LAAOS III) trial as well as the left atrial appendage exclusion concomitant to structural heart procedures (Atlas) study may evaluate the role of left atrial appendage exclusion in patients without a history of AF but it increased risk for its development postoperatively.[74]

INVESTIGATIONAL DEVICES

Several devices are currently in clinical trials and may provide additional options and improved results with endocardial left atrial appendage occlusion. These include the Amplatzer amulet (Abbott, Inc., Austin, TX), the Lariat suture delivery system (Sentre-Heart, Palo Alto, CA), the Coherex WaveCrest occlusion system (Biosense Webster,

Irvine, CA), and the LAmbre left atrial appendage closure system (Lifetech Scientific, Shenzen, China).[79]

NONPHARMACOLOGIC THERAPY FOR ATRIAL FIBRILLATION
Catheter-Based Therapy

Catheter ablation for AF is the most widely performed electrophysiologic procedure. It is generally used as a second-line treatment strategy in patients who have failed anti-arrhythmic therapy for rhythm or rate management and remain symptomatic. Recent guidelines have made His treatment in paroxysmal AF a class I indication, for persistent AF a class IIa recommendation, and for patients with longstanding persistent AF a class IIb recommendation.[1]

Ablation for paroxysmal AF is based on the elimination of initiating electrical triggers, the majority of which come from the pulmonary veins in humans.[13] Electrical pulmonary vein isolation (PVI) has become a highly effective treatment for paroxysmal AF compared with medical therapy.[80,81] The 2 most common energy sources used for PVI include radiofrequency ablation navigated by electroanatomic mapping systems and cryoballoon technology. These have proven to be equally efficacious in multiple trials and 3 recent meta-analyses.[82–84] Advantages of the cryoballoon ablation include shorter procedural time, a shorter learning curve, and less operator dependence, possibly leading to better reproducibility.[85–87] Serious complications associated with catheter-based AF ablation include cardiac perforation, and tamponade, stroke, atrio-esophageal fistula, and pulmonary vein stenosis are uncommon.[88] Recurrent AF is generally related to pulmonary vein reconnection, either incomplete scarring of the initial ablation injury or healing that allows electrical communication between the trigger site and the atrium.

Catheter-based management of persistent or longstanding persistent AF requires a different strategy, with the addition of substrate modification in the left atrium in addition to PVI. Despite multiple ablations, results tend to be less favorable.[89] Results in very large left atria, patients with structural heart disease, patients with multiple comorbidities, and patients with no-pulmonary vein triggers tend to be less favorable. Early recurrence during the first 3 months after the procedure (blanking period) also portend less favorable outcomes. New developments and technologies in the form of novel energy sources, multielectrode ablating catheters, lesion visualization technologies, and development of a radiofrequency balloon catheter may lead to improved results in more complex disease and more widespread utilization of ablation technology in the treatment of AF.[89]

Surgical Therapy

Surgical therapy for AF is commonly performed at the time of otherwise indicated cardiac surgery (concomitant treatment), as a stand-alone procedure in complex AF, such as longstanding persistent AF where medical therapy or catheter-based therapy has proven to be ineffective, or as a hybrid procedure in conjunction with endovascular ablation as a single-stage or multistage hybrid procedure.

The first clinical ablation procedure for AF was performed 1997 by Dr James Cox. Termed the Maze I procedure, it was the culmination of robust laboratory and clinical work by a multidisciplinary team that continues today. The group reported its first series in 1991 and continued to refine the procedure over the years.[90] The classic cut-and-sew Maze III became the standard of care in surgical ablation for many years.[91] With continued modification and the addition of new energy sources, Damiano and colleagues used a combination of radiofrequency energy and cryoablation to develop what is now the Cox-Maze IV.[92,93] Continued refinements and improved outcomes have been reported.[94,95] A minimally invasive approach was recently described with equal efficacy and decreased morbidity and hospital stay.[96]

Concomitant Therapy

Patients presenting for cardiac surgery often have a diagnosis of AF, whether it is related to the primary pathologic condition or independent of it. Gammie and colleagues[97] report the incidence of AF in patients having mitral valve surgery, and the Society of Thoracic Surgeons database was approximately 30%. The same study showed an incidence of 14% in patients undergoing aortic valve surgery and 6% in patients undergoing coronary artery bypass (CAB) surgery. The diagnosis of AF increases the morbidity and mortality of any cardiac surgical procedures and reduces the long-term survival.[98] It would stand to reason that the opportunity to treat AF at the time of cardiac surgery would be an opportunity to positively impact short- and long-term morbidity and mortality for patients.

Despite a growing consensus regarding the importance of concomitant ablation of AF at the time of cardiac surgery, consensus regarding lesion sets and energy sources has not been as readily achieved. During mitral procedures, an open left atrium facilitates directly by atrial ablation creating a more complete Maze-type lesion set with bilateral PVI, posterior left atrial wall isolation, as well as mitral isthmus and left atrial appendage lesions.[99,100] Recent experience has suggested that a left atrial lesion set alone may be similarly effective but with fewer complications, including need for pacemaker implantation.[101] Although bipolar radiofrequency ablation clamps have become the most effective means of ensuring transmural lesion sets, more recently, cryoablation has emerged as an effective alternative to radiofrequency energy in creating concomitant ablation lines. In addition to creating reproducible, electrically silent ablation lines, it can be used judiciously in proximity to coronary arteries and valve tissue without injury.[4]

Rates of concomitant treatment have improved recently, but opportunities remain. In a recent report from the STS database, concomitant surgical ablation for AF was performed in patients undergoing mitral valve operations in 68.4%, those undergoing aortic valve replacement in 39.3%, and those having isolated CAB in 32.8%.[98] The same study showed a reduction in relative risk (RR) of 30-day mortality (RR, 0.92) and stroke (RR, 0.84). Some have suggested that the resistance by some surgeons to open the left atrium at the time of closed left atrial procedures, such as AVR and coronary artery bypass grafting, has resulted in the low application of concomitant ablation and those procedures. Surgeons performing concomitant ablation should remember that lesion sets should be burden specific. PVI alone is an effective strategy in the treatment of paroxysmal atrial fibrillation, but nonparoxysmal AF requires more complex lesion sets for substrate modification. Use of epicardial ablation techniques could help bridge that gap and improve the treatment of concomitant AF in patients undergoing AVR and CAB.[102–104]

Results after concomitant surgical ablation for AF at the time of mitral valve surgery have demonstrated clinical effectiveness and restoration of sinus rhythm without increase in operative morbidity or mortality and may improve long-term survival.[99,105,106] Similar data have been reported in patients undergoing concomitant ablation for aortic valve and coronary disease.[107–109] These results have led to a class I indication for concomitant surgical ablation for AF at the time of mitral operations to restore sinus rhythm (class I, level a) and the time of aortic valve replacement, isolated coronary bypass, and aortic valve replacement plus coronary bypass graft operations to restore sinus rhythm (class I, level B nonrandomized).[1,4] New advances in ablation technology may further reduce the surgical impact of additional concomitant therapy, therefore increasing its utilization.

STAND-ALONE SURGICAL THERAPY AND HYBRID THERAPY
Thoracoscopic Approach

Although the ablation principles described above developed by Cox, Damiano, and colleagues remain the basis for all surgical ablation, the invasive nature of the procedure and to an extent its complexity have limited its acceptance and application in treating isolated AF without concomitant structural disease (lone AF). Initial attempts to perform epicardial ablation on the beating heart were performed through unilateral thoracoscopy.[110] As technology and experience grew, the procedure matured to its current form, which is performed via bilateral thoracoscopy. The use of the bipolar radiofrequency clamp provides extremely effective bilateral PVI. Unipolar devices for creating epicardial lines of ablation have been better than point-to-point radiofrequency ablation but continue to have limitations regarding their ability to perform reliable transmural lines. This realization has led to the development of a hybrid procedure where the above lesion sets are augmented by endocardial mapping and ablation of incomplete portions of lesion sets to approximate the lesion sets performed in the Maze III procedure. The addition of left atrial appendage ligation with the previously described AtriClip, which provides not only mechanical but also electrical isolation across the base of left atrial appendage, completes the procedure. This can be performed as a same-day hybrid procedure or in a staged fashion with surgical ablation first and touchup catheter ablation once the surgical lines have matured.[111] The importance of close collaboration in an AF heart team approach like that used in structural heart procedures has been described.[110,112]

Several reports of safe and effective treatment of complex AF using epicardial radiofrequency energy as a stand-alone surgical procedure have been reported.[113–116] As experiences have grown, its safe and effective use in a high-risk subgroup of patients has recently been described.[117,118] Durable results have recently been described with a unilateral left thoracoscopic approach.[119]

Several randomized trials and meta-analyses have documented improved superior results from thoracoscopic ablation compared with catheter ablation for maintenance of sinus rhythm in patients with persistent and longstanding persistent AF.[120–124] As a result, recent guidelines report surgical ablation for symptomatic AF in the absence of structural heart disease that is refractory to class I/III antiarrhythmic drugs or catheter-based therapy BEING reasonable as a primary stand-alone procedure to restore sinus rhythm (class IIa, level B).[4]

Subxiphoid Approach

A same-day subxiphoid epicardial approach to surgical ablation with subsequent endocardial PVI has been described[125,126]; although initially performed as a transabdominal transdiaphragmatic approach to the pericardial space, it is not performed with a simple subxiphoid incision and the use of a suction-based radiofrequency ablation catheter. This creates continuous intersecting linear lesions across the posterior wall of the left atrium. Lesions around the pulmonary veins bilaterally can be variably achieved. Because of this limitation, the surgical lesion set may not be stand-alone and may be arrhythmogenic. It is generally performed as a same-day hybrid procedure with endocardial ablation, including PVI. Reports of safety and efficacy have been promising.[127,128] Recent publication of the CONVERGE clinical trial showed superior effectiveness of this hybrid convergent procedure compared with catheter ablation in patients with persistent longstanding persistent AF.[129] Recently, left thoracoscopy has been added to this procedure to allow epicardial left atrial appendage ligation. No current data exist comparing this subxiphoid approach with the previously described thoracoscopic approach.

Additional Considerations after Surgical Treatment of Atrial Fibrillation

Perioperative care and postoperative care of patients undergoing surgical and hybrid ablation therapy are similar. As with all ablation procedures, a blanking period of 3 months must pass before assessment of the success of an ablation procedure. To help maintain sinus rhythm until ablation lines heal, patients are generally administered a class I or class III antiarrhythmic drug such as amiodarone or sotalol. Effective rhythm monitoring is key to the evaluation of the success of an ablation procedure and imperative in determining the ability to safely discontinue antiarrhythmic therapy and anticoagulation. Wellness guidelines suggest 24-hour Holter monitoring is adequate to assess occult AF recurrence; the author has tended to rely on more vigorous rhythm monitoring. He has favored implanting an internal loop recorder preoperatively in all patients to assess the AF burden preoperatively and monitor the success of rhythm management perioperatively and postoperatively. The battery and these devices generally last about 3 years, providing excellent long-term follow-up. Management of left atrial appendage has been previously described and is routinely used at the time of any surgical ablation procedure whether it be concomitant or stand alone. After surgical ablation for AF, anticoagulation therapy is reasonable if safe until durable sinus rhythm can be documented. After cardiac surgery, safe administration of warfarin may not be possible. Low-dose Eliquis has recently been substituted with excellent safety and efficacy in these high-risk patients. Perioperative and postoperative echocardiography to ensure complete left atrial appendage ligation is important.[1–3]

BEYOND ATRIAL FIBRILLATION
Atrial Flutter

Atrial flutter is a reentrant supraventricular arrhythmia with an atrial rate generally between 250 and 350 bpm. An intact atrioventricular (AV) node protects the ventricle from these rates; a healthy AV node is commonly conducted 2 to 1 out of rate of 140 to 160 bpm. In the face of AV nodal conduction delays, higher rates of AV block (3–1, 4–1, or variable conduction) can be observed.

Intravenous ibutilide and oral dofetilide are effective at chemical cardioversion. If chemical cardioversion cannot be achieved, electrical cardioversion is generally successful. For recurrent and drug-resistant atrial flutter, endocardial ablation is extremely effective.

DEVICES AND LEADS IN THE TREATMENT OF ARRHYTHMIAS: UPDATE FOR THE SURGEON
Cardiovascular Implantable Electrical Devices and Perioperative Management

Cardiovascular implantable electrical devices (CIEDs) are routine treatment for a wide variety of bradycardic and tachycardic arrhythmias. A basic understanding of their function is important for the surgeon in the perioperative management of these devices and problems associated with their use.

Pacemakers in the Treatment of Bradycardia

Moderate pacemakers consist of a pulse generator, which contains the battery and electronics as well as the leads, which are usually implanted transvenously to connect the generator to the myocardium to allow sensing of electrical activity as well as the delivery of energy to polarize (pace in) the myocardium.[130] Today's leads are generally active-fixation types, which allow an early, stable connection with the myocardium until healing and fixation occur. Epicardial leads are an option when an endocardial access is not possible. Indication for device implantation includes symptomatic bradycardia, sinus node dysfunction with bradycardia, advanced second- or third-degree AV block, and neurocardiogenic syncope.

Pacing Modes

Pacing modes are generally described with a 5-letter code, as seen in **Table 4**, and summarized as follows:

First position: Chamber paced
Second position: Chamber sensed
Third position: Device response-demand vs asynchronous pacing
Fourth position: Rate response
Fifth position: Biventricular pacing/resynchronization therapy

COMMON PACING MODES
Demand Pacing

Demand pacing can occur in the atrium or the ventricle. If the sensed heart rate drops below a preset level, the device will trigger pacing at that level. Common modes include AAI pacing, which is demand pacing in the atrium only; VVI pacing, which is demand pacing in the ventricle only; and DDD pacing, which is demand pacing in both the atria and the ventricle. DDD pacing is the most common demand pacing mode when the sinus node is intact, but AV conduction is impaired.

Asynchronous Pacing

In synchronous pacing, the device is at a set rate independent of sensing. This most commonly used for overdrive pacing in situations whereby the device may be inhibited by electromechanical inhibition (EMI), and asynchronous pacing modes include AOO, which is asynchronous pacing in the atrium only, VOO which is asynchronous pacing in the ventricular cavity only, and DOO pacing, which is a synchronous pacing in both atria and the ventricle.

Rate Response Mode

DDDR pacing is a demand pacing in both atria and ventricle associated with the ability of the generator to respond to an increase in physiologic demand and provide appropriate increased chronotropic response.

Table 4
Pacing modes

Pacing Chamber	Sensing Chamber	Device Response	Rate Response	LV Pacing
O = none	O = none	O = none	O = none	O = none
A = atrium	A = atrium	I = inhibited	R = rate modulation	A = atrium
V = ventricle	V = ventricle			V = ventricle
D = dual	D = dual	D = dual		D = dual

Internal Cardiac Defibrillator and the Management of Tachycardia Arrhythmias

An internal cardiac defibrillator (ICD) is a CIED that can detect and treat malignant ventricular arrhythmias. In addition, all ICDs are programmed with the ability to treat bradycardic arrhythmias like a pacemaker. Generally implanted endocardially, subcutaneous leads are now available. Indications for ICD insertion include a history of ventricular tachycardia or ventricular fibrillation or conditions associated with sudden cardiac death, such as long QT syndrome, Brugada syndrome, arrhythmogenic RV dysplasia, or infiltrative cardiomyopathy.[131–133] They are also indicated as the primary prevention of sudden cardiac death in patients with hypertrophic cardiomyopathy or in patients with nonischemic or ischemic cardiomyopathy with an ejection fraction less than 35%[131–136]

Resynchronization Therapy

Resynchronization therapy uses biventricular pacing to resynchronize myocardial contraction in patients with advanced heart failure and ventricular conduction delay, and it often leads to significant symptomatic improvement and improved clinical outcomes.[137] The addition of an endocardial lead placed through the coronary sinus is used to pace the left ventricle. When coronary sinus access is not available or feasible, left ventricular epicardial lead placement can be performed through a small left anterolateral thoracotomy. Optimal lead placement is generally high on the lateral wall.

PERIOPERATIVE DEVICE MANAGEMENT

Current recommendations from the American Society of Anesthesiology and the AHA/HRS strongly recommend individualized treatment with recommendations from the patient's own CIED team or another available CIED team to give the operative team recommendations for the perioperative management of the device.[138] They have stressed less reliance on industry-employed allied health professionals, placing them in a position of medical responsibility to provide independent prescriptive recommendations, which is generally beyond the scope of their practice.[7,139] As such, a basic knowledge of devices and settings is necessary for the surgeon to participate in perioperative device management. This begins with an understanding of the device in place, the date and the time of its implant, the indications for its placement, and the current settings and pulse generator reserve. Instructions on specific devices are beyond the scope of this text but have recently been published for each of the major manufacturers and are included in the references for completeness.[140–143]

Electromechanical Interference

For the surgeon, EMI related to electrocautery use is by far the most common source of potential CIED dysfunction. Unipolar energy used to cut or coagulate at the surgical site passes from there to a grounding pad. This EMI sensed by a ventricular pacing electrode can be misinterpreted by the device as intrinsic cardiac activity, resulting in interruption of the device leading to bradycardia and asystole. When sensed by an atrial lead, it may result in the device responding to what it senses is increased atrial activity with a subsequent rapid ventricular pacing rate up to the program to limit. When sensed by an ICD lead, EMI could be misinterpreted as ventricular tachycardia or ventricular fibrillation and lead to a therapeutic defibrillator discharge. Other risks of EMI include program reset to nominal modes and pulse generator damage.[131,132] The risk of deleterious EMI depends on the location of the surgical site and the grounding pad. It is highest for cardiac and thoracic procedures, followed by head and neck, shoulder, and upper-extremity procedures and less in abdominal and pelvic procedures. The risk for EMI is minimal for hip and lower-extremity procedures.[144]

Other Means of Mitigating Electromechanical Inhibition

Aside from distance, other techniques can be used to mitigate the effects of EMI perioperatively. Relocating grounding pads to allow minimized current interaction with the device can mitigate the disruption of EMI. The use of bipolar cautery creates local rather than distant EMI, which is less likely to disrupt pacemaker function. Short bursts of unipolar activity (<4 seconds, with >2 seconds pause between bursts) can lower risk of EMI. In addition, the use of lower electrocautery settings, on nonblended cutting current, and the use of ultrasonic cutting devices, such as a harmonic scalpel, may mitigate interference with a CIED.

Manipulating Pacemaker Settings

Placing a magnet over the device will inhibit antitachycardic therapy and an ICD. Understanding the magnet mode response for a particular device is important. Alternatively, reprogramming and targeting cardiac functions of an ICD can be performed preoperatively. It is important in that circumstance to have an external defibrillator available. Reprogramming a pacemaker placed for bradycardic diagnoses to an asynchronous mode will guard against EMI problems. In addition, rate response mode should be turned off to prevent problematic increases in heart rate. Devices should be returned to their preoperative mode settings postoperatively.

Surgical Considerations and Complications

Surgeons may be called on to manage various complications related to CIEDs. Several are outlined in later discussion.

Pocket Management

Management of the CIED pocket may involve a standard postsurgical issue, such as wound healing, bleeding, infection, and mechanical issues. Early, aggressive treatment is important, as delays in managing these complications can lead to contamination and infection of the pocket and the device, resulting in its need for removal.

Bleeding from either the pocket itself or the endovascular insertion site can lead to significant hematoma development. Occasionally this can be managed with pressure bandages and cessation of anticoagulation. Should a difficult hematoma develop, these are best treated early and aggressively with intraoperative exploration, hematoma removal, appropriate hemostasis, and secure closure. This aggressive approach is less likely to result in late infection.

Occasionally, the position of a subclavicular CIED pocket may be inadequate. Pain with movement, abrasion against the clavicle, and irritation from clothing or seat belts have all been experienced. If this cannot be managed with more conservative measures, operative exploration and translocation of the device to a subpectoral position may provide relief.[145] This will complicate subsequent generator changes for battery end-of-life, as additional dissection will be required to gain access to the generator.

If infection occurs, devices or leads become exposed, or the surgeon is uncomfortable managing these issues, referral to a specialist and complex lead management and device management are recommended.

COMPLEX LEAD MANAGEMENT AND LASER LEAD EXTRACTION
Risks of Abandoned Leads

In the past, it was standard practice when endocardial leads failed to leave them in place and add new leads. Recent evidence has suggested that this practice is potentially harmful, and it has become less common.[146] Capping and leaving leads in place can lead to increased risk of infection, particularly at device changes.[147] Abandoned leads are more difficult to remove later, can lead to increased risk of venous occlusion either in the subclavian vein or in the superior vena cava (SVC) with clinical sequelae, as well as increased risk of tricuspid regurgitation with resultant AF or right-sided heart failure. In addition, most old leads are MRI incompatible, limiting patient access to this increasingly important diagnostic modality.

Infection and Cardiovascular Implantable Electrical Devices
Indications for lead removal

Indications for lead removal are summarized in **Table 5**.[148,149] Class I indications include device infection, endocarditis, gram-positive bacteremia, subclavian vein or SVC stenosis, or occlusion that leads to thromboembolic events or prevents implantation of a necessary lead and life-threatening arrhythmias related to retained leads.

Procedural details

Extraction devices help release an endovascular lead from encapsulating fibrotic tissue on major vascular or cardiac structures. These risks are higher in older leads and ICD leads compared with pacemaker leads. The development of an Excimer laser system for lead extraction has shown significant benefits in improving procedural success in reducing vascular cardiac injury compared with previously used mechanical systems.[150]

Heretofore, endovascular injury in the SVC or at the cavoatrial junction often resulted in significant morbidity and mortality. The development of a bridge occlusion

Table 5		
Summary of significant lead removal indications		
Category	**Indications**	**Class**
Infection	Pocket infection	I
	Occult gram-positive bacteremia	I
	Cold gram-negative bacteremia	IIa
Chronic pain	Severe chronic pain	IIa
Thrombosis/venous stenosis	Ipsilateral occlusion without contralateral contraindication	IIa
Functional leads	Due to design or failure, may pose immediate threat	I
	Risk of interference with device operation	IIb
	Due to design or failure poses potential future threat	IIb
	Functional leads not being used (ICD upgrade)	IIb
	Need MRI with no other imaging options	IIb
Nonfunctional leads	Implant would require >4 leads on 1 side	
	or >5 leads through SVC	IIa
	Need MRI with no other imaging options	IIa
	Nonfunctional lead at device/lead procedure	IIb

balloon has provided a new level of safety for lead extraction. Placed through the common femoral vein under fluoroscopic guidance, this can be deployed at the cavoatrial junction should a vascular injury occur in that area, one of the most common and deadly sites of vascular injury during lead removal. Clinical scenarios where significant vascular injury is higher and placement of the bridge balloon prophylactically should be considered for Ariane ICD lead removal, when multiple leads are present, with older leads, in the face of low left ventricular ejection fraction. Its use has resulted in a significant decrease in the perioperative morbidity and mortality of lead extraction. With proper deployment, the survival rate of SVC tear was recently reported at 91.7% compared with historical data of 56% survival.[151]

Procedural risks and outcomes

Current data suggest a 97.7% clinical success rate for extraction with current laser technology. These studies are also associated with a 0.28% mortality and 1.4% procedural major complication rate.[152] Carrillo and colleagues[149,153] recently presented data showing significant improvement in morbidity and mortality related to use of a bridge occlusion balloon in the SVC should injuries occur there.

NEW DEVELOPMENTS/FUTURE DIRECTIONS

Practice evolution and technological advances will inevitably lead to favorable change in the guideline-directed therapy discussed above. Advances in antiarrhythmic therapy and anticoagulation, including the reliable ability to reverse anticoagulation, are likely. A second-generation Watchman device and several other endocardial left atrial appendage closure devices are in clinical trials. Anticipated clinical trials regarding routine left atrial appendage ligation during cardiac surgery will likely affect the standard of care. Investigation into new energy sources for endocardial and epicardial surgical ablation will continue to make improvements in outcomes.

CLINICS CARE POINTS

- Atrial fibrillation is independently associated with significantly increased morbidity and mortality.

- Postoperative atrial fibrillation has unique mechanisms of initiation and provides special challenges for treatment.

- Concomitant surgical ablation for atrial fibrillation can be performed without additional morbidity and mortality.

- Nonpharmacologic left atrial appendage management offers an alternative to standard anticoagulation for stroke risk reduction.

- Hybrid therapies for stand-alone ablation of atrial fibrillation are safe and effective.

- Abandoned cardiovascular implantable electrical device leads lead to increased complications.

- Laser lead extraction is associated with improved procedural success and reduced vascular and cardiac injury compared with previously used systems.

DISCLOSURE

The author discloses a consultant relationship with Atricure, Inc.

REFERENCES

1. Calkins H, Hindricks G, Cappato R, et al. 2017 HRS/EHRA/ECAS/APHRS/SOL-AECE expert consensus statement on catheter and surgical ablation of atrial fibrillation. Heart Rhythm 2017;14(10):e275–444.

2. Hindricks G, Potpara T, Dagres N, et al. 2020 ESC guidelines for the diagnosis and management of atrial fibrillation developed in collaboration with the European Association for Cardio-Thoracic Surgery (EACTS). Eur Heart J 2020;42: 373–498.

3. Andrade JG, Aguilar M, Atzema C, et al. 2020 Canadian Cardiovascular Society/Canadian Heart Rhythm Society comprehensive guidelines for the management of atrial fibrillation. Can J Cardioliol 2020;36:1847–948.

4. Badwar V, Rankin JS, Dasmiano RJ, et al. The Society of Thoracic Surgeons 2017 clinical practice guidelines for the surgical treatment of atrial fibrillation. Ann Thorac Surg 2017;103:329–41.

5. January CT, Wann LS, Calkins H, et al. 2019 AHA/ACC/HRS focused update of the 2014 AHA/ACC/HRS guidelines for the management of patients with atrial fibrillation: a report of the American College of Cardiology/American Heart Association task force on clinical practice guidelines and the Heart Rhythm Society in collaboration with the Society of Thoracic Surgeons. Circulation 2019;140(2): e125–51.

6. Calkins H, Kuck KH, Cappato R, et al. 2012 HRS/EHRA/ECAS expert consensus statement on catheter and surgical ablation of atrial fibrillation: recommendations for patient selection, procedural techniques, patient management and follow-up, definitions, endpoints, and research trial design. Heart Rhythm 2012;9(4):632–96.

7. Crossley GH, Poole JE, Rozner MA, et al. The Heart Rhythm Society (HRS)/American Society of Anesthesiologists (ASA) expert consensus statement on the perioperative management of patients with implantable defibrillators, pacemakers and arrhythmia monitors: facilities and patient management. Heart Rhythm 2011;9(7):1114–54.

8. Kusumoto FM, Schoenfeld MH, Wilkoff MH, et al. 2007 HRS expert consensus statement on cardiovascular implantable electronic device lead management and extraction. Heart Rhythm 2017;14(12):e503–51.

9. Issa ZF, Miller JM, Zipes DP, et al. Atrial fibrillation. In: Clinical arrhythmology and electrophysiology. Philadelphia (PA): Elsevier; 2019. p. 433–4.

10. Benjamin EJ, Munter P, Alonso A, et al. American Heart Association Council on Epidemiology and Prevention Statistics Committee and Stroke Statistics Subcommittee. Heart disease and stroke statistics-2019 update: a report from the American Heart Association. Circ 2019;139:e56–528.

11. Chung SS, Havmoeller R, Narayanen K, et al. Worldwide epidemiology of atrial fibrillation: a global burden of disease 2010 study. Circ 2014;129:837–47.

12. Chung MK, Refaat M, Shen WK, et al. Atrial fibrillation. JACC council perspectives. JACC 2020;75(14):1689–713.

13. Haissaguerre M, Jais P, Shah DC, et al. Spontaneous initiation of atrial fibrillation by ectopic beats originating in the pulmonary veins. N Engl J Med 1998;339(10): 659–66.

14. Kazui T, Henn MC, Watanabe Y, et al. The impact of 6 weeks of atrial fibrillation on left atrial and ventricular structure and function. J Thorac Cardiovasc Surg 2015;150:1602–8.

15. Kotecha D, Chudasama R, Lane DA, et al. Atrial fibrillation and heart failure due to reduced versus preserved ejection fraction: a systematic review and meta-analysis of death and adverse outcomes. Int J Cardiol 2016;203:606–66.

16. Ferrari F, Santander IRMF, Stein R. Digoxin in atrial fibrillation: an old topic revisited. Curr Cardiol Rev 2020;16:141–6.

17. Shah MS, Tsadok MA, Jackevicius CA, et al. Relation of digoxin use in atrial fibrillation and the risk of all-cause mortality in patients > 65 years of age with versus without heart failure. Am J Cardiol 2014;114:401–6.

18. Van Gelder IC, Groenveld HF, Crijins HJ, et al. RACE II Investigators. Lenient versus strict rate control in patients with atrial fibrillation. N Engl J Med 2010; 362(15):1363–73.

19. Van Gelder IC, Hagens VE, Bosker HA, et al. Rate Control versus Electrical Cardioversion for Persistent Atrial Fibrillation Study Group. A comparison of rate control and rhythm control in patients with recurrent persistent atrial fibrillation. N Engl J Med 2002;347(23):1834–40.

20. Roy D, Talajic M, Nattel S, et al. Atrial Fibrillation and Congestive Heart Failure Investigators. Rhythm control versus rate control for atrial fibrillation and heart failure. N Engl J Med 2008;358(25):2667–77.

21. Hagens VE, Ranchor AV, Van Sonderen E, et al. RACE Study Group. Effective of rate or rhythm control on quality of life in persistent atrial fibrillation: results from the Rate Control versus Electrical Cardioversion (RACE) Study. J Am Coll Cardiol 2004;43(2):241–7.

22. Kelly JP, DeVore AD, Wu J, et al. Rhythm control versus rate control in patients with atrial fibrillation and heart failure with preserved ejection fraction: insights from Get with the Guidelines-Heart Failure. J Am Heart Assoc 2019;8(24): e011560.

23. Lowres N, Mulcahy G, Jin K, et al. Incidence of postoperative atrial fibrillation recurrence in patients discharged in sinus rhythm after cardiac surgery: a systematic review and meta-analysis. Interact Cardiovasc Thorac Surg 2018;26: 504–11.

24. Dobrev D, Aguilar M, Heijman J, et al. Postoperative atrial fibrillation: mechanisms, manifestations and management. Nat Rev Cardiol 2019;16:417–36.

25. Echahidi N, Pibarot P, O'Hara G, et al. Mechanisms, prevention, and treatment of atrial fibrillation after cardiac surgery. J Am Coll Cardiol 2008;51:793–801.

26. Gillinov AM, Bagiella E, Moskowitz AJ, et al. Rate control versus rhythm control for atrial fibrillation after cardiac surgery. NEJM 2016;374:1911–21.

27. Amar D. Postthoracotomy atrial fibrillation. Curr Opin Anaesthesiol 2007; 20:43–7.

28. Philip I, Berroeta C, Leblanc I. Perioperative challenges of atrial fibrillation. Curr Opin Anaesthesiol 2014;27:344–52.

29. Lin MH, Kamel H, Singer DE, et al. Perioperative/postoperative atrial fibrillation and risk of subsequent stroke and/or mortality. Stroke 2019;50:1364–71.

30. AlTurki A, Marafi M, Proietti R, et al. Major adverse cardiovascular events associated with postoperative atrial fibrillation after noncardiac surgery: a systematic review and meta-analysis. Circ Arrhythm Electrophysiol 2020;13:e007437.

31. Mathew JP, Fontes ML, Tudor IC, et al. Investigators of the Ischemia Research and Education Foundation, Multicenter Study of Perioperative Ischemia Research Group. A multicenter risk index for atrial fibrillation after cardiac surgery. JAMA 2004;291:1720–9.

32. Villareal RP, Hariharan R, Liu BC, et al. Postoperative atrial fibrillation and mortality after coronary artery bypass surgery. J Am Coll Cardiol 2004;43:742–8.

33. Lee SH, Kang DR, Uhm JS, et al. New-onset atrial fibrillation predicts long-term newly developed atrial fibrillation after coronary artery bypass graft. Am Heart J 2014;167:593–600.

34. Konstantino Y, Zelnik Yovel D, Friger MD, et al. Postoperative atrial fibrillation following coronary artery bypass graft surgery predicts long-term atrial fibrillation and stroke. Isr Med Assoc J 2016;18:744–8.

35. Cardinale D, Sandri MT, Colombo A, et al. Prevention of atrial fibrillation in high-risk patients undergoing lung cancer surgery: the PRESAGE Trial. Ann Surg 2016;264:244–51.

36. Ojima T, Nakamori M, Nakamura M, et al. Randomized clinical trial of landiolol hydrochloride for the prevention of atrial fibrillation and postoperative complications after oesophagectomy for cancer. Br J Surg 2017;104:1003–9.

37. Arsenault KA, Yusuf AM, Crystal E, et al. Interventions for preventing postoperative atrial fibrillation in patients undergoing heart surgery. Cochrane Database Syst Rev 2013;CD003611.

38. Ozaydin M, Icli A, Yucel H, et al. Metoprolol vs. carvedilol or carvedilol plus N-acetyl cysteine on post-operative atrial fibrillation: a randomized, double-blind, placebo-controlled study. Eur Heart J 2013;34:597–604.

39. O'Neal JB, Billings FT 4th, Liu X, et al. Effect of preoperative beta-blocker use on outcomes following cardiac surgery. Am J Cardiol 2017;120:1293–7.

40. Zhu J, Wang C, Gao D, et al. Meta-analysis of amiodarone versus beta-blocker as a prophylactic therapy against atrial fibrillation following cardiac surgery. Intern Med J 2012;42:1078_1087.

41. Auer J, Weber T, Berent R, et al. Study of Prevention of Postoperative Atrial Fibrillation. A comparison between oral antiarrhythmic drugs in the prevention of atrial fibrillation after cardiac surgery: the pilot study of prevention of postoperative atrial fibrillation (SPPAF), a randomized, placebo-controlled trial. Am Heart J 2004;147:636–43.

42. Imazio M, Brucato A, Ferrazzi P, et al. Colchicine for prevention of postpericardiotomy syndrome and postoperative atrial fibrillation: the COPPS-2 randomized clinical trial. JAMA 2014;312(10):1016–23.

43. Benjamin EJ, Wolf PA, D'Agostino RB, et al. Impact of atrial fibrillation on the risk of death: the Framingham Heart Study. Circ 1998;98:946–52.

44. Lin HJ, Wolf PA, Kelly-Hayes M, et al. Stroke severity and atrial fibrillation. The Framingham Study. Stroke 1996;27:1760–4.

45. Ferro JM. Cardioembolic stroke: an update. Lancet Neurol 2003;2(3):177–88.

46. Boston Area Anticoagulation Trial for Atrial Fibrillation Investigators. The effect of low-dose warfarin on the risk of stroke in patients with nonrheumatic atrial fibrillation. NEJM 1990;323:1505–11.

47. Ezekowitz MD, Bridgers SL, James KE, et al. Warfarin in the prevention of stroke associated with nonrheumatic atrial fibrillation. Veterans Affairs stroke prevention in nonrheumatic atrial fibrillation investigators. NEJM 1992;327(20):1406–12.

48. Connoly SJ, Laupacis A, Gent M, et al. Canadian atrial fibrillation anticoagulation (CAF A) study. J Am Coll Cardiol 1991;18(2):349–55.

49. Gage BF, Waterman AD, Shannon W, et al. Validation of clinical classification schemes for predicting stroke: results from the National Registry of Atrial Fibrillation. JAMA 2001;285:2864–70.

50. Lip GYH, Nieuwloat R, Pistero R, et al. Refining clinical risk stratification for predicting stroke and thromboembolism in atrial fibrillation using a novel risk factor-

based approach: the Euroheart Survey on Atrial Fibrillation. Chest 2010;137: 263–72.

51. Atrial fibrillation investigators. Echocardiographic predictors of stroke in patients with atrial fibrillation: a prospective study of 1066 patients from 3 clinical trials. Arch Intern Med 1998;185:1316–20.

52. Dibiase L, Santangell P, Anselmimo M, et al. Does the left atrial morphology correlate with risk of stroke in patients with atrial fibrillation? Results from a multi-center study. J Am Coll Cardiol 2012;60:535–8.

53. Zabalgoita M, Halpern JL, Pearce LA, et al. Stroke Prevention in Atrial Fibrillation III Investigators. Transesophageal echocardiographic correlates of clinical risk of thromboembolism in nonvalvular atrial fibrillation. J Am Coll Cardiol 1998; 31:1622–6.

54. Seeno K, Proletti M, Lane DA, et al. Evaluation of the HAS-BLED, ATRIA, and ORBIT bleeding risk scores in patients with atrial fibrillation taking warfarin. AM J Med 2016;129:600–7.

55. Albers GW, Dalen JE, Lauparis A, et al. Antithrombotic therapy in atrial fibrillation. Chest 2001;119(Suppl 1):194S–206S.

56. Connoly SJ, Ezekowitz MD, Yusuf S, et al. Dabigatran versus warfarin in patients with atrial fibrillation. NEJM 2009;301:1139–51.

57. Patel MR, Mahaffey KW, Garg J, et al. Rivaroxaban versus warfarin in nonvalvular atrial fibrillation. NEJM 2011;365:883–91.

58. Granger CB, Alexander JH, McMurray JJV, et al. Apixaban versus warfarin in patients with atrial fibrillation. NEJM 2011;365:981–92.

59. Giugliano RP, Ruff CT, Braunwald E, et al. Edoxaban versus warfarin in patients with atrial fibrillation. NEJM 2013;369:2093–104.

60. Doukatis JD, Spyropoulas AC, Kaatz S, et al. Bridge investigators. Perioperative bridging anticoagulation in patients with atrial fibrillation. NEJM 2015;373: 823–33.

61. Ayoub K, Nairooz R, Almomani A, et al. Perioperative heparin bridging in atrial fibrillation patients requiring temporary interruption of anticoagulation. Evidence from meta-analysis. J Stroke Cerebrovasc Dis 2016;25:2215–21.

62. Steffel J, Verkamme P, Potpara TS, et al. The 2018 European Heart Rhythm Association practical guide on the use of a non-vitamin K antagonist oral anticoagulation in patients with atrial fibrillation: executive summary. Europace 2018; 20(8):1231–42.

63. Connoly S, Crowther M, Eikenboom JW, et al. Full study report of Andexanet alpha for bleeding associated with factor Xa inhibitors. NEJM 2009;380:1326–35.

64. Levy JH, Doukatis J, Weitz JI, et al. Reversal agents for non-vitamin K antagonist oral anticoagulation. Nat Rev Cardiol 2019;15:273–81.

65. Blackshear JL, Odell JA. Appendage obliteration to reduce stroke in cardiac surgical patients with atrial fibrillation. Ann Thorac Surg 1996;61:755–9.

66. Sharma S, Devine W, Anderson RH, et al. The determination of atrial arrangement by examination of appendage morphology in 1842 heart specimens. Br Heart J 1988;60:227–31.

67. Cabrera JA, Saremi F, Sanchez-Quintana D. Left atrial appendage: anatomy and imaging landmarks pertinent to percutaneous transcatheter occlusion. Heart 2014;100:1636.

68. Wang Y, Dibiase L, Horton RP, et al. left atrial appendage studied by computed tomography to help planning for appendage closure device placement. J Cardiovasc Electrophysiol 2010;21:973–82.

69. Yaghi S, Chang A, Akiki R, et al. The left atrial appendage morphology is associated with embolic stroke subtypes using a simple classification system: a proof of concept study. J Cardiovasc Comput Tomography 2020;14(1):27–33.
70. Murtaza G, Turazam MK, Della Rocca DG, et al. Risks and benefits of removal of the left atrial appendage. Curr Cardiol Rep 2020;22(11):129.
71. Dibiase L, Burkhardt JD, Mohantz P, et al. Left atrial appendage: an underrecognized trigger site of atrial fibrillation. Circ 2010;122(2):109–18.
72. Friedman DJ, Black-Maier EW, Barnett AS, et al. Left atrial appendage electrical isolation for treatment of recurrent atrial fibrillation: a meta-analysis. JACC Clin Electrophysiol 2014;4(1):112–20.
73. Lakireddy D, Sridhar Maharkali A, Kanmarthareddy A, et al. Left atrial appendage ligation and ablation for persistent atrial fibrillation: the LAA LA-AF registry. JACC Clin Electrophysiol 2015;1(3):153–60.
74. Edgerton JR. Current state of surgical left atrial appendage exclusion: how and when. Card Electrophysiol Clin 2020;12:109–55.
75. Reddy VY, Sievert H, Halperin J, et al. Percutaneous left atrial appendage closure versus warfarin for atrial fibrillation: a randomized clinical trial. JAMA 2014;32(19):1988–98.
76. Reddy VY, Doshi SK, Kar S, et al. 5-year outcomes after left atrial appendage closure: from the PREVAIL and PROTECT-AF trials. JACC 2017;70(24):2964–75.
77. Salzberg SP, Plass A, Emmert MY, et al. Left atrial appendage clip occlusion: early clinical results. J Thorac Cardiovasc Surg 2010;139(5):1269–74.
78. Ailawadi G, Gerdisch MW, Harvey RL, et al. Exclusion of left atrial appendage with a novel device: early results of a multicenter trial. J Thorac Cardiovasc Surg 2011;142:102–9.
79. Caliskan E, Cox JL, Holmes DR, et al. Interventional and surgical occlusion of the left atrial appendage. Nat Rev Cardiol 2017;14:727–43.
80. Hahalati A, Biancari F, Nielson JC, et al. Radiofrequency ablation versus antiarrhythmic drug therapy as first-line treatment of symptomatic atrial fibrillation: systematic review and meta-analysis. Europace 2015;17:370–8.
81. Asad ZA, Yausif A, Khan MS, et al. Catheter ablation versus medical therapy for atrial fibrillation: a systematic review and meta-analysis of early clinical trials. Circ Arrhythm Electrophysiol 2019;12(9):e007414.
82. Patel N, Patel K, Shenoy A, et al. Cryoablation for the treatment of atrial fibrillation: a meta-analysis. Curr Cardiolrev 2019;15:230–8.
83. Murray M, Arnold A, Youn is M, et al. Cryoballoon versus radiofrequency ablation for paroxysmal atrial ablation: a meta-analysis of randomized controlled trials. Clin Res Cardiol 2018;107(8):658–69.
84. Chen YH, Lu ZY, Xiang Y, et al. Cryoablation versus radiofrequency ablation for treatment of paroxysmal atrial fibrillation: a systematic review and meta-analysis. Europace 2017;19:784–94.
85. Kuck KH, Brugada J, Furnkranz A, et al. On behalf of the FIR ED and ICE investigators. Cryoballoon or radiofrequency ablation for paroxysmal atrial fibrillation. NEJM 2016;324:2235–45.
86. Luik A, Radzewitz A, Kieser M, et al. Cryoballoon versus open irrigated radiofrequency ablation in patients with paroxysmal atrial fibrillation: the prospective randomized, controlled, noninferiority FREEZE AF study. Circ 2015;132:1311–9.
87. Vogt J, Heintze J, Gutleben KJ, et al. Long-term outcomes after cryoballoon pulmonary vein isolation: results from a prospective study in 605 patients. JACC 2013;61:1707–12.

88. Gupta A, Perera T, Ganesan A, et al. Complications of catheter ablation of atrial fibrillation: a systematic review. Circ arrhythmia Electrophysiol 2013;6(6): 1082-8.

89. Parameswaran R, Al-Kaisez AM, Kalman JM, et al. Catheter ablation for atrial fibrillation: current indications and evolving technologies. Nat Rev Cardiol 2021;18(3):210-25.

90. Cox JL, Boineau JP, Schessler RB, et al. Successful surgical treatment of atrial fibrillation. Review and clinical update. JAMA 1991;266:1976-80.

91. Cox JL, Schessler RB, Lappas DG, et al. An 8-1/2-year clinical experience with surgery for atrial fibrillation. Ann Surg 1996;224:267-75, 2008; 85: 909-275.

92. Gaynor SL, Diodato MD, Prassad SM, et al. A prospective single-center clinical trial of a modified Cox maze procedure with bipolar radiofrequency ablation. J Cardiovasc Thorac Surg 2004;128:535-42.

93. Mokadam NA, McCarthy PM, Gillinov AM, et al. A prospective multicenter trial of bipolar radiofrequency ablation for atrial fibrillation: early results. Ann Thorac Surg 2004;78:1665-70.

94. Damiano RJ, Schwartz FH, Bailey MS, et al. the Cox-Maze for procedure: predictors of late recurrence. J Cardiovasc Thorac Surg 2011;141:113-21.

95. Cheema FH, Younus MJ, Pasha A, et al. effective modification to simplify the right atrial lesion set of the Cox-cryomaze. Ann Thorac Surg 2013;96:330-2.

96. Lawrence CP, Hen MC, Miller JR, et al. A minimally base of Cox-Maze for procedure is as effective as sternotomy while decreasing major morbidity and hospital stay. J Cardiovasc Thorac Surg 2014;148:955-62.

97. Gammie JS, Haddad M, Milford-Beland S, et al. Atrial fibrillation corrective surgery: lessons from the Society of Thoracic Surgery National Cardiac Database. Ann Thorac Surg 2008;85:909-14.

98. Badhwar V, Rankin JS, Ad N, et al. Surgical ablation of atrial fibrillation in the United States: trends and propensity matched outcomes. Ann Thorac Surg 2017;104:493-500.

99. Barrett SD, Ad N. Surgical ablation as treatment for the elimination of atrial fibrillation: a meta-analysis. J Cardiovasc Thorac Surg 2006;131:1029-35.

100. Melo J, Santiago T, Aguiar C, et al. Surgery for atrial fibrillation in patients with mitral valve disease: results at 5 years from the international registry of atrial fibrillation surgery. J Cardiovasc Thorac Surg 2008;135:863-9.

101. Saint LL, Damiano RJ, Cuculich PS, et al. Incremental risk of the Cox-Maze IV procedure for patients with atrial fibrillation undergoing mitral valve surgery. J Cardiovasc Thorac Surg 2013;146:1072-7.

102. Edgerton JR, Jackman WM, Mack MJ. A new epicardial lesion set for minimal access left atrial maze: the dialysis lesion set. Ann Thorac Surg 2009;88(5): 1655-7.

103. Edgerton JR, Jackman WM, Mahoney, et al. Totally thoracoscopic surgical ablation of persistent AF and longstanding persistent atrial fibrillation using the "Dallas" lesion set. Heart Rhythm 2009;6(12 Suppl):S64-70.

104. Lockwood D, Nakagawa H, Peyton MD, et al. Linear left atrial lesions in minimally invasive surgical ablation of persistent atrial fibrillation: techniques for assessing conduction block across surgical lesions. Heart Rhythm 2009;6(12 Suppl):S50-63.

105. Gillinov AM, Gelijns AC, Paraides MK, et al. Surgical ablation of atrial fibrillation during mitral-valve surgery. N Engl J Med 2015;372(15):1399-409.

106. Rankin JS, He X, O-Brien SM, et al. The Society of Thoracic Surgeons risk model for operative mortality after multiple valve surgery. Ann Thorac Surg 2013;95(4): 1484–90.
107. Malaisrie SC, Lee R, Kruse J, et al. Atrial fibrillation ablation in patients undergoing aortic valve replacement. J Heart Valve Dis 2012;21(3):350–7.
108. Cherniavsky A, Kareva Y, Pak I, et al. Assessment of results of surgical treatment for persistent atrial fibrillation during coronary artery bypass grafting using implantable loop recorders. Interact Cardiovasc Thorac Surg 2014;18:727–31.
109. Yoo JS, Kim JB, Ro SK, et al. Impact of concomitant surgical atrial fibrillation ablation in patients undergoing aortic valve replacement. Circ J 2014;78(6): 1364–71.
110. LaMeir M. New technologies and hybrid surgery for atrial fibrillation. Ramdan Maimonides Med J 2013;4(3):1–8.
111. Richardson TD, Shoemaker MB, Whalen SP, et al. Staged versus simultaneous thoracoscopic hybrid ablation for persistent atrial fibrillation does not affect time to recurrence of atrial arrhythmia. J Cardiovasc Electrophysiol 2016;27:428–34.
112. Salzberg SP, Zerm J, Wyss C, et al. AF Heart Team" guided indication for stand-alone thoracoscopic left atrial appendage ablation and left atrial appendage closure. J Atrial Fib 2019;1:1–7.
113. Vos LM, Bentala M, Geruzebrock GSC, et al. Long-term outcome after totally thoracoscopic ablation for atrial fibrillation. J Cardiovasc Electrophysiol 2020; 31:40–5.
114. Ni B, Wang Z, Gu W, et al. Thoracoscopic left atrial appendage exclusion plus ablation for atrial fibrillation to prevent stroke. Semin Throrac Surg 2020;33:61–7.
115. Maesen B, Pison L, Vroomen M, et al. Three-year follow-up of hybrid ablation for atrial fibrillation. Eur J Cardiothorac Surg 2018;53(Supp 1):26–32.
116. Van Laar C, Kelder J, vanPutte BP. The totally thoracoscopic Maze procedure for the treatment of atrial fibrillation. Interact Cardiovasc Thorac Surg 2017;24: 102–11.
117. Phan K, Pison L, Wang N, et al. Effectiveness and safety of simultaneous hybrid thoracoscopic and endocardial catheter ablation of atrial fibrillation in the obese and nonobese patient. J Thorac Dis 2017;9(9):3087–96.
118. Kim HR, Joeng DS, Kwon HJ, et al. Totally thoracoscopic ablation in patients with atrial fibrillation and left ventricular dysfunction. JTCVS Tech 2021; 20(8):60–6.
119. deAsmundis C, Varnavas V, Siera J, et al. 2-year follow-up of a 1 stage left uni-lateral thoracoscopic epicardial and transcatheter endocardial ablation for persistent and longstanding persistent atrial fibrillation. J Interv Card Electro-physiol 2020;50(3):333–43.
120. Yi S, Lu X, Wang W, et al. Thoracoscopic surgical ablation or catheter ablation for patients with atrial fibrillation? A systematic review and meta-analysis of ran-domized control trials. Interact Cardiovasc Thorac Surg 2020;31:763–73.
121. Wang TKM, Liao YW, Wamg MTM, et al. Catheter vs thoracoscopic ablation for atrial fibrillation: meta-analysis of randomized trials. J Arrhythmia 2020;36: 789–93.
122. Haldar S, Khan HR, Boyalla V, et al. Catheter ablation versus thoracoscopic sur-gery ablation and long stay persistent atrial fibrillation: CASA-AF randomized control trial. Eur Heart J 2020;41(47):4471–80.
123. Castella M, Kotacha D, van Laar C, et al. Thoracoscopic versus catheter abla-tion for atrial fibrillation: long-term follow-up of the F AST randomized trial. Euro-pace 2019;21:746–53.

124. Phan K, Phan S, Thiagalingam A, et al. Thoracoscopic surgical ablation versus catheter ablation for atrial fibrillation. Eur J Cardiothorac Surg 2016;49:1044–51.
125. Gehi AK, Mounsey JP, Pursell I, et al. Hybrid epicardial-endocardial ablation using a pericardioscopic technique for the treatment of atrial fibrillation. Heart Rhythm 2013;10(1):22–8.
126. Gersak B, Pernat A, Robic B, et al. Low rate of atrial fibrillation recurrence verified by implantable loop recorder monitoring following a convergent epicardial and endocardial ablation of atrial fibrillation. J Cardiovasc Electrophysiol 2012; 23:1059–66.
127. Maclean E, Yap J, Saberwal B, et al. The convergent procedure versus catheter ablation alone in longstanding persistent atrial fibrillation: a single center, propensity-matched cohort study. Int J Cardiol 2020;303:49–53.
128. Ellis CR, Badhwar N, Tschopp D, et al. Subxiphoid hybrid epicardial-endocardial atrial fibrillation ablation and LAA ligation: initial Sub-X Hybrid Maze Registry results. JACC Clin Electrophysiol 2020;6(13):1603–15.
129. De Lurgio DB, Crossen KJ, Gill J, et al. Hybrid convergent procedure for the treatment of persistent and longstanding persistent atrial fibrillation: results of the CONVERGE clinical trial. Circ Arrhythm Electrophysiol 2020;13(12): e009288.
130. Mulpuru SK, Madhaven M, McLeod CJ, et al. Cardiac pacemakers: function, troubleshooting, and management. JACC 2017;69(2):211–35.
131. Kadish A, Dyer A, Daubert JP, et al. Prophylactic defibrillator implantation in patients with nonischemic dilated cardiomyopathy. N Eng J Med 2004;350:2151–8.
132. Moss AJ, Zareba W, Hall WJ, et al. Prophylactic implantation of a defibrillator in patients with a myocardial infarction and reduced ejection fraction. N Eng J Med 2002;346:877–83.
133. Bardy GH, Lee KL, Mark DB, et al. Amiodarone or an implantable cardioverter-defibrillator for congestive heart failure. N Eng J Med 2005;352:225–37.
134. Rozner MA. Cardiac implantable electrical devices. In: Kaplan JA, editor. Kaplan's cardiac anesthesia: for cardiac and noncardiac surgery. Philadelphia (PA): Elsevier; 2016. p. 1663.
135. Brugada P, Geelen P. Some electrocardiographic patterns predicting sudden cardiac death that every doctor should recognize. Acta Cardiol 1997;52: 473–84.
136. Maron BJ, Shen WK, Link MS, et al. Efficacy of implantable cardio converter-defibrillators for the prevention of sudden death in patients with hypertrophic cardiomyopathy. N Eng J Med 2000;342:365–73.
137. Katbeh A, Van Camp G, Barbato E, et al. Cardiac resynchronization therapy optimization: a comprehensive approach. Cardiology 2019;142:116–27.
138. American Society of Anesthesiologists. Practice advisory for the perioperative management of patients with cardiac implantable electronic devices: pacemakers and implantable cardioverter-defibrillators: an update report by the American Society of Anesthesiologists Task Force on Perioperative Management of Patients with Cardiac Implantable Electronic Devices. Anesthesiology 2011;114:247–61.
139. Lindsey BD, Estes NA III, Maloney JD, et al. Heart Rhythm Society policy statement update: recommendations on the role of Industry Employed Allied Professionals (IEAPs). Heart Rhythm 2008;5:8–10.
140. Cronin B, Essandoh MK. Perioperative interrogation of St Jude cardiovascular implantable electronic devices: a guide for anesthesiologists. J Cardiothorac Vasc Anesth 2018;32:982–1000.

141. Cronin B, Birghersdotter U, Essandoh MK. Perioperative interrogation of Boston Scientific cardiovascular implantable electronic devices: a guide for anesthesiologists. J Cardiothorac Vasc Anesth 2019;33:1076–89.

142. Cronin B, Dalia A, Sandoval K, et al. Perioperative interrogation of Biotronik cardiovascular implantable electronic devices: a guide for anesthesiologists. J Cardiothorac Vasc Anesth 2019;33:3427–36.

143. Cronin B, Dalia A, Hguyen QS, et al. Perioperative interrogation of Medtronic cardiovascular implantable electronic devices: a guide for anesthesiologists. J Cardiothorac Vasc Anesth 2020;34:2465–75.

144. Cronin B, Essadoh MK. Update on cardiovascular implantable electronic devices for anesthesiologists. J Cardiothorac Vasc Anesth 2018;32:1871–84.

145. Hesselson AB. A simple technique for relocating chronic CI ED leads to a subpectoral position for relief of erosion and pain. Pacing Clin Electrophysiol 2018; 41(7):834–8.

146. Pokorney SD, Mi X, Lewis RK, et al. Outcomes associated with extraction versus capping and abandoning pacing and defibrillator leads. Circulation 2017; 136(15):1387–95.

147. Boyle TA, Uslan DZ, Prutkin JM, et al. Impact of abandoned leads on cardiovascular implantable electronic device infections: a propensity matched analysis of MEDIC (multicenter electrophysiologic device infection cohort). JACC Clin Electrophysiol 2018;4(2):209–11.

148. Wilkoff BL, Love CJ, Byrd GH, et al. transvenous lead extraction: Heart Rhythm Society expert consensus on facilities, training, indications, and patient management. Heart Rhythm 2009;6(7):1085–104.

149. Carrillo RG, Tsang DC, Azarafiy R, et al. Multi-year evaluation of compliant endovascular balloon in treating superior vena cava tears during transvenous lead extraction EHRA late breaking trial. March 2018;19.

150. Okamura H. Lead extraction using a laser system: techniques, efficacy, and limitations. J Arrhythmia 2016;32:279–82.

151. Wazni, O, Epstein LM, Carrillo RG, et al. Lead extraction in the contemporary setting: the Lexicon study: a multicenter observational retrospective study of consecutive laser lead extractions, JACC 55: 579-586.

152. Kusumoto FM, Schoenfeld MH, Wilkoff BL. 2017 HRS expert consensus statement on cardiovascular implantable electronic device lead management and extraction. Heart Rhythm 2017;14(12):e503–51.

153. Bashir J, Carrillo RG. Cardiac and vascular injury sustained during transvenous lead extraction. Card Electrophysiol Clin 2018;10:651–7.

Endobronchial Therapies for Diagnosis, Staging, and Treatment of Lung Cancer

Sameer K. Avasarala, MD[a], Otis B. Rickman, DO[b],*

KEYWORDS

- Flexible bronchoscopy • Endobronchial ultrasound • Rigid bronchoscopy
- Central airway obstruction • Lung cancer staging

KEY POINTS

- Bronchoscopy is an essential diagnostic and therapeutic tool for the management of lung cancer.
- Peripheral bronchoscopy and endobronchial ultrasound are minimally invasive, safe procedures that can provide critical information for both lung cancer diagnosis and staging.
- A variety of tools can be paired with traditional white light bronchoscopy to enhance imaging, lesion localization, and biopsy acquisition.
- Rigid bronchoscopy is an important tool in the management of central airway obstruction, a variety of techniques can be used to provide rapid relief.

INTRODUCTION

Lung cancer is the leading cause of cancer-related mortality in the United States. Although lung cancer screening programs have shown success with early-stage diagnosis, most patients still present with manifestations of late-stage disease.[1] Radiographically, early-stage lung cancer can present as ground-glass opacities or pulmonary nodules. Late-stage lung cancer often presents with stigmata of metastatic disease. Bronchoscopy has been proven to be an essential tool in diagnosing, staging, and treating lung cancer. It is a safe procedure that can be performed under moderate sedation or general anesthesia. Data have proven that the implementation of advanced diagnostic bronchoscopic procedures reduces the rate of benign resections within thoracic surgery.[2] In addition, central airway obstruction treated with rigid

[a] Division of Pulmonary, Critical Care and Sleep Medicine, University Hospitals – Case Western Reserve University School of Medicine, 11100 Euclid Avenue, Bolwell 6th, Floor, Cleveland, OH 44106, USA; [b] Division of Allergy, Pulmonary and Critical Care Medicine, Department of Thoracic Surgery, Vanderbilt University Medical Center, T-1218 Medical Center North, 1161 21st Avenue South, Nashville, TN 37232, USA
* Corresponding author.
E-mail address: otis.rickman@vumc.org
Twitter: @SKAvasarala (S.K.A.)

Surg Clin N Am 102 (2022) 393–412
https://doi.org/10.1016/j.suc.2022.01.004
0039-6109/22/© 2022 Elsevier Inc. All rights reserved.
surgical.theclinics.com

bronchoscopy has improved essential health care utilization and patient-centric metrics.[3] This article outlines the instruments that can be used within bronchoscopy for the management of lung cancer. The devices are categorized broadly into diagnostic and therapeutic groups; further subdivision is based on mechanical or technological attributes.

DIAGNOSTIC PROCEDURES
Imaging

Standard white light bronchoscopy
White light bronchoscopy (WLB) is a valuable tool for assessing the appearance of the endoluminal anatomy. It is the foundation for all other bronchoscopic procedures. With WLB, lesions affecting the central, lobar, and segmental airways are easily seen. Depending on the size of the bronchoscope that is used, later-generation bronchi can also be visualized. Advances in engineering have allowed for the development of smaller diameter bronchoscopes less than 3 mm in size.[4]

The airway examination is vital to any bronchoscopic procedure, including the management of lung cancer. It is estimated that 13% of all new lung cancer diagnoses will have malignant central airway obstruction[5] (**Fig. 1**). The occult nature of endoluminal disease limits the usefulness of standard WLB. It is estimated that less than one-third of carcinoma in situ and 69% of microinvasive tumors can be seen on WLB alone.[6] Imaging adjuncts such as narrow-band imaging (NBI), autofluorescence bronchoscopy (AFB), and optical coherence tomography (OCT) have been developed or are currently under investigation. These modalities are helpful in the assessment of airway disease that is not visible on WLB.

Narrow-band imaging
Narrow-band imaging has been proposed to better evaluate early, invasive lung cancer within the visible endobronchial tree. The use of NBI enhances the endobronchial microvascular tree. Two narrow wavebands of light irradiate the visualized tissue. The green narrow-band (530–550 nm) is absorbed by hemoglobin in the submucosal blood vessels; the blue narrow band (390–445 nm) is absorbed by superficial mucosal layer capillaries.[7] A prospective study of 22 patients showed that NBI was superior to WLB in identifying dysplasia or malignancy within the airway. In addition to identifying areas

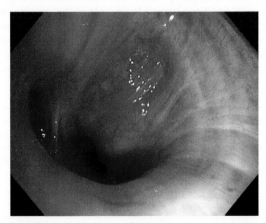

Fig. 1. White light bronchoscopy showing abnormal mucosa and vasculature in a patient with clear evidence of endobronchial disease. This lesion is localized in the left lower lobe; histopathological analysis later revealed squamous cell carcinoma.

of abnormal tissue, data suggest that NBI can be used to differentiate histologic cancer types. In a prospective study of patients with endoscopically visible, biopsy-confirmed tumors, distinct pathologic vascular patterns seen on NBI were associated with cancer subtypes. A dotted pattern of vascularity was highly suggestive of adenocarcinoma, while tortuous and abrupt-ending blood vessels were suggestive of squamous cell carcinoma.[8] Another prospective study showed that NBI could be useful in the evaluation of lung cancer extension. In a study of 106 patients with suspected lung cancer, the use of NBI led to a change in treatment decisions in 14 patients. The change in treatment was due to higher specificity and sensitivity for assessing endoscopic lung cancer extent compared with WLB.[9] Several commercially produced bronchoscopes and endoscopy systems include NBI as a standard option.

Autofluorescence

Autofluorescence bronchoscopy is based on the concept of tissue fluorescence. Tissue fluorescence provides visual clues regarding intracellular chemical changes and the electronic structure of absorption chromophores.[10] Normal respiratory tissue fluoresces green when exposed to the violet-blue light spectrum (400–450 nm). In diseases with metaplasia, dysplasia, or carcinoma in situ, green autofluorescence is lost, and the tissues impart a red-brown color. The red-brown color is primarily due to cancer cells' increased epithelial thickness and vascularity.[7] A meta-analysis that reviewed 14 studies showed that the pooled sensitivity of AFB was higher than WLB for the detection of lung cancer and preneoplastic lesions (0.90 vs 0.66). However, the specificity of WLB was higher than that of AFB (0.69 vs 0.56).[11] The higher sensitivity and lower specificity of AFB (with WLB) compared with WLB alone was again demonstrated in a meta-analysis by Sun and colleagues.[12]

Specialized equipment is required to perform AF.[13] Over the years, several systems have been introduced into the market.[14] One meta-analysis suggests that NBI has a higher sensitivity, specificity, and diagnostic odds ratio in the evaluation of premalignant lesions when compared with AFB.[15]

Optical coherence tomography

Optical coherence tomography is an advanced imaging modality that showcases near-microscopic resolution assessment of tissue architecture.

To examine the area of interest, the OCT catheter is introduced through the bronchoscope's working channel. High-resolution images in real-time are generated using near-infrared light; tissue structures can be imaged with a resolution of ±10 to 15 μm and a depth of 2 to 3 mm.[16] OCT allows for cross-sectional imaging of the structures surrounding the airways. The image that is reproduced is like a radial probe endobronchial ultrasound (RP-EBUS) generated image. Instead of ultrasound waves, OCT uses scattered light to generate images. It has been studied in various pulmonary diseases: obstructive airway diseases, malignancy, interstitial lung diseases, and pulmonary vascular disease.[17] For now, OCT bronchoscopy is considered investigational.

Pathologic Sample Acquisition

Endobronchial

There are a variety of ways endobronchial samples can be obtained via traditional bronchoscopy. However, some modalities are more valuable than others in the context of lung cancer diagnosis.

The simplest forms of sample acquisition are bronchial washings (BW) and bronchoalveolar lavage (BAL). A BAL involves the instillation and aspiration of sterile isotonic saline via a wedged flexible bronchoscope. The tip of the bronchoscope is wedged in a segmental or subsegmental airway. The instilled volume should be suffi-cient to reach the alveoli. A BAL samples the alveoli and the small airways.

Both BW and BAL can provide some information about inflammation, infection, or malignancy. BAL is a commonly performed procedure, and it samples the alveoli. It is usually used in concerns for an infectious etiology and has poor sensitivity for malignancy. Historically, it was thought that the routine collection of washings increased the sensitivity of bronchoscopy for the diagnosis of malignancy. Howev-er, a large retrospective study evaluated 667 bronchial cytologic specimens, and the malignancy sensitivity was 14.7%.[18] Interestingly, only one washing specimen (0.2%) showed malignant cells that were not captured by other samples acquired during the procedure. The sensitivity for BAL or BW for malignancy is low; 43% is reported in the American College of Chest Physicians Guidelines for the diag-nosis and management of lung cancer.[19] Although BW and BAL samples may pro-vide cytologic samples showing malignant cells, additional cell characteristics are often unable to be ascertained. These characteristics are of utmost importance in the current landscape of cancer therapeutics. A differentiation between nonsmall cell lung cancer (NSCLC) and small cell lung cancer can often be made from pos-itive BAL or BW.[19]

Similarly, a bronchial brush can be used to obtain endobronchial cytologic samples by rubbing the instrument against diseased mucosa. In visible endobronchial tumors, biopsies and brushings have been shown to provide helpful information. In a prospec-tive study of 86 patients who had visible endobronchial abnormalities and underwent sequential washing, brushing, and biopsy of the endobronchial lesion, brushing and biopsy showed the best concordance for lung cancer (78%).[20]

Transbronchial needle aspiration (TBNA) has become a mainstay for sampling endobronchial and peripheral lesions. A variety of needles can be used to sample visible endoscopic lesions and acquire a tissue diagnosis. In peripheral bronchos-copy, an aspirating needle was the most common first tool used in a large prospective study that assessed electromagnetic navigation bronchoscopy (ENB).[21] In the 300 cases in which rapid onsite examination yielded a malignant diagnosis, the aspirating needle was the first used in 49.5% of cases.

Advanced Bronchoscopy

Thin bronchoscope

It is believed that thin or ultrathin bronchoscopes are advantageous over standard-sized bronchoscopes in peripheral bronchoscopy. The smaller bronchoscopes can travel more distal in the airway, which was thought to allow better localization. This belief, however, has not been well represented in data. A prospective multicenter ran-domized control study showed there was no statistical difference in diagnostic yield between standard bronchoscopy (6.0 mm outer diameter) with fluoroscopy or thin bronchoscope (4.2 mm outer diameter) with RP-EBUS (37% vs 49%).[22]

Radial probe endobronchial ultrasound

Radial probe endobronchial ultrasound is an essential tool within bronchoscopy, espe-cially peripheral bronchoscopy. The RP-EBUS probe can be passed through the work-ing channel of a bronchoscope to acquire a 360° grey-scale image of surrounding structures[23] (**Fig. 2**). A systematic review that analyzed data of 57 procedures that used RP-EBUS showed that the overall weighted diagnostic yield for RP-EBUS was 70.6%.[24] None of the studies included in this systematic review used additional advanced guidance techniques such as ENB or virtual bronchoscopic navigation

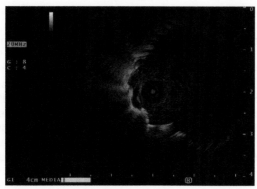

Fig. 2. Radial probe endobronchial ultrasound is commonly used in peripheral bronchoscopy to localize lesions. The probe is passed through a bronchoscope's working channel, extended working channel, or a guide sheath. Well-localized lesions provide a concentric radial probe endobronchial ultrasound image.

(VBN). Although RP-EBUS has been around since 2002, it is still an essential tool in peripheral bronchoscopy and is often incorporated into the sampling process.

Computer-assisted navigational bronchoscopy: electromagnetic navigation bronchoscopy, virtual bronchoscopic navigation

Virtual bronchoscopic navigation relies on generating a static bronchoscopic road map that the bronchoscopist can follow. The process relies on the matching of the virtual images with the WLB images. Then, based on the series of displayed virtual images, the bronchoscope is guided under direct vision into the sampling area.[25]

A systematic review that included 32 studies estimated the pooled sensitivity, specificity, and area under the curve (95% confidence interval) of VBN to be 0.80 (0.76–0.83), 0.65 (0.56–0.73), and 0.81 (0.78–0.85), respectively.[26]

Electromagnetic navigation bronchoscopy was first introduced into the market in the early 2000s.[27] A variety of systems currently exist on the market. Due to a variance in definition, the reported diagnostic yield varies greatly. The 2 most extensive data series in ENB are from the AQuIRE Registry and NAVIGATE studies. Data from the AQuIRE Registry showed poor diagnostic yield with ENB use: 38.5% for EMN alone and 47.1% for ENB combined with RP-EBUS.[28] The prospective multicenter NAVIGATE study showed a 12-month diagnostic yield of 73%, and the median lesion size was 20.0 mm.[29] Studies that used ENB bronchoscopy systems with digital tomosynthesis correction for CT-Body divergence showed diagnostic yields ranging between 77.4 and 83.[30–32]

Robotic-assisted bronchoscopy

Currently, 2 robotic-assisted bronchoscopy platforms are on the market: MONARCH Platform by Auris Health© (Redwood City, CA, USA) and Ion Endoluminal System by Intuitive Surgical© (Sunnyvale, CA, USA). The reported advantage of both systems is precision control in the periphery.

Monarch

The MONARCH Platform was cleared for use by the United States Food and Drug Administration in March 2018. Rojas-Solano and colleagues[33] used the system to sample 15 parenchymal lesions, a malignant diagnosis was found in 9 patients. There were no significant adverse events noted. The system was also successfully used to diagnose 97% of nodules (n = 77) among 8 human cadaveric lungs.[34] A retrospective study that assessed the platform across academic and community medical centers in the United States revealed a diagnostic yield ranging between 69.1% and 77%. One-hundred and sixty-seven lesions among 165 patients were included in this study, and navigation was successful in 88.6% of cases. Navigation success was defined as either diagnostic tissue on final pathology or an abnormal RP-EBUS signal.[35]

A multicenter, prospective clinical trial that assessed the successful navigation of the system and the incidence of device or procedure-related adverse effects has been completed. Fifty-five patients were enrolled across five centers, and lesion localization rate was 96.2%, pneumothorax rate was 3.7%, one needed a chest tube.[36]

Ion

The Ion robotic bronchoscopy platform uses a fully articulating 3.5 mm outer diameter catheter to access difficult-to-reach nodules.[36] The working channel diameter is 2.0 mm. The system is designed to allow direct visualization during only a portion of the navigation process; after a specific depth is reached, the visualization probe must be removed. For real-time orientation and feedback, the rest of the navigation process is dependent on the system's shape sensing technology. A single-arm, single-center study (29 patients) has shown high rates of reaching the target (96.6% success) and an overall diagnostic yield of 79.3% (88% for malignancy).[37] All lesions in this study were ≤12.3 mm in size, and 41.4% did not have a bronchus sign present. Another study that evaluated successful navigation rates between ultrathin bronchoscopy with RP-EBUS, EMN bronchoscopy, and the Ion platform showed that the robotic system outperformed the other modalities with a successful navigation rate of 100%.[38] Preliminary results from a prospective multicenter study using the Ion system (ClinicalTrials.gov Identifier: NCT03893539) showed that the system is safe to use, with no adverse event or pneumothorax requiring intervention during the sampling of 74 nodules.[39]

A single-center, prospective study of 131 cases with the Ion platform (targeting 159 pulmonary lesions) showed that the overall diagnostic yield was 81.7%, the overall complication rate was 3.0%, and the pneumothorax rate was 1.5%.[40] Another single-center observational study that combined the Ion platform with cone-beam CT guidance showed an overall diagnostic yield of 86% among 59 nodules that were biopsied.[41]

Linear endobronchial ultrasound

Linear endobronchial ultrasound (also known as convex probe endobronchial ultrasound [CP-EBUS]) has been a revolutionary tool in thoracic medicine. It is an important tool in the diagnosis and staging of lung cancer. The use of CP-EBUS allows for minimally invasive sampling of suspicious lymph nodes and central pulmonary lesions (**Fig. 3**). Additionally, CP-EBUS can also be used to access and sample extrathoracic sites such as the adrenal glands.[42,43]

The European Society of Thoracic Surgeons and the American College of Chest Physicians recommend that suspicious mediastinal lymphadenopathy be evaluated by EBUS TBNA, endoscopic ultrasound fine-needle aspiration, or a combined approach.[44,45] In a prospective study that evaluated surgical patients with CT, PET, and EBUS-TBNA before surgery, the sensitivity, and specificity of EBUS-TBNA (92.3/100%) were higher than chest CT (76.9%/55.3%) or PET (80%/70.1%) for accurately staging the mediastinum.[46] Additionally, EBUS-TBNA has been helpful in sampling lesions around the central airways and may not be seen on WLB.[47–49]

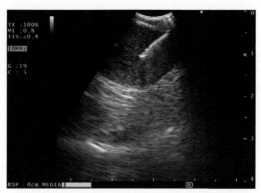

Fig. 3. Linear endobronchial ultrasound allows for real-time sampling of structures that can be visualized via the airway or esophagus. Unlike radial probe endobronchial ultrasound, tool-in-lesion (such as the sampling needle within a lymph node) can be confirmed.

Endobronchial ultrasound transbronchial needle injection (EBUS-TBNI) has been used to access and inject therapeutic agents into lymph nodes with malignant involvement. The first series of EBUS-TBNI was published by Hohenforst-Schmidt and colleagues[50] in 2013. In this study, EBUS-TBNI was used to inject cisplatin analogs directly into affected lymph nodes.

THERAPEUTIC PROCEDURES

The endoluminal approach can also be used to deliver therapeutics within the airways and lung parenchyma. A variety of tools can be used to destroy a tumor or abnormal tissue. In the central airways, this tissue can cause central airway obstruction, bleeding, or recurrent lower respiratory tract infections. In the periphery, imaging evidence of abnormal tissue may represent a malignancy or a lesion with a high probability of being malignant. Endoluminal therapeutic tools can be classified in a variety of ways, including their area of use.

Central Airway Ablation

Thermal modalities
Heat-based therapeutics. Heat-based therapies are commonly used within the visible airways. Both contact and noncontact forms exist. The tissue destruction delivered by hot therapies is immediate. Endobronchial fire is a rare event but a risk with the use of heat-based therapies. Therefore, careful attention must be paid to the fraction of inspired oxygen being delivered to the patient, and it should not exceed 0.40.[51]

Laser
Laser is a commonly used airway ablative tool. It is a method of delivering light energy that is noncontact, which gets absorbed and converted into heat energy. There are a variety of lasers that can be used for therapeutic procedures within the airway. Each type of laser has specific characteristics which must be kept in mind when choosing the correct device. The laser, power output, and laser fiber distance to tissue greatly impact the interaction between the laser and the target tissue.[52] In general, the Nd:YAP laser is best suited for coagulation, while the CO2 laser (more commonly used in Otorhinolaryngology) is best for precise cutting.[53] Other lasers commonly used lasers include Nd:YAG, Ho:YAG, and KTP. Data support the use of lasers in the context of malignant central airway obstruction. One of the largest series with

lasers was published by Cavaliere and colleagues[54] in 1988. One thousand patients were treated with the Nd:YAG laser. In the group with malignant airway obstruction (649), an improvement in airway diameter was achieved 92% of the time. It should be kept in mind that although Nd:YAG laser offers excellent tissue vaporization and vasoconstriction, the depth of penetration is more profound than other lasers and heat-based modalities.[55]

Electrosurgery

Electrocautery is a contact method of heat-based thermal ablation. High frequency, alternating electrical current passes through a probe, which generates heat. Its penetration depth is variable and is affected by the type of probe used to deliver the heat (blunt-tipped probe, knife, snare, or hot forceps). It is an excellent tool to achieve tissue destruction and hemostasis. Electrocautery can be delivered through various tools that are generally re-useable: blunt probe (semi-rigid or flexible), knife, snare, or hot biopsy forceps[56] (**Fig. 4**).

Argon plasma coagulation

Argon plasma coagulation (APC) is a noncontact heat-based thermal modality used to achieve tissue destruction or hemostasis (**Fig. 5**). With APC, argon gas flows out of the distal end of the catheter; the argon gas follows the path of least resistance.[55] This gas conducts a high-frequency monopolar current, which causes thermal effects.

It is an excellent tool for achieving rapid hemostasis. However, due to its noncontact nature, there are some challenges when using APC for debulking. A unique risk with APC is the creation of a gas embolism. Gas embolism is a rare but severe complication that can lead to shock, cardiac arrest, stroke, and death.[57] Avoidance of direct mucosal contact may mitigate the risk.

Cold-Based Therapeutics

Two primary modalities of applying cryotherapy within the airways exist: spray cryotherapy (SCT) and contact probe cryotherapy. Both depend on the generation of extreme cold to cause cell death. Immediate injury is caused by extra-and intracellular ice crystal formation. In SCT, the extracellular matrix is preserved. Delayed tissue injury is caused by local vasoconstriction, thrombosis, and immune-mediated cell

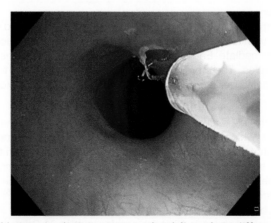

Fig. 4. Thermal ablation via electrocautery can be delivered via different interfaces; one example is the needle knife. Activation of the circuit heats the knife and allows for precise cuts into abnormal areas of the airways, such as subglottic stenosis.

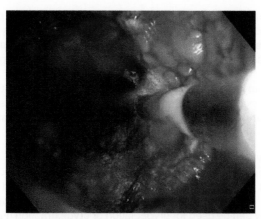

Fig. 5. Argon plasma coagulation is a noncontact mode of thermal ablation. Argon gas emits from the distal end of the catheter; an electrical charge activates the gas. Argon plasma coagulation is being used to destroy recurrent respiratory papillomatous lesions.

death.[58] Intracellular water content determines cryosensitivity; tumor, skin, mucous membranes, nerves, granulation tissue, and endothelium are cryosensitive due to their high water content.[59] Achieving a lower temperature, faster freezing rate, slower thaw rate, repeated freeze–thaw cycles, and a smaller target tissue volume enhances the cryotherapy effect.

Spray cryotherapy

In SCT, liquid nitrogen is delivered via a catheter through the working channel of a bronchoscope. Flash freezing at −196°C occurs. The system comprises a 7 Fr catheter connected to a container with liquid nitrogen and machinery to regulate flow, all within a self-contained console (**Fig. 6**). It is mainly used to treat benign airway strictures but can also be used to manage endoluminal malignancies. A unique risk of SCT is the development of a pneumothorax, Liquid nitrogen changes into a gas after it is sprayed onto tissue. This liquid to gas transformation results in a 700-fold increase

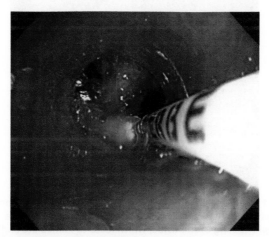

Fig. 6. Spray cryotherapy delivers liquid nitrogen to the target tissue via the use specialized catheter. This liquid nitrogen causes flash freezing at −196°C.

in volume which can lead to barotrauma from the high intrathoracic pressure if there is inadequate means for the gas to escape. The other unique risk is hypoxemia secondary to nitrogen displacement.[60] Therefore, an adequate sized airway device must be used to allow passive egress of expanding gas.[61] Akin to APC, a gas embolism can also occur.

Spray cryotherapy application should not occur too distally, as the liquid nitrogen can easily be trapped and cause a pneumothorax. In a case series that included 37 patients that underwent 80 procedures with SCT, it proved to be safe. Only 3 complications occurred, all of which were transient hypoxia.[60]

Contact probe cryotherapy

The contact cryoprobe has several applications within diagnostic and therapeutic bronchoscopy. At present, probes come in 4 sizes: 1.1, 1.7, 1.9, and 2.4 mm.[62] In general, the 1.9 mm or 2.4 mm probes are used for therapeutic applications. Contact probe cryotherapy can be used for cryoablation or cryoextraction (**Fig. 7**). In cryoablation, the cryoprobe makes direct contact with the abnormal tissue. The cryoprobe is activated in the region of interest for 30 to 60 seconds, followed by thawing. This freeze–thaw cycle can be repeated several times, which leads to delayed tissue destruction.[63] The necrotic tissue can then be debulked during a follow-up bronchoscopy. Similarly, cryoextraction or cryorecanalization can be performed. In this method, the probe contacts lesion for 3 to 5 seconds, and then the tumor-probe and flexible bronchoscope are removed en-bloc rapidly.[64]

Brachytherapy

The principle of brachytherapy is radiation application directly into the tumor area. It can be combined with other treatment modalities, such as external beam radiotherapy (EBRT)—brachytherapy is considered when EBRT is not an option. Few randomized controlled trials assessing endobronchial brachytherapy exist.[65] Like photodynamic therapy (PDT), a delayed response typically takes 2 to 3 weeks. The central tenant of brachytherapy is the concentrated delivery of radiation to the tumor. It is commonly performed as an outpatient procedure.

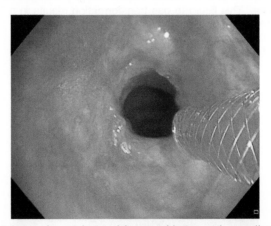

Fig. 7. The contact cryoprobe can be used for cryoablation and cryoadhesion. Unlike spray cryotherapy, the probe must be in direct contact with the target tissue. Activation of the catheter causes rapid cooling of the tissue, which leads to immediate and late cell death effects. For example, a cryoprobe is used to debulk stent-generated granulation tissue in a patient with tracheobronchomalacia.

In summary, a flexible polyurethane catheter is guided into the airway under bron-choscopic visualization to the area of interest. Once the position has been confirmed, the catheter is secured into place and loaded with radioactive beads. Within bron-choscopy, brachytherapy is mainly used as a treatment option for NSCLC. It can be used in conjunction with EBRT.[66] The most typical indication is early-stage lung can-cer confined to the airway lumen. However, it can be used as a method of salvage therapy in locally recurrent or residual disease. Risks of brachytherapy include hemop-tysis, fistula formation, and bronchial stenosis.

Most brachytherapy data are limited to retrospective reports. Aumont-le Guilcher M and colleagues. reported a series of 226 patients with NSCLC with no extra bronchial spread were treated with endobronchial brachytherapy. A 3-month response rate of 93.6% was noted, the 5-year survival rate was 29%.[67] Similarly, Soror T and col-leagues. reported a series of 126 patients with endobronchial recurrence of NSCLC.[68] The 3-month local response rate was 86.5%. Of note, 12.7% of patients in this series died from massive hemoptysis. Endobronchial brachytherapy has been combined with other ablative modalities as an adjunct. A Cochrane meta-analysis assessed the effectiveness of palliative endobronchial brachytherapy with EBRT or other alter-native endoluminal modalities for symptom control and survival benefit in patients with NSCLC.[69] Fourteen randomized controlled trials were included. Overall, it was concluded that EBRT alone was more effective for palliation than endobronchial brachytherapy alone.

For lung cancer, brachytherapy can be delivered endobronchial via a catheter or percutaneously via radioactive seed implantation. Based on the American Brachyther-apy Society, the indications for endobronchial therapy are restricted to specific sce-narios: (1) sole therapy for small-sized peripheral lung cancer in nonoperable patients or those with localized bronchial carcinoma, (2) therapy for those with small, central, early lung cancer, (3) central carcinoma in situ or precancerous lesions, or (4) posttransplant benign endobronchial lesions.[70]

The most severe complication of endobronchial brachytherapy is the development of an airway fistula, which may lead to fatal hemoptysis. Radiation bronchitis and bron-chial stenosis are other known complications that can occur.[71]

Photodynamic therapy

Both brachytherapy and PDT are forms of ablation that have found a use for treating early lung cancer. With PDT, a photosensitizing agent is given systematically. It achieves a higher concentration in tumor cells. Cell damage and death are triggered by the delivery of a direct light application via a probe that is positioned bronchoscopi-cally. This light is of a specific wavelength and matches the absorption band of the drug. The photodynamic reaction drives cell necrosis. The latter is dependent on the generation of oxygen-dependent cytotoxic agents and the release of singlet-oxy-gen.[72] There are several photosensitizers on the market, the most commonly used ones being that of the porphyrin family.[73] Photofrin (porfimer sodium) (Pinnacle Bio-logics Incorporated, Bannockburn, IL, U.S.A.) is an intravenous injection at 2 mg/kg. Maximum tissue concentration is reached in about 24 to 48 hrs. Photosensitizer con-centration occurs in malignant cells, skin, liver, and spleen.[74]

Light wavelength matching with the absorption band of the photosensitizer is essen-tial. The activation of porphyrin-based photosensitizers occurs in the red region of the spectrum, 620 nm.[75] The argon/dye laser is the most frequently used activator. The light is typically delivered via the working channel of a flexible bronchoscope 48 hours after the injection of the photosensitizer. A "clean-up" bronchoscopy is usually per-formed one to 2 days after light application. Re-illumination can be performed around

1 week after the sensitizer injection. PDT can be used for malignant central airway obstruction (it will not provide immediate relief) and radiographically occult lung cancer. Data support a favorable safety profile, with a 30-day mortality rate of 1%.[74] Skin sensitization is a unique concern; sun exposure may have to be avoided for several weeks.[7] Contraindications to PDT include porphyria, aerodigestive tract fistulas, tumor erosion into blood vessels, and critical malignant central airway obstruction that requires immediate airway enlargement. In addition, porfimer sodium can cause fetal harm, and caution must be taken in patients with renal or hepatic impairment (due to slower drug clearance).[76] PDT is also expensive due to the cost of porfimer sodium, which is estimated to cost $6600 for 140 mg (doses at 2 mg/kg body weight).[77]

Mechanical destruction

Mechanical destruction of airway lesions can be accomplished in a variety of ways. The simplest form is using the rigid bronchoscope to core through lesions that are causing central airway obstruction. Coring allows quick recanalization of the airway, the barrel of the rigid bronchoscope pressed against the diseased airway allows for tamponade and partial control of any bleeding that may have been caused by coring (**Fig. 8**).

Additionally, a variety of tools can be used to excise the lesion from the airway. Excision usually involves a combination of forceps (flexible or rigid) to grasp tissue and remove it from the airway. The room provided by the rigid barrel allows for multiple tools and devices such as the microdebrider.

In various benign or malignant airway diseases, endobronchial stents can be used to maintain airway patency. A variety of stents are currently on the market. The stents range from simple straight silicone stents to more complex designs such as hybrid stents, and even patient-specific 3D printed stents[78] (**Figs. 9** and **10**). However, it is vital to keep in mind that, in general, stenting should be seen as a temporary option until definitive therapy can take place.

Peripheral Airway Ablation

Brachytherapy

Much like brachytherapy can be used endoscopically to treat lesions that affect the airway wall, endoscopic brachytherapy has also been used to treat peripheral lung

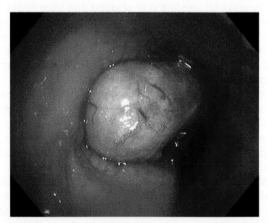

Fig. 8. The distal end of the rigid tracheoscope or bronchoscope barrel can be used to core lesions in central airways. The lip of the distal end of the rigid bronchoscope is used to engage the edge of the abnormal tissue to free it from the walls of the airway lumen.

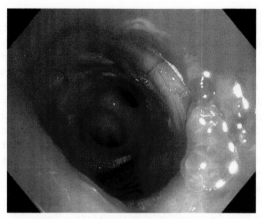

Fig. 9. A straight silicone stent is a popular type of stent used for the management of central airway disease. It can be used in a variety of disease states. A silicone stent is used to maintain the patency of the left main stent in a patient with lung transplant anastomotic complication.

lesions. In a feasibility study of a patient with nonoperable NSCLC, navigational bronchoscopy was used to localize the lesion, place a 6 Fr brachytherapy catheter in the tumor, and then deliver high-dose-rate brachytherapy.[79] The patient tolerated the treatment with the catheter in situ for 5 days. Histologic follow-up showed complete remission.

Microwave and radiofrequency ablation

Radiofrequency (RF) ablation and microwave (MV) ablation have been studied as treatment modalities for local ablative therapy in patients with peripherally located lung malignancies.[80] One of the latest research topics within bronchoscopy and lung cancer is the application of bronchoscopic MV therapy for the ablation of early-stage cancer. In theory, it is an alternative to stereotactic body radiation therapy for those deemed to be unfit or unwilling to undergo surgical resection. Most of the

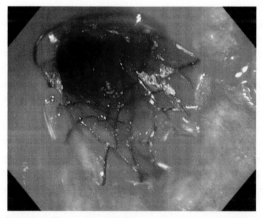

Fig. 10. Self-expanding metallic stents are also commonly used to treat airway narrowing. For example, a BONASTENT Bronchial stent (Thoracent, Huntington, NY, USA) is used to maintain the patency of the left main stem.

published literature is centered around animal studies. In 2019, Yuan and colleagues[81] reported their experience with bronchoscopic ablation with MW in 12 in vivo ablations of porcine lung. No intraprocedural complications were noted to occur. In 2020, Sebek and colleagues[82] reported their experience with the ablation of lung parenchyma of three pigs. No pneumothoraxes or significant airway bleeding was observed. Additional research is taking place using accelerant gel and MV ablation.[83] The most significant published study is the one by Chan and colleagues. They published their retrospective single-center experience using EMN guided bronchoscopy MW ablation in a hybrid OR.[84] Thirty lung nodules among 25 patients were treated. Technical success was noted to be 100%. A Complication rates were low: pain (13.3%), pneumothorax requiring intervention (6.67%), postablation reaction (6.67%), pleural effusion (3.33%), and hemoptysis (3.33%).

Within bronchoscopy, RF ablation has been studied and reported less than MV ablation. A systematic review showed that the 1-year control rate for RF ablation was 77% and was 97% for stereotactic body radiation therapy.[85]

In addition to bronchoscopic MV and RF ablation, feasibility studies have been published regarding the delivery of PDT to treat peripheral lesions.[85–88] Other modalities that have also been studied for the ablation of peripheral lung tumors include bronchoscopic thermal vapor ablation. Thus far, it has only been used and ex vivo human lungs. Ferguson and colleagues reported the use of BTVA among 10 human lungs. Further studies are needed to assess the safety and clinical efficacy.[89]

SUMMARY

Bronchoscopy is an invaluable procedure in the management of lung cancer. It allows for a minimally invasive approach to acquire tissue samples and intervene on cancer-related airway pathologies such as obstruction, stenosis, and hemoptysis. Depending on the procedure being performed, it can serve a role in diagnosis, treatment, or both. Overall, bronchoscopy has been proven to be safe and effective. The next phase of research is centered around peripheral ablation. If found to be safe and effective, it will open yet another frontier for this critical tool.

CLINICS CARE POINTS

- When assessing for the presence of endobronchial disease, NBI can be used as a complementary modality to WLB inspection.
- Even if malignant cells are identified on BW or BAL, additional samples must be obtained as important cell characteristics cannot be determined on the washings or lavage.
- No heat-based ablation therapy has been proven to be better than the other; selection should be based on local expertise, equipment availability, and anatomic specifics of the area that is being ablated.
- If airway tumor debulking is urgently needed and the Fio_2 cannot be reduced to an acceptable level, cryoextraction with a contact cryoprobe can be considered.
- Although effective for treating malignant endoluminal disease, PDT should not be considered as a primary modality to provide immediate airway obstruction relief.

DISCLOSURE

The authors have nothing to disclose.

REFERENCES

1. de Koning HJ, van der Aalst CM, de Jong PA, et al. Reduced lung-cancer mortality with volume CT screening in a randomized trial. N Engl J Med 2020; 382(6):503–13.
2. Polcz ME, Maiga AW, Brown LB, et al. The impact of an interventional pulmonary program on nontherapeutic lung resections. J Bronchology Interv Pulmonol 2019; 26(4):287–9.
3. Colt HG, Harrell JH. Therapeutic rigid bronchoscopy allows level of care changes in patients with acute respiratory failure from central airways obstruction. Chest 1997;112(1):202–6.
4. Avasarala SK, Gillaspie EA, Maldonado F. Rigid versus flexible bronchoscopy. In: Turner JJF, Jain P, Yasufuku K, et al, editors. From thoracic surgery to interventional pulmonology: a clinical guide. Manhattan: Springer International Publishing; 2021. p. 1–17.
5. Daneshvar C, Falconer WE, Ahmed M, et al. Prevalence and outcome of central airway obstruction in patients with lung cancer. BMJ Open Respir Res 2019;6(1): e000429.
6. Andolfi M, Potenza R, Capozzi R, et al. The role of bronchoscopy in the diagnosis of early lung cancer: a review. J Thorac Dis 2016;8(11):3329–37.
7. Ernst A, Herth FJ. Principles and practice of interventional pulmonology. New York: Springer Science & Business Media; 2012.
8. Zaric B, Perin B, Stojsic V, et al. Relation between vascular patterns visualized by narrow band imaging (NBI) videobronchoscopy and histological type of lung cancer. Med Oncol 2013;30(1):374.
9. Zaric B, Becker HD, Perin B, et al. Narrow band imaging videobronchoscopy improves assessment of lung cancer extension and influences therapeutic strategy. Jpn J Clin Oncol 2009;39(10):657–63.
10. Feller-Kopman D, Lunn W, Ernst A. Autofluorescence bronchoscopy and endobronchial ultrasound: a practical review. Ann Thorac Surg 2005;80(6): 2395–401. https://doi.org/10.1016/j.athoracsur.2005.04.084.
11. Chen W, Gao X, Tian Q, et al. A comparison of autofluorescence bronchoscopy and white light bronchoscopy in detection of lung cancer and preneoplastic lesions: a meta-analysis. Lung Cancer 2011;73(2):183–8.
12. Sun J, Garfield DH, Lam B, et al. The value of autofluorescence bronchoscopy combined with white light bronchoscopy compared with white light alone in the diagnosis of intraepithelial neoplasia and invasive lung cancer: a meta-analysis. J Thorac Oncol 2011;6(8):1336–44.
13. Crymes T, Fish R, Smith D. Autofluorescence bronchoscopy definition autofluorescence bronchoscopy is a broncho-scopic procedure in which a blue light rather than a white light is employed for illumination, and prema. Chest 2003; 123:1701.
14. Herth FJF, Ernst A, Becker HD. Autofluorescence bronchoscopy – A comparison of two systems (LIFE and D-light). Respiration 2003;70(4):395–8.
15. Iftikhar IH, Musani AI. Narrow-band imaging bronchoscopy in the detection of premalignant airway lesions: a meta-analysis of diagnostic test accuracy. Ther Adv Respir Dis 2015;9(5):207–16.
16. Huang D, Swanson EA, Lin CP, et al. Optical coherence tomography. Science 1991;254(5035):1178–81.

17. Goorsenberg A, Kalverda KA, Annema J, et al. Advances in optical coherence tomography and confocal laser endomicroscopy in pulmonary diseases. Respiration 2020;99(3):190–205.

18. Girard P, Caliandro R, Seguin-Givelet A, et al. Sensitivity of cytology specimens from bronchial aspirate or washing during bronchoscopy in the diagnosis of lung malignancies: an update. Clin Lung Cancer 2017;18(5):512–8.

19. Rivera MP, Mehta AC, Wahidi MM. Establishing the diagnosis of lung cancer: diagnosis and management of lung cancer, 3rd ed: american college of chest physicians evidence-based clinical practice guidelines. Chest 2013;143(5 Suppl):e142S–65S.

20. Soler TV, Isamitt DD, Carrasco OA. [Yield of biopsy, brushing and bronchial washing through fiberbronchoscopy in the diagnosis of lung cancer with visible lesions]. Rev Med Chil 2004;132(10):1198–203. https://doi.org/10.4067/s0034-98872004001000006. Rendimiento de la biopsia, cepillado y lavado bronquial por fibrobroncoscopia en el diagnóstico de cáncer pulmonar con lesiones visibles endoscópicamente.

21. Gildea TR, Folch EE, Khandhar SJ, et al. The impact of biopsy tool choice and rapid on-site evaluation on diagnostic accuracy for malignant lesions in the prospective: multicenter navigate study. J Bronchology Interv Pulmonol 2021;28(3): 174–83.

22. Tanner NT, Yarmus L, Chen A, et al. Standard bronchoscopy with fluoroscopy vs thin bronchoscopy and radial endobronchial ultrasound for biopsy of pulmonary lesions: a multicenter, prospective, randomized trial. Chest 2018;154(5):1035–43.

23. Avasarala SK, Aravena C, Almeida FA. Convex probe endobronchial ultrasound: historical, contemporary, and cutting-edge applications. J Thorac Dis 2019;12(3): 1085–99.

24. Ali MS, Trick W, Mba BI, et al. Radial endobronchial ultrasound for the diagnosis of peripheral pulmonary lesions: a systematic review and meta-analysis. Respirology 2017;22(3):443–53.

25. Asano F, Matsuno Y, Tsuzuku A, et al. Diagnosis of peripheral pulmonary lesions using a bronchoscope insertion guidance system combined with endobronchial ultrasonography with a guide sheath. Lung Cancer 2008;60(3):366–73.

26. Qian K, Krimsky WS, Sarkar SA, et al. Efficiency of electromagnetic navigation bronchoscopy and virtual bronchoscopic navigation. Ann Thorac Surg 2020; 109(6):1731–40.

27. Cicenia J, Avasarala SK, Gildea TR. Navigational bronchoscopy: a guide through history, current use, and developing technology. J Thorac Dis 2020;12(6): 3263–71.

28. Ost DE, Ernst A, Lei X, et al. Diagnostic yield and complications of bronchoscopy for peripheral lung lesions. results of the AQuIRE registry. Am J Respir Crit Care Med 2016;193(1):68–77.

29. Folch EE, Pritchett MA, Nead MA, et al. Electromagnetic navigation bronchoscopy for peripheral pulmonary lesions: one-year results of the prospective, multicenter navigate study. J Thorac Oncol 2019;14(3):445–58.

30. Katsis J, Roller L, Aboudara M, et al. Diagnostic yield of digital tomosynthesis-assisted navigational bronchoscopy for indeterminate lung nodules. J Bronchology Interv Pulmonol 2021;28(4):255–61.

31. Aboudara M, Roller L, Rickman O, et al. Improved diagnostic yield for lung nodules with digital tomosynthesis-corrected navigational bronchoscopy: Initial experience with a novel adjunct. Respirology 2020;25(2):206–13.

32. Avasarala SK, Roller L, Katsis J, et al. Sight unseen: diagnostic yield and safety outcomes of a novel multimodality navigation bronchoscopy platform with real-time target acquisition. Respiration 2021;101(2):166–73.

33. Rojas-Solano JR, Ugalde-Gamboa L, Machuzak M. Robotic bronchoscopy for diagnosis of suspected lung cancer: a feasibility study. J Bronchology Interv Pulmonol 2018;25(3):168–75.

34. Chen AC, Pastis NJ, Machuzak MS, et al. Accuracy of a robotic endoscopic system in cadaver models with simulated tumor targets: access study. Respiration 2020;99(1):56–61.

35. Chaddha U, Kovacs SP, Manley C, et al. Robot-assisted bronchoscopy for pulmonary lesion diagnosis: results from the initial multicenter experience. BMC Pulm Med 2019;19(1):243.

36. Chen AC, Pastis NJ Jr, Mahajan AK, et al. Robotic bronchoscopy for peripheral pulmonary lesions: a multicenter pilot and feasibility study (BENEFIT). Chest 2021;159(2):845–52.

37. Fielding DIK, Bashirzadeh F, Son JH, et al. First human use of a new robotic-assisted fiber optic sensing navigation system for small peripheral pulmonary nodules. Respiration 2019;98(2):142–50. https://doi.org/10.1159/000498951.

38. Yarmus L, Akulian J, Wahidi M, et al. A Prospective randomized comparative study of three guided bronchoscopic approaches for investigating pulmonary nodules: the PRECISION-1 study. Chest 2019. https://doi.org/10.1016/j.chest.2019.10.016.

39. Folch EE, Pritchett M, Reisenauer J, et al. A prospective, multi-center evaluation of the clinical utility of the ion endoluminal system -experience using a robotic-assisted bronchoscope system with shape-sensing technology. A110 advances in interventional pulmonology. American Thoracic Society 2020;201:A2719. American Thoracic Society International Conference Abstracts.

40. Kalchiem-Dekel O, Connolly JG, Lin IH, et al. Shape-sensing robotic-assisted bronchoscopy in the diagnosis of pulmonary parenchymal lesions. Chest 2021. https://doi.org/10.1016/j.chest.2021.07.2169.

41. Benn BS, Romero AO, Lum M, et al. Robotic-Assisted navigation bronchoscopy as a paradigm shift in peripheral lung access. Lung 2021;199(2):177–86.

42. Christiansen IS, Ahmad K, Bodtger U, et al. EUS-B for suspected left adrenal metastasis in lung cancer. J Thorac Dis 2020;12(3):258–63.

43. Crombag LM, Annema JT. Left adrenal gland analysis in lung cancer patients using the endobronchial ultrasound scope: a feasibility trial. Respiration 2016;91(3):235–40.

44. Detterbeck FC, Lewis SZ, Diekemper R, et al. Executive summary: diagnosis and management of lung cancer, 3rd ed: american college of chest physicians evidence-based clinical practice guidelines. Chest 2013;143(5 Suppl):7s–37s.

45. De Leyn P, Dooms C, Kuzdzal J, et al. Revised ESTS guidelines for preoperative mediastinal lymph node staging for non-small-cell lung cancer. Eur J Cardiothorac Surg 2014;45(5):787–98.

46. Yasufuku K, Nakajima T, Motoori K, et al. Comparison of endobronchial ultrasound, positron emission tomography, and CT for lymph node staging of lung cancer. Chest 2006;130(3):710–8.

47. Zhao H, Xie Z, Zhou ZL, et al. Diagnostic value of endobronchial ultrasound-guided transbronchial needle aspiration in intrapulmonary lesions. Chin Med J (Engl) 2013;126(22):4312–5.

48. Verma A, Jeon K, Koh WJ, et al. Endobronchial ultrasound-guided transbronchial needle aspiration for the diagnosis of central lung parenchymal lesions. Yonsei Med J 2013;54(3):672–8.

49. Nakajima T, Yasufuku K, Fujiwara T, et al. Endobronchial ultrasound-guided transbronchial needle aspiration for the diagnosis of intrapulmonary lesions. J Thorac Oncol 2008;3(9):985–8.

50. Hohenforst-Schmidt W, Zarogoulidis P, Darwiche K, et al. Intratumoral chemotherapy for lung cancer: re-challenge current targeted therapies. Drug Des Devel Ther 2013;7:571–83.

51. Akhtar N, Ansar F, Baig MS, et al. Airway fires during surgery: management and prevention. J Anaesthesiol Clin Pharmacol 2016;32(1):109–11.

52. Chaddha U, Hogarth DK, Murgu S. Bronchoscopic ablative therapies for malignant central airway obstruction and peripheral lung tumors. Ann Am Thorac Soc 2019;16(10):1220–9.

53. Miller RJ, Murgu SD. Bronchoscopic resection of an exophytic endoluminal tracheal mass. Ann Am Thorac Soc 2013;10(6):697–700.

54. Cavaliere S, Foccoli P, Farina PL. Nd:YAG laser bronchoscopy. A five-year experience with 1,396 applications in 1,000 patients. Chest 1988;94(1):15–21.

55. Mahajan AK, Ibrahim O, Perez R, et al. Electrosurgical and laser therapy tools for the treatment of malignant central airway obstructions. Chest 2020;157(2):446–53.

56. Tremblay A, Marquette CH. Endobronchial electrocautery and argon plasma coagulation: a practical approach. Can Respir J 2004;11(4):305–10.

57. Folch EE, Oberg CL, Mehta AC, et al. Argon plasma coagulation: elucidation of the mechanism of gas embolism. Respiration 2021;100:1–5.

58. Mazur P. The role of intracellular freezing in the death of cells cooled at supraoptimal rates. Cryobiology 1977;14(3):251–72.

59. DiBardino DM, Lanfranco AR, Haas AR. Bronchoscopic cryotherapy. Clinical applications of the cryoprobe, cryospray, and cryoadhesion. Ann Am Thorac Soc 2016;13(8):1405–15.

60. Browning R, Turner JF Jr, Parrish S. Spray cryotherapy (SCT): institutional evolution of techniques and clinical practice from early experience in the treatment of malignant airway disease. J Thorac Dis 2015;7(Suppl 4):S405–14.

61. O'Connor JP, Hanley BM, Mulcahey TI, et al. N(2) gas egress from patients' airways during LN(2) spray cryotherapy. Med Eng Phys 2017;44:63–72.

62. Administration USFD. ERBECRYO 2 cryosurgical unit and accessories: ERBECRYO 2 cryosurgical unit; erbe flexible cryoprobe. Silver Spring, Maryland: U.S. Food & Drug Administration; 2020. Available at: https://www.accessdata.fda.gov/cdrh_docs/pdf19/K190651.pdf. Accessed 05/26/2020.

63. Mahmood K, Wahidi MM. Ablative therapies for central airway obstruction. Semin Respir Crit Care Med 2014;35(6):681–92.

64. Schumann C, Hetzel M, Babiak AJ, et al. Endobronchial tumor debulking with a flexible cryoprobe for immediate treatment of malignant stenosis. J Thorac Cardiovasc Surg 2010;139(4):997–1000.

65. Stewart A, Parashar B, Patel M, et al. American brachytherapy society consensus guidelines for thoracic brachytherapy for lung cancer. Brachytherapy 2016;15(1):1–11.

66. Qiu B, Jiang P, Ji Z, et al. Brachytherapy for lung cancer. Brachytherapy 2021;20(2):454–66.

67. Aumont-le Guilcher M, Prevost B, Sunyach MP, et al. High-dose-rate brachyther-apy for non-small-cell lung carcinoma: a retrospective study of 226 patients. Int J Radiat Oncol Biol Phys 2011;79(4):1112–6.

68. Soror T, Kovács G, Fürschke V, et al. Salvage treatment with sole high-dose-rate endobronchial interventional radiotherapy (brachytherapy) for isolated endobron-chial tumor recurrence in non-small-cell lung cancer patients: a 20-year experi-ence. Brachytherapy 2019;18(5):727–32.

69. Reveiz L, Rueda JR, Cardona AF. Palliative endobronchial brachytherapy for non-small cell lung cancer. Cochrane Database Syst Rev 2012;12:Cd004284.

70. Ernst A, Herth FJF. *Principles and Practice of interventional pulmonology.* Text. 1st edition. New York : Imprint: Springer; 2013. p. 732.

71. Nag S, Kelly JF, Horton JL, et al. Brachytherapy for carcinoma of the lung. Oncology (Williston Park) 2001;15(3):371–81.

72. Vergnon JM, Huber RM, Moghissi K. Place of cryotherapy, brachytherapy and photodynamic therapy in therapeutic bronchoscopy of lung cancers. Eur Respir J 2006;28(1):200–18.

73. Allison RR, Downie GH, Cuenca R, et al. Photosensitizers in clinical PDT. Photo-diagnosis Photodynamic Ther 2004;1(1):27–42. https://doi.org/10.1016/S1572-1000(04)00007-9.

74. Kidane B, Hirpara D, Yasufuku K. Photodynamic therapy in non-gastrointestinal thoracic malignancies. Int J Mol Sci 2016;17(1):135.

75. Mang TS. Lasers and light sources for PDT: past, present and future. Photodiag-nosis Photodynamic Ther 2004;1(1):43–8.

76. Pereira SP, Ayaru L, Ackroyd R, et al. The pharmacokinetics and safety of por-fimer after repeated administration 30-45 days apart to patients undergoing photodynamic therapy. Aliment Pharmacol Ther 2010;32(6):821–7.

77. Porfimer sodium. Drug Bank Online 2021. Available at: https://go.drugbank.com/drugs/DB00707. Accessed 09/08/2021.

78. Avasarala SK, Freitag L, Mehta AC. Metallic endobronchial stents: a contempo-rary resurrection. Chest 2019;155(6):1246–59.

79. Harms W, Krempien R, Grehn C, et al. Electromagnetically navigated brachyther-apy as a new treatment option for peripheral pulmonary tumors. Strahlenther On-kol 2006;182(2):108–11.

80. Olive G, Yung R, Marshall H, et al. Alternative methods for local ablation-interventional pulmonology: a narrative review. Transl Lung Cancer Res 2021; 10(7):3432–45.

81. Yuan HB, Wang XY, Sun JY, et al. Flexible bronchoscopy-guided microwave abla-tion in peripheral porcine lung: a new minimally-invasive ablation. Transl Lung Cancer Res 2019;8(6):787–96.

82. Sebek J, Kramer S, Rocha R, et al. Bronchoscopically delivered microwave abla-tion in an in vivo porcine lung model. ERJ Open Res 2020;6(4). https://doi.org/10.1183/23120541.00146-2020.

83. Maxwell AWP, Park WKC, Baird GL, et al. Effects of a thermal accelerant gel on microwave ablation zone volumes in lung: a porcine study. Radiology 2019; 291(2):504–10.

84. Chan JWY, Lau RWH, Ngai JCL, et al. Transbronchial microwave ablation of lung nodules with electromagnetic navigation bronchoscopy guidance-a novel tech-nique and initial experience with 30 cases. Transl Lung Cancer Res 2021;10(4): 1608–22.

85. Bi N, Shedden K, Zheng X, et al. Comparison of the effectiveness of radiofre-quency ablation with stereotactic body radiation therapy in inoperable stage i

non-small cell lung cancer: a systemic review and pooled analysis. Int J Radiat Oncol Biol Phys 2016;95(5):1378–90.

86. Musani AI, Veir JK, Huang Z, et al. Photodynamic therapy via navigational bronchoscopy for peripheral lung cancer in dogs. Lasers Surg Med 2018;50(5): 483–90.

87. Chen KC, Lee JM. Photodynamic therapeutic ablation for peripheral pulmonary malignancy via electromagnetic navigation bronchoscopy localization in a hybrid operating room (OR): a pioneering study. J Thorac Dis 2018;10(Suppl 6): S725–30.

88. Usuda J. Photodynamic therapy for peripheral lung cancers using composite-type optical fiberscope of 1.0 mm in diameter. B80-J interventional pulmonology in thoracic oncology. Am Thorac Soc 2017;195:A7637.

89. Ferguson JS, Henne E. Bronchoscopically Delivered thermal vapor ablation of human lung lesions. J Bronchology Interv Pulmonol 2019;26(2):108–13.

Surgical Management of Pneumothorax and Pleural Space Disease

Andrew P. Dhanasopon, MD, Justin D. Blasberg, MD, MPH,
Vincent J. Mase Jr, MD*

KEYWORDS

- Pneumothorax • Spontaneous pneumothorax • Empyema • Pleurodesis
- Pleural effusion

KEY POINTS

- Some patients with primary spontaneous pneumothorax may be safely managed nonoperatively in an ambulatory setting, whereas nearly all patients with secondary spontaneous pneumothoraces require an intervention.
- As an empyema progresses through its stages from exudative, to fibropurulent, to organizational, successful treatment strategies also require escalation from tube thoracostomy plus or minus intrapleural fibrinolytics to operative decortication.
- In the coronavirus disease 2019 (COVID-19) era, proper personal protective equipment and modification of technique is warranted for interventions on patients with COVID-19 with pleural space diseases.

SPONTANEOUS PNEUMOTHORAX

Introduction

Spontaneous pneumothoraces occur without trauma, injury, or precipitating event and are classified as either primary or secondary. Distinguishing between these 2 processes is important because of differences in management and outcomes. Primary spontaneous pneumothorax (PSP) is caused by no apparent lung disease, whereas secondary spontaneous pneumothorax (SSP) is the result of a known underlying process, such as emphysema, cystic fibrosis, lung cancer, interstitial pneumonitis, and other infectious processes of the lung.[1] Regardless of cause, if left undiagnosed and untreated, the accumulation of air in the pleural space potentially leads to tension pneumothorax, leading to a decrease in venous return, low preload, and cessation of cardiac output, resulting in hemodynamic catastrophe.[2]

Division of Thoracic Surgery, Yale School of Medicine, Yale University School of Medicine, PO Box 208062, New Haven, CT 06520-8062, USA
* Corresponding author.
E-mail address: vincent.mase@yale.edu

Surg Clin N Am 102 (2022) 413–427
https://doi.org/10.1016/j.suc.2022.03.001
surgical.theclinics.com

The prevalence and incidence of all types of spontaneous pneumothorax is higher in men than in women by approximately 6-fold. Within the PSP group, which constitutes ~85% of all cases, average patient age is 35 ± 18 years, and most do not have a documented history of underlying or concurrent lung disease.[2,3] In 1 international review of studies including men and women, average patient characteristics included height of 73 cm (5 feet 8 inches), an average body mass index (BMI0 of 20.3, and a history of smoking, confirming the general observation that patients tend to be taller, leaner men.[4] In contrast, patients with SSP constitute ~15% of cases, and the incidence in men is approximately 3-fold higher than in women, where the average patient age is 53 ± 20 years.[2,3] Cigarette smoking seems to significantly increase the risk of pneumothorax in men by 22-fold and women by 9-fold.[1,5] In 1 study of pneumothorax recurrences after nonoperative management, patients who quit smoking after their first episode of pneumothorax have a 40% risk of recurrence, whereas those who continued to actively smoke had a 70% risk of recurrence.[6]

Clinical Presentation

Although patients present with a variety of complaints, there is a constellation of symptoms that should raise a clinician's suspicion for pneumothorax. In a review by Mendogni and colleagues,[7] 69% of patients with PSP present with pleuritic chest pain as their main complaint and 55% dyspnea. A presentation of tension pneumothorax, which represents the most dangerous and potentially fatal consequence of air under pressure in the pleural space, constituted 16% of cases.[8] Aside from clinical assessment, the first and most sensitive diagnostic imaging modality is chest radiograph (CXR). Computed tomography (CT) scans can be performed for clinically stable patients with uncertain CXR findings or known/anticipated complex lung parenchyma architecture, more commonly identified in patients with SSP. Depending on the guideline as detailed later, the size of a pneumothorax can be measured from the apex of the chest to the cupola of the lung (American College of Chest Physicians [ACCP]), or from the lateral chest wall to the edge of the lung as measured at the hilum (British Thoracic Society [BTS]).

Although parenchymal lung diseases underlie the cause of pneumothorax in patients with SSP, an understanding of the pathophysiology causing PSP has continued to evolve. PSP has traditionally been ascribed to an increased basilar relative to apical pressure gradient in the lung, especially in tall patients, favoring the development and rupture of subpleural blebs. However, pathologic review has identified widespread inflammatory, elastofibrosing processes leading to an increase in porosity of the visceral pleural in a significant number of patients (10–20 mm in diameter).[5] This phenomenon helps explain the high success rate of talc poudrage even without bleb resection.[5]

Clinical Management Guidelines for primary spontaneous pneumothorax and secondary spontaneous pneumothorax

The primary goals when managing both PSP and SSP are (1) to remove air from the pleural space when necessary, and (2) to prevent the recurrence of pneumothorax. Two major consensus guidelines from the ACCP (2001)[9] and the BTS (2011)[10] are appropriate evidence-based guidelines to guide clinical decision making in both PSP and SSP, with varying degrees of escalating interventions, including observation for small pneumothoraces, image-guided drain placement in a semielective setting, bedside procedures without image guidance, and definitive surgical treatments including both minimally invasive and open options (**Fig. 1; Tables 1** and **2**). Excluded

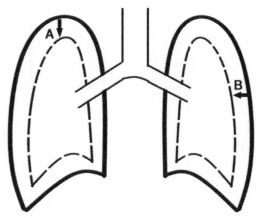

Fig. 1. Pneumothorax size measured according to (A) ACCP guidelines, apex-to-cupola distance (small, <3 cm; large, ≥3 cm), and (B) BTS guidelines, at hilum (small, ≤2 cm; large, >2 cm).

from these recommendations are patients who present with tension pneumothorax and/or bilateral pneumothorax that require expeditious chest drain insertion before any other consideration, which is consistent with best practice.

Although ACCP and BTS guidelines are generally consistent, the major difference in management is large PSP (without tension physiology): BTS (2010) recommends ambulatory management using needle aspiration and consideration of discharge with appropriate follow-up, whereas ACCP recommends hospital admission with tube insertion (up to 22 Fr). The more modern pigtail catheter kits and Heimlich valves enabled a French group (Voisin and colleagues[11]) to study ambulatory management of large PSP in select patients. From 2007 to 2011, patients with large PSP (and SSP) were managed with pigtail catheters with a 1-way valve. Patients with stable imaging were discharged and followed in the office every 2 days. Of 132 patients (110 primary, 22 secondary), 103 were exclusively managed as outpatients, with full pneumothorax resolution by day 2 or 4, and a mean catheter duration of 3.4 days. In this study, the 1-year recurrence rate was 26%. With estimated mean cost savings of $926 (up to 2 outpatient visits, 1 CXR) compared with $4276 for a chest tube and hospital admission over 4 days, this protocol was assessed to be both safe and effective in the management of uncomplicated PSP and SSP cases.

Over the years, debate over ambulatory management has continued. In a recent study from the United Kingdom (Hallifax and colleagues[12]), adult patients (16–55 years old) with symptomatic PSP were randomized to either an ambulatory device or standard guideline-based management (aspiration, standard chest tube insertion, or both). A total of 236 patients were randomized to ambulatory care (n = 117) versus standard care (n = 119). Of these patients, 110 (47%) had adverse events (pain, tube displacement, hematoma, and so forth), including 64 (55%) ambulatory care and 46 (39%) standard care patients. Of the 110 adverse events, 14 were considered serious and occurred only in the patients who received ambulatory care (8 were related to the intervention: enlarging pneumothorax; asymptomatic pulmonary edema; and device malfunctioning, leaking, or dislodging). Therefore, in the appropriate setting, ambulatory management of PSP may reduce the patient and health system burden of hospitalization, and this strategy may be used safely and effectively in select patient populations.

Table 1
Management guidelines for primary spontaneous pneumothorax

	Small and Clinically Stable	Large and Clinically Stable ± SX	Large and Unstable	Removal	Persistent AL	Recurrence Prevention
BTS 2010	• Observe and DC • If SX: NA (14–16 G)/chest drain (8–14 Fr), water seal	• NA (14–16 G) and DC • If not resolved, chest drain (8–14 Fr)	• Any chest drain	—	• >3-5 d: surgery vs medical pleurodesis (talc/doxycycline)	• Prior/bilateral pneumothorax • Persistent AL • At risk patients: pilots, divers • Resect blebs, mechanical pleurodesis/pleurectomy
ACCP 2001	• Observe (3–6 h) and DC (f/u 12 h–2 d)	• Small (≤14 Fr) or moderate (16–22 Fr) tube, water seal	• Moderate (16–22 Fr) or larger	• No AL >4 h ± clamp trial • CXR (5–12 h after no AL)	• >4 d: surgery vs medical pleurodesis (talc/doxycycline)	• As above

Abbreviations: DC, discharge; f/u, follow-up; SX, symptomatic; NA, needle aspiration; AL, air leak.

Table 2
Management guidelines for secondary spontaneous pneumothorax

	Small and Clinically Stable	Large and Clinically Stable ± SX	Large and Unstable	Removal	Persistent AL	Recurrence Prevention
BTS 2010	• NA (14–16 G)/chest drain (8–14 Fr) - water seal • If SX: chest drain (8–14 Fr)	• Chest drain (8–14 Fr)	• Any chest drain	—	• >2 d: surgery vs medical pleurodesis (talc/doxycycline)	• After first occurrence • Resect blebs, mechanical pleurodesis/ pleurectomy
ACCP 2001	• NA/small chest tube (≤14 Fr), water seal	• Moderate chest tube (16–22 Fr)	• Large chest tube (24–28 Fr)	• No AL >5–12 h ± clamp trial • CXR (13–23 h after no AL)	• >5 d: surgery vs medical pleurodesis (talc/doxycycline)	• As above

Management in the Coronavirus Disease 2019 Era

Special consideration is warranted for interventions on pneumothorax patients with coronavirus disease 2019 (COVID-19) given the mode of transmission of the severe acute respiratory syndrome coronavirus-2 (SARS-CoV-2) virus and the aerosolizing nature of the procedure. Proper preparation, personal protective equipment, and modified techniques are critical to minimizing exposure to health care personnel. For example, at our institution, we use an in-line viral particle filter between the patient's tube and the drainage system and strict suction instead of water seal to minimize the escape of SARS-CoV-2 from the chest tube system.[13]

In consideration of limiting exposure of otherwise healthy patients to COVID-19 and reducing the health system burden in order to flex resources for such patients, this is an important time to consider the use of safe, ambulatory strategies for the management of pneumothorax. At our institution, we have had success with ambulatory management in select patients. For patients who present with small pneumothoraces (<2-cm apex-to-cupola distance without lateral component) and clinical stability, observed in the emergency department with repeat CXR at 4 hours with outpatient follow-up has been a safe alternative to admission. For patients with large pneumothoraces (≥2-cm apex-to-cupola distance without lateral component), a chest tube is inserted (20–24 Fr in the event beside talc slurry is considered) and placed on suction. At 48 hours, if there has been no air leak, consideration is made for water seal and/or clamp trial for at least 4 hours before removing. At 48 hours, if there is a persistent air leak, surgery is recommended to facilitate cessation of the air leak and to expedite the patient's ultimate discharge from the hospital. Our institutional experience is that patients with an air leak greater than 48 hours are less likely to stop leaking within 4 to 5 days, favoring surgical escalation of care. The most common operative technique is video-assisted thoracoscopic surgery (VATS), bleb resection, and talc or mechanical pleurodesis.

EMPYEMA
Introduction

Empyema has been documented for centuries but the mainstay of treatment objectives has remained unchanged: to stop ongoing infection and facilitate reexpansion of the lung. However, the treatments to achieve these objectives have evolved over time. In the preantibiotic era, the tools were limited to drainage either with or without a tube; much of management was driven by the Empyema Commission of 1918.[14] The treatments options have now evolved to include antibiotics; a spectrum of drainage options that are surgical, nonsurgical, image guided, and non–image guided; as well as the use of fibrinolytics.

The well-documented phenomenon of a parapneumonic effusion associated with pneumonia progressing to empyema is the most common mechanism. There are other causes of empyema, including lung cancer, postsurgical, esophageal disease related, and extension from sources outside the chest (eg, Ludwig angina). The focus of this review is on the more common scenario because it is the one most often encountered. The tenets of treatment remain the same for any of the causes of empyema but, just like in a parapneumonic effusion, managing the underlying cause needs to be addressed to ensure resolution.

The 3 phases of empyema were first described in 1962.[15] In 1968, there was a better understanding of pleural fluid analysis.[16] Dr Light[17] published his observations in 1972 and the first reference to Light's criteria can be identified in 1989.[18] Now our understanding of the pathophysiologic process is better understood because of an appreciation of the biochemical cascade of events (**Fig. 2**; Villena Garrido and colleagues[19]).

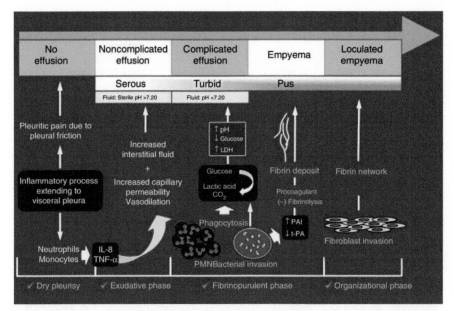

Fig. 2. Empyema biochemical cascade of events. IL, interleukin; t-PA, tissue plasminogen activator; PMN, polymorphonuclear leukocytes; PAI, plasminogen activator inhibitor;TNF, tumor necrosis factor. (*From* Villena Garrido V, Cases Viedma E, Fernández Villar A, et al. Recommendations of diagnosis and treatment of pleural effusion. Update. Arch Bronconeumol 2014; 50(6):235-49. English, Spanish; with permission.)

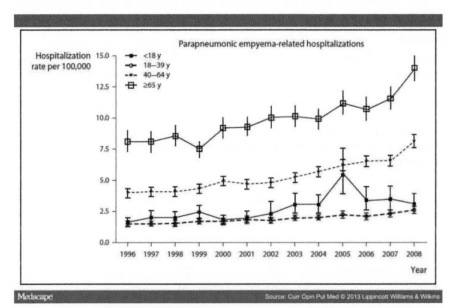

Fig. 3. Trends in parapneumonic empyema-related hospitalization in the United States 1996 to 2008. (*From* Grijalva CG, Zhu Y, Nuorti JP, Griffin MR. Emergence of parapneumonic empyema in the USA. Thorax 2011; 66(8):663-8; with permission.)

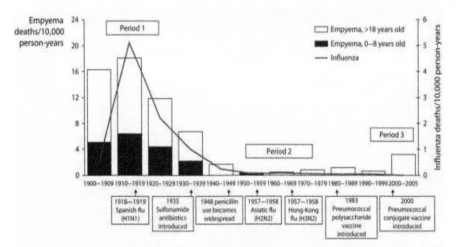

Fig. 4. History of empyema over the last century. (*From* Burgos J, Falcó V, Pahissa A. The increasing incidence of empyema. Curr Opin Pulm Med 2013;19(4):350-6; with permission.)

However, despite our better understanding and description of the sequence of events, the risk of mortality for empyema has been unchanged and, in certain patient[21] demographics, trending up (**Figs. 3** and **4**).

Diagnostic modalities are helpful in determining whether pleural fluid is a transudate or exudate. However, clinically, there is not a reliable test or fluid analysis to confidently determine empyema stage or the best treatment option. The paradox of which treatment option for empyema is ideal is now more confusing given there are more choices. Therefore, this article outlines our understanding of the different stages and the varied treatment options that can be used.

Diagnosis

We have found the triphasic nature of progression to be helpful but the time course or sequence of progression to not be consistent from patient to patient. There is a triad of factors that seems to affect the time course: patient innate immune capabilities, bacterial virulence, and rapidity and appropriateness of treatment (**Fig. 5**). As a general principle, when an empyema progresses and becomes more organized, the nonoperative management success rates are lower and operative complications are higher. The implication here is that timeliness of treatment and rapidity of responding to a clinical change are critical.

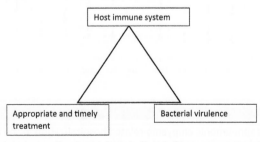

Fig. 5. Empyema triangle; predominant factors that influence severity of disease in patients with empyema.

The American Association for Thoracic Surgery (AATS) Expert Consensus Guidelines on Empyema (Shen and colleagues[20]) recommend to "Obtain pleural fluid culture specimens during aspiration or drainage procedures." Imaging studies include CXR, pleural ultrasonography (US), and chest CT. Chest CT with intravenous contrast helps to distinguish an intraparenchymal versus extraparenchymal fluid collection. PET CT has limited utility in pleural space infections.

Pleural fluid analysis remains an important determinant of the ongoing physiologic process. Sampling can be done via thoracentesis or at the time of placement of a tube thoracostomy. Frank pus does not require additional analysis other than cultures to speciate the organism and to help with antibiotic management.

Numbers that Matter

Roughly 175 mL of fluid is needed to cause blunting of the costophrenic sulcus on a CXR.[22] Of the 1 million patients hospitalized with pneumonia each year, up to 40% have an associated effusion. From 5% to 10%, or roughly 32,000, of these progress to empyema annually in the United States.[23] Timely and appropriate management of this patient population is paramount for reduced length of stay, improved outcomes, and reduced morbidity.

Identifying the bacterial pathogen based solely on pleural fluid is only possible in about 50% of cases.[24] Waiting for speciation or identification to proceed to the next step in management tends to delay necessary treatment. Empiric antibiotics should be adjusted based on historical prevalence of known organisms specific to the relevant institution.

There is a late mortality associated with pleural infection; the 1-year, 3-year, and 5-year mortality is 15%, 24%, and 30% respectively. A subgroup of patients have a history of chronic medical illness and therefore the management of the acute empyema should strongly consider the overall frailty of the patient and tolerance of surgical procedures to avoid pitfalls associated with this disease entity.

Tube Thoracostomy

The AATS expert consensus guidelines on empyema[20] recommend that, if infection is proved at a prior thoracentesis, tube thoracostomy should be performed to drain the pleural space. Tube thoracostomy allows drainage and is effective for the treatment of empyema. For stage I disease, there is a likelihood that tube thoracostomy drainage is sufficient and definitive treatment. For stage II disease, if drainage of the fluid can be achieved before fibrinous septations and there can be some sort of lung apposition to the chest wall, and if other important conditions are favorable (ie, early stage of disease, low bacterial virulence, patient immunocompetent), drainage alone may be sufficient and no additional interventions are needed. In cases where this is not the case, a trial of fibrinolytics via the tube thoracotomy or surgical decortication may be indicated. For stage III disease, the risk of complication (ie, parenchymal damage) of a nonimaged or bedside chest tube placement increases because of the organized phase and because the lung can be fixed in place because of the inflammatory process. For later-stage disease, imaged-guided drainage is a better option.

The optimal chest tube size was evaluated in a prospective nonrandomized study of more than 400 patients, with primary end points being death or need for thoracic surgery.[25] Serious and adverse events were also evaluated. In a logistic regression analysis, there was no difference in progression to death or need for thoracic surgery based on chest tube size. Although there were some confounding issues, this study lends support to smaller tubes being noninferior to larger-bore chest tubes, the caveat being that, with smaller tubes, routine flushing is paramount to prevent clogging and allow continued drainage.[26]

The risk of bleeding or intraparenchymal injury with bedside chest tube placement is less than 2%. This risk is further reduced with imaging adjuncts such at US.

Fibrinolytics

Stage II (fibrinopurulent phase) empyema is associated with the deposition of fibrin, which is the predominant component of the underlying biochemical cascade of events. This deposition leads to septations and loculated fluid that go on to set the conditions for rind formation and lung entrapment in stage III. The instillation of fibrin degrading products for nonoperative management has been a strategy for many decades now. The use of fibrinolytics is a tradeoff: its use can avoid the need for surgery but, if unsuccessful, can delay definitive treatment.

There are 7 randomized controlled trials evaluating the use of fibrinolytics as an adjunct to the management of empyema (**Table 3**). The 2 larger trials that are often cited are the MIST1 and MIST2 trials.

The MIST1 trial evaluated the instillation of streptokinase compared with placebo in 430 patients. Although there was an increase in pleural drainage there was no impact on study end points such as avoidance of surgery, hospital stay, and mortality.[25]

The MIST 2 trial evaluated the instillation of intrapleural tissue plasminogen activase (tpa) (10 mg) with or without DNase (5 mg). The primary outcome was reduction of opacification on CXR. There were 4 treatment arms: tpa/DNase, tpa/placebo, DNase/placebo, placebo/placebo. The regimen consisted of sequential instillation of drug with a dwell time of 1 hour for each enzyme. There was an increase in pleural drainage as well as a statistical impact on need for surgery, hospital stay, and mortality for the tpa/DNase arm.[24] In this analysis, extending treatment beyond the 3 days was not shown to be beneficial.

The risk of bleeding with instillation of intrapleural enzymes ranges in the literature from 0% to 5%. Mitigating strategies such as using partial dose, single agent, or holding anticoagulation are reasonable but not founded specifically in available evidence.

The challenge with understanding the role of fibrinolytic therapy within these studies is the confounding variables that might affect the clinical end points, including the patient population, comorbid conditions, length of nonoperative management, and readmission for treatment failure. Furthermore, most fibrinolytic studies view failure as progression to surgery. There is clearly a subset of patients in whom fibrinolytic therapy is beneficial but there are no long-term studies that assess long-term outcomes such as trapped lung, PFTs, or functional status. These outcomes have yet to be defined.

Video-assisted Thoracoscopic Surgery Drainage and Decortication

Once a decision to operate is made, there are 4 key goals of the operation: (1) safe entry into the thoracic cavity; (2) establishing a thoracic domain or an operative space to have adequate visualization; (3) removal of infected tissue/fluid; (4) reexpansion of the lung. The ability to achieve these 4 goals is used as a guide to determine when there is a need to convert from a minimally invasive to an open approach.

Improved outcomes associated with minimally invasive decortication have lowered the threshold from which the authors consider operative intervention. Of the patients that are treated for empyema, roughly one-third require a surgical procedure. The mortality data for empyema are high at roughly 6% to 11%; however, nonoperatively managed empyema mortality has been reported as high as 15%.[27]

Table 3
Summary of randomized control trials for intrapleural fibrinolytics

Study	Sample Size	Enzyme	Mean Age (y)	Mean Drain Size	End Point	Duration of Treatment	Notes
Tuncozgur[28]	49	Streptokinase	33.0	30 Fr	Resolution of symptoms	5 d	—
Diacon[29]	53	Streptokinase	39.0	26 Fr	Clinical treatment success; need for referral to surgery	7 d	Frank pus aspirated in 81%; 2 patients died
Misthos[30]	127	Streptokinase (250,000 IU)	46.0	30 Fr	Successful drainage	3 d	—
Thommi[31]	108	Alteplase (25 mg)	64.0	28 Fr	40% reduction in surgery	3 d	—
MIST 1	454	Streptokinase (250,000 Units)	60.0	12 Fr	Death or need for surgical drainage at 3 mo	3 d	—
MIST 2	210	Tpa and DNase	60.0	15 Fr	Change in pleural opacity	3 d	—
Bedat[32]	93	Urokinase vs tpa/DNase	61.5	12 Fr	Need for second intervention	3 d	—

tpa, tissue plasminogen activase.

The decision to convert to an open approach is based on 3 factors: (1) if any of the 4 operative goals cannot be achieved minimally invasively; (2) unable to tolerate lung isolation or periods of apnea; and (3) intraoperative complication (ie, bleeding, diaphragm injury).

Our Institutional Algorithm

Our practice is to approach patients with empyema in a multidisciplinary fashion, including a thoracic surgeon, thoracic interventional pulmonary service, pulmonologist, and primary service. We have found upfront discussion before thoracentesis for diagnosis is helpful for purposes of determining whether placement of a thoracostomy tube in addition to fluid sampling will shorten the time to the definitive treatment and prevent multiple procedures.

There are some general concepts. Rather than thinking of what treatment option is best, the authors view the treatment options along a continuum (**Fig. 6**), and, if used appropriately, the goal is to identify the nonresponders such that we shift to VATS drainage and decortication in a timely fashion. The appropriate antibiotics are started as soon as possible. The patient's overall status is important to determine the success of any intervention, and the clinical indicators we find the most helpful are fever, white blood cell count, chest wall pain (not chest tube insertion pain), malaise, and procalcitonin. There are only a few patients who present either in extremis or shock (tachycardic, and so forth) where surgical exploration for source control is needed immediately. For these patients, we typically start thoracoscopically. A follow-up chest CT scan after treatment is not needed to document complete resolution; if the patient clinically is improving and there is a small rim of pleural fluid, pleural thickening, or focus of air, this generally resolves over time.

For the patients that are not in this category, we have found that a short period of nonoperative management with tube thoracostomy plus or minus intrapleural enzyme is a successful strategy to identify the nonresponders that will ultimately require surgical intervention.

For patients with a small, moderate, or large effusion with a high degree of clinical suspicion for empyema, a bedside chest tube is placed for drainage and the fluid is sent for analysis. For patients with complicated effusions with a high degree of clinical suspicion, an image-guided pigtail is placed.

If there is improvement in opacification with lung reexpansion after chest tube placement, we typically do not add intrapleural enzymes and follow the patient clinically with daily complete blood count and CXR. However, if there is inadequate drainage or restricted expansion, a 3-day trial of bedside intrapleural DNase/tpa is initiated. It has been our experience that, after the first 2 instillations of enzymes, the drainage amount and character is an indicator to the success of enzymatic

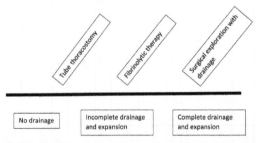

Fig. 6. Continuum of clinical response for varying treatments of empyema and a visual stepwise strategy for escalation of treatment options from minimally invasive to surgery.

therapy. For example, after intrapleural enzyme treatment, if 500 mL egresses from the tube, subsequent treatments will also be effective. Also, for example, after enzymatic treatment, if 20 mL egresses, additional treatment will likely not be effective.

For many patients, a tube thoracotomy is placed within 24 hours of consult. At the time of tube thoracostomy, we have a discussion with the patient regarding the potential need for surgery in 3 to 4 days. This accomplishes the following: (1) the patient has some time to process this information because this is usually a nonelective setting, and (2) a hard line is made about the timeline for nonoperative management. We have found the latter to be effective in reducing length of stay and appropriately identifying those patients who respond to nonoperative treatment and do not require surgery.

SUMMARY

Pneumothorax and pleural-based disease are ancient maladies with a rich history of management strategies, but the basic tenets of surgical goals and objectives have been consistent for centuries. Pneumothorax presents in both the outpatient and inpatient setting with escalating levels of intervention from simple observation to surgical exploration with 2 surgical goals: pleural symphysis and prevention of recurrence. Empyema, typically seen in the inpatient setting, requires an understanding of the patients' immune status, virulence of the organism, and timeliness of treatment to determine what management tools (tube thoracostomy, fibrinolytics, surgical exploration) are needed to achieve the surgical goals of removal of infected fluid/tissue and reexpansion of the lung.

CLINICS CARE POINTS

Pearls
- When evaluating a patient with a pneumothorax, it is important to accurately determine whether it is a primary versus secondary pneumothorax, because initial management differs.
- When performing either mechanical or chemical pleurodesis for recurrent spontaneous pneumothorax, it is imperative to work to obtain visceral and parietal pleural symphysis to prevent recurrence.
- When a thoracentesis rules in empyema in addition to appropriate antibiotics; a tube thoracostomy is usually required for drainage.
- When assessing a patient for surgical management of an empyema, look for malnutrition and any evidence of pulmonary hypertension.

Pitfalls
- Chest radiograph can often underrepresent the degree or size of the pneumothorax.
- Chest radiograph or any diagnostic imaging is not needed for treatment of a patient presenting with tension pneumothorax.
- Avoid prolonged nonoperative management of an empyema; 3 to 4 days of nonoperative management without success usually requires escalation of treatment.
- When using fibrinolytic therapy, look for generous chest tube drainage after the initial treatment and avoid continued instillation if drainage does not increase because additional treatments are a point of diminishing returns.

DISCLOSURE

The authors have nothing to disclose.

REFERENCES

1. Kucharczuk J. Ch. 46: "The role of VATS pleurodesis in the management of initial primary spontaneous pneumothorax". In: Ferguson MK, editor. Difficult decisions in thoracic surgery. 2nd edition. Springer; 2011. p. 401–7.
2. Cerfolio RJ. Ch.130:" Pneumothorax and Pneumomediastinum. In: Sugarbaker DJ, et al, editors. Sugarbaker's Adult Chest Surgery, 3e. McGraw Hill; 2020.
3. Aragaki-Nakahodo A. Management of pneumothorax: an update. Curr Opin Pulm Med 2022;28(1):62–7.
4. Ghisalberti M, et al. Age and Clinical Presentation for Primary Spontaneous Pneumothorax. Heart Lung Circ 2020;29(11):1648–55.
5. Plojoux J, et al. New insights and improved strategies for the management of primary spontaneous pneumothorax. Clin Respir J 2019;13(4):195–201.
6. Sadikot RT, et al. Recurrence of primary spontaneous pneumothorax. Thorax 1997;52(9):805–9.
7. Mendogni P, et al. Epidemiology and management of primary spontaneous pneumothorax: a systematic review. Interact Cardiovasc Thorac Surg 2020;30(3): 337–45.
8. Yoon JS, et al. Tension pneumothorax, is it a really life-threatening condition? J Cardiothorac Surg 2013;8:197.
9. Baumann MH, et al. AACP Pneumothorax Consensus Group. Management of spontaneous pneumothorax: an American College of Chest Physicians Delphi consensus statement. Chest 2001;119(2):590–602.
10. MacDuff A, et al. BTS Pleural Disease Guideline Group. Management of spontaneous pneumothorax: British Thoracic Society Pleural Disease Guideline 2010. Thorax 2010;65(Suppl 2): ii18–31.
11. Voisin F, et al. Ambulatory management of large spontaneous pneumothorax with pigtail catheters. Ann Emerg Med 2014;64(3):222–8.
12. Hallifax RJ, et al. Ambulatory management of primary spontaneous pneumothorax: an open-label, randomised controlled trial. Lancet 2020;396(10243): 39–49.
13. Dhanasopon, et al. Chest Tube Drainage in the Age of COVID-19. In Van Rhee JA, ed. Physician Assistant Clinical Surgery. Elsevier, 2021;6:2, 261-265.
14. Tung J, Carter D, Rappold J. Empyema commission of 1918-Impact on acute care surgery 100 years later. J Trauma Acute Care Surg 2019;86(2):321–5.
15. Statement of the Subcommittee on Surgery, "Management of Nontuberculous Empyema. Am Rev Resp Dis 1962;85:935.
16. Holten K. Diagnostic value of some biochemical pleural fluid examinations. Scand J Respir Dis Suppl 1968;63:121–6.
17. Light RW, Macgregor MI, Luchsinger PC, et al. Pleural effusions: the diagnostic separation of transudates and exudates. Ann Intern Med 1972;77(4):507–13.
18. Scheurich JW, Keuer SP, Graham DY. Pleural effusion: comparison of clinical judgment and Light's criteria in determining the cause. South Med J 1989; 82(12):1487–91.
19. Villena Garrido V, Cases Viedma E, Fernández Villar A, et al. Recommendations of diagnosis and treatment of pleural effusion. Update. Arch Bronconeumol 2014; 50(6):235–49. English, Spanish.
20. Shen KR, Bribriesco A, Crabtree T, et al. The American Association for Thoracic Surgery consensus guidelines for the management of empyema. J Thorac Cardiovasc Surg 2017;153(6):e129–46.

21. Burgos J, Falcó V, Pahissa A. The increasing incidence of empyema. Curr Opin Pulm Med 2013;19(4):350–6.
22. Colins JD, Burwell D, Furmanski S, et al. Minimal detectable pleural effusions. A roentgen pathology model. Radiology 1972;105(1):51–3.
23. Ahmed RA, Marrie TJ, Huang JQ. Thoracic empyema in patients with community-acquired pneumonia. Am J Med 2006;119(10):877–83.
24. Rahman NM, Maskell NA, West A, et al. Intrapleural use of tissue plasminogen activator and DNase in pleural infection. N Engl J Med 2011;365(6): 518–26.
25. Rahman NM, Maskell NA, Davies CW, et al. The relationship between chest tube size and clinical outcome in pleural infection. Chest 2010;137(3):536–43.
26. Maskell NA, Davies CW, Nunn AJ, et al. First Multicenter Intrapleural Sepsis Trial (MIST1) Group. U.K. Controlled trial of intrapleural streptokinase for pleural infection. N Engl J Med 2005;352(9):865–74. Erratum in: N Engl J Med. 2005;352(20): 2146.
27. Farjah F, Symons RG, Krishnadasan B, et al. Management of pleural space infections: a population-based analysis. J Thorac Cardiovasc Surg 2007;133(2): 346–51.
28. Tuncozgur B, Ustunsoy H, Sivrikoz MC, et al. Intrapleural urokinase in the management of parapneumonic empyema: a randomised controlled trial. Int J Clin Pract 2001;55(10):658–60.
29. Diacon AH, Theron J, Schuurmans MM, et al. Intrapleural streptokinase for empyema and complicated parapneumonic effusions. Am J Respir Crit Care Med 2004;170(1):49–53.
30. Misthos P, Sepsas E, Konstantinou M, et al. Early use of intrapleural fibrinolytics in the management of postpneumonic empyema. A prospective study. Eur J Cardiothorac Surg 2005;28(4):599–603.
31. Thommi G, Shehan JC, Robison KL, et al. A double blind randomized cross over trial comparing rate of decortication and efficacy of intrapleural instillation of alteplase vs placebo in patients with empyemas and complicated parapneumonic effusions. Respir Med 2012;106(5):716–23.
32. Bédat B, Plojoux J, Noel J, et al. Comparison of intrapleural use of urokinase and tissue plasminogen activator/DNAse in pleural infection. ERJ Open Res 2019; 5(3):00084–2019.

Interventional Therapies for Acute Pulmonary Embolism

Asishana A. Osho, MD, MPH[a], David M. Dudzinski, MD[b],*

KEYWORDS

- Pulmonary embolism • Catheter intervention • Thrombolysis
- Catheter-directed thrombolysis • Catheter-directed embolectomy
- Surgical pulmonary embolectomy • Interventional therapy
- Pulmonary embolism response team (PERT)

KEY POINTS

- Risk stratification based on society guidelines is a critical step in tailoring management regimens for patients presenting with acute pulmonary embolism (PE); however, as not all scenarios are covered it is incumbent on the clinician to individualize the approach to the patient.
- There is a paucity of comparative outcomes data to guide the selection of interventional therapies in patients with intermediate and high-risk acute PE.
- Pulmonary embolism response teams (PERT), which include the combined expertise of cardiac surgeons, interventional cardiologists, and interventional radiologists, should be considered for multi-disciplinary decision making for patients with intermediate and high-risk acute PE.

INTRODUCTION

Acute pulmonary embolism (PE) is a leading cause of modern cardiovascular morbidity and mortality. While both acute PE and acute coronary syndrome (ACS) both reflect arterial occlusion syndromes, PE usually represents a thromboembolic phenomenon while ACS represents thrombosis *in situ* due to atherosclerotic plaque rupture. ACS treatment has progressed over recent decades from thrombolytic-based to targeted endovascular intervention, relying on millions of patient-years of randomized data. The endovascular "open-artery" approach is being actively applied to PE in contemporary practice, but there is a paucity of rigorous data. This article reviews the multiple contemporary interventional modalities for acute PE available to clinicians.

[a] Division of Cardiac Surgery, Massachusetts General Hospital, Cox 6, 55 Fruit Street, Boston, MA 02114, USA; [b] Cardiac Intensive Care Unit, Department of Cardiology, Heart Center Intensive Care Unit, Massachusetts General Hospital, Blake 254, 55 Fruit Street, Boston, MA 02114, USA
* Corresponding author.
E-mail address: ddudzinski@partners.org
Twitter: @criticalecho (A.A.O.); @mghhearthealth; @mghhcicu (D.M.D.)

Surg Clin N Am 102 (2022) 429–447
https://doi.org/10.1016/j.suc.2022.02.004
0039-6109/22/© 2022 Elsevier Inc. All rights reserved.

surgical.theclinics.com

NATURE OF THE PROBLEM

Fundamentally, PE is an intraluminal obstruction in the pulmonary arterial (PA) tree, most commonly due to the translocation of a dislodged deep venous thrombus (DVT) from elsewhere in the systemic venous circulation. Annually there are approximately 900,000 new diagnoses of venous thromboembolism (VTE) in the United States, and more than 200,000 PE-related admissions.[1] The significant public health burden is underscored by the fact that PE is the third most common cause of cardiovascular mortality behind myocardial infarction and stroke.[2,3] These statistics are driven by 15% to 20% rates of in-hospital mortality for patients admitted with acute PE,[4,5] with short-term mortality in high-risk PE greater than 50%.[6–8]

PRESENTATION AND NATURAL HISTORY OF PULMONARY EMBOLISM

Acute PE may manifest with a wide range of symptoms including dyspnea, tachypnea, hemoptysis, or pleuritic pain. Symptoms of PE may be protean, including anxiety or syncope,[9] requiring clinicians to consider PE in diverse presentations and to maintain an appropriate index of suspicion for the diagnosis. In more severe cases of acute PE, patients present with right ventricular strain, hemodynamic compromise, or hypoxia. Although most patients with PE also have concomitant DVTs, not all have symptoms attributable to extremity venous thrombosis.[10] Severity of PE somewhat correlates with the extent of clots and obstruction of the PA, but mechanical obstruction is merely one facet of the physiology of PE.[11] Humoral factors generated due to downstream ischemia and inflammatory messengers produced by neutrophils and platelets, exacerbate pulmonary vasoconstriction and thus contribute to progressive hemodynamic instability.[12]

The natural history of PE varies by the severity of disease, with the degree of right ventricular overload and hypoxemia correlating with prognosis. In general, mortality associated with untreated PE is estimated to range between 20% and 30%,[5] but this statistical decreases when the diagnosis is made early with timely initiation of interventions. One in 5 patients with VTE will have recurrent disease within 5 years, with slightly higher rates in patients with unidentified or uncorrectable provoking factors.[13]

A major contemporary challenge of acute PE is to identify patients who will experience short-term cardiopulmonary deterioration, so that PE-debulking interventions can be used specifically for this subgroup.[14] Identifying this subgroup has been challenging because most of the patients who have a cardiopulmonary reserve to withstand the insult of the initial acute PE, autolysis of clots begins within days, once the natural fibrinolytic system is mobilized.[15] Full resolution of clots can be observed as early as 2 weeks after diagnosis, with most requiring between 30 and 60 days depending on the extent of disease.[5] A notable percentage of patients (15%–30%) have persistent thrombus a year after initial diagnosis. In approximately 3% of PE survivors, clot within the PA results in the development of chronic thromboembolic pulmonary hypertension (CTEPH), though this rate may be underestimated.[13] CTEPH diagnosis and management, including interventions such as balloon pulmonary angioplasty and pulmonary thromboembolectomy, exceeds the scope of this review of acute PE.

DIAGNOSIS OF ACUTE PULMONARY EMBOLISM

Given the somewhat nonspecific constellation of signs and symptoms associated with VTE, maintaining a high index of suspicion is critical to early diagnosis and treatment.[1] Increased risks for developing VTE include immobilized patients (ie surgery or trauma), malignancy, cigarette use, women in the early postpartum period, and inherited clotting disorders or thrombophilia.

Whether the clinical presentation is suspicious for PE or undertaken for protean chest symptoms, the diagnostic evaluation will already typically have included chest radiography (may show peripheral oligemia or infarction), electrocardiogram (may show right heart strain), and echocardiography (may demonstrate right heart dilation and strain, abnormal interventricular septal geometry, and elevated right heart pressures).[1,16] Contemporary definitive diagnosis is by computed tomography angiography (CTA). Less commonly magnetic resonance angiography (MRA) or pulmonary angiography is used, though all provide detailed information about the PA. CTA is generally ubiquitous in hospitals and available at any hour of the day. However, in hemodynamically unstable patients, CTA may not be feasible. Instead, one must rely on clinical gestalt, biomarkers, or echocardiography to render inferences about underlying pathology.[16] In general, echocardiography will demonstrate right heart abnormalities with a sensitivity of 50% to 80% in significant PE.

RISK CLASSIFICATION OF PULMONARY EMBOLISM AND GENERAL TREATMENT PRINCIPLES

Most clinical classifications of acute PE stratify patients based on the severity of the consequences of the PE, integrating imaging findings and associated hemodynamic impacts.[1,14,16–18] Terminology varies somewhat among major society guidelines, but generally, patients are divided into 3 major groups based on the risk of short-term PE-related mortality. The American Heart Association (AHA) stratifies PE into massive, submassive, and low-risk[19,20] while the European Society of Cardiology (ESC) endorses high-risk, intermediate-risk, and low-risk categories[21]; the latter categorization seems more commonly used in contemporary practice. Clinicians should be aware of the lack of standardization and variable terminology in the PE field which limits the generalizability of any particular investigation result, as various trials have used diverse definitions and characterizations. Another classification scheme is the Pulmonary Embolism Severity Index (PESI) score–including the "simplified" version sPESI. PESI estimates risk based on age, comorbidities, vital signs, and RV function, and can discriminate which acute PE patients can be treated without admission to the hospital[20] (**Fig. 1**).

Some patients with acute PE may initially present with cardiac arrest or cardiogenic shock, and represent the highest risk strata ("catastrophic PE"), and merit immediate interventional therapies and hemodynamic support.[14,22] Other patients with high-risk acute PE are at significant risk for cardiac arrest and mortality due to hemodynamic compromise. Significant hypotension (systolic blood pressure < 90 mm Hg, or decline $\geq$ 40 mm Hg), tachycardia, and elevation in central venous pressures are hallmarks of acute high-risk PE with associated severe hypoxemia (Pao_2 < 50 mm Hg) and indicia of systemic malperfusion; malignant ventricular rhythms and paradoxic bradycardia also evince high-risk PE.[19,21] Patients will generally demonstrate greater than 50% PA occlusion and significant right ventricular strain. Importantly acute high-risk PE remains a clinical diagnosis, even if findings on cardiovascular imaging seem discordant. Early circulatory and ventilatory support is critical in acute high-risk PE. Where cardiogenic shock persists or progresses despite optimal critical care support and early initiation of therapeutic anticoagulation, consideration must be given to advanced reperfusion and debulking therapies, as described subsequently. Extracorporeal membrane oxygenation (ECMO) and other mechanical circulatory support (MCS) modalities may support perfusion while clot is lysed, and pulmonary blood flow improved. The urgency of early recognition and management of patients who present with acute

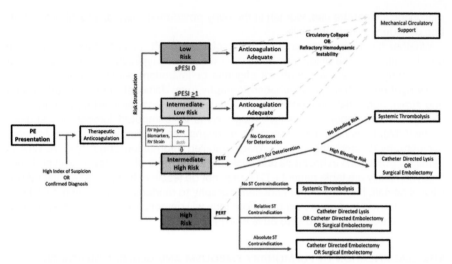

Fig. 1. Treatment algorithm for acute pulmonary embolism stratified by patient risk at presentation. Caption: PE, pulmonary embolism; PERT, pulmonary embolism response team; RV, right ventricular; sPESI, simplified Pulmonary Embolism Severity Index; ST, systemic thrombolysis.

high-risk PE is underscored in the associated mortality statistics – 10% of fatalities for acute high-risk PE occur within the first hour after the presentation, and up to 80% occur within the first 2 hours.[6–8,23] Early critical care to prevent circulatory arrest is paramount as survival is invariably worse if cardiopulmonary resuscitation (CPR) was required at any point in the clinical trajectory.

Patients with intermediate-risk PE are initially normotensive but characterized by clinical indicia of severity (eg, sPESI score ≥1) including imaging and biomarker evidence of right ventricular dysfunction.[21] Patients may also exhibit moderate hypoxemia (Pao$_2$ 50mm Hg-65 mm Hg on ambient air), though not definitionally required. Imaging evaluation may show occlusion of 30% to 50% of the PA, and right ventricular strain. ESC guidelines further stratify intermediate-risk patients into intermediate-high and intermediate-low, based on the presence of both or one of the RV dysfunctions (echocardiogram) and RV injuries (serum markers including natriuretic peptide, indicating ventricular dilatation, and troponin, indicating myocardial ischemia) (see **Fig. 1**).[1,16,19,21]

Minor or low-risk phenotypes constitute most PE presentations. Patients may be asymptomatic and incidentally identified on imaging but may present with typical PE symptoms. These patients have typically exhibited normotension and normal heart rates and would be expected to have no evidence of RV strain on imaging or biomarkers. Imaging evaluation would generally demonstrate less than 30% occlusion of the PA (ie distal rather than central emboli).[21]

MEDICATIONS FOR THE TREATMENT OF ACUTE PULMONARY EMBOLISM

Specific strategies for hemodynamic and respiratory support for patients with acute PE are beyond the scope of this review. Intravenous fluid management, inotropes, and vasopressors, and possibly pulmonary vasodilators, all play roles in the initial stabilization of PE, though the evidence base for these interventions is limited and often depends on local practice individualized to the patient's hemodynamic status.[1,21,24,25]

Therapeutic Anticoagulation

Rapid initiation and achievement of therapeutic anticoagulation is the most essential part of medical management for patients with PE. Indeed, parenteral anticoagulation should be started before confirming the diagnosis, if clinical suspicion is high and bleeding risk is low.[1] Intravenous unfractionated heparin is the initial agent in many cases of intermediate or high-risk PE, and it provides some flexibility in patients who may need downstream interventional or surgical therapy. Patients are transitioned to enteral or subcutaneous anticoagulants as they stabilize and progress in their recovery. Consideration of the specific agents used for initial anticoagulation in hemodynamically stable patients and for long term anticoagulation in patients with PE is beyond the scope of this interventional review.[1,18,26] Most guidelines recommend at least 3 months of therapeutic anticoagulation with consideration for extended (6–12 months) or indefinite therapy in patients who have medical predispositions to recurrent PEs, increased burden of embolic disease, or unclear etiology of PE; there is a growing trend toward indefinite anticoagulation for first PE without clear etiologic risk factor, given high rates of recurrence.[26,27]

Systemic Thrombolysis

In patients with PE with hemodynamic instability (high risk), systemic thrombolysis (ST) is often used in the absence of contraindications.[1] Where indicated, ST could be initiated even in the setting of ongoing evaluation for procedural therapies, noting, however, that ST may be considered a relative contraindication to subsequent surgical embolectomy, at least in the short term. Other relative indications for ST include right heart thrombi (thrombus-in-transit), and intermediate-risk PE with features portending higher risk of cardiopulmonary decompensation, including vital sign trend, severity of RV strain, and impaired gas exchange.[1] Compared with therapeutic anticoagulation alone, ST is associated with increased bleeding complications, notably intracranial hemorrhage (ICH).[20,21,26] Contraindications to ST include[1]:

- Absolute
  - Active bleeding,
  - History of ICH,
  - Recent ischemic stroke,
  - Recent head trauma,
  - Central nervous system surgery,
  - Known structural brain disease such as arteriovenous malformation, neoplasms, or aneurysms.
- Relative
  - Existing coagulopathy or platelet dysfunction,
  - Pregnancy,
  - Recent internal bleeding (ie gastrointestinal),
  - Recent major surgery,
  - History of uncontrolled systemic hypertension,
  - Advanced age.

In patients with acute, high-risk PE, ST has been shown to reduce PE-related mortality and PE recurrence compared with therapeutic anticoagulation alone.[28] In patients with relative contraindications, reduced dose regimens of ST may be used, although the evidence base is less robust.[29] Use of ST in intermediate-high-risk PE is somewhat less straightforward as data from PEITHO suggest a decrease in short-term hemodynamic deterioration (1.6% vs 5.0%, odds ratio 0.30, $P = .002$), but not all-cause mortality (1.2% vs 1.8%, odds ratio 0.65, $P = .42$), at the cost of higher risks of major extracranial bleeding (odds ratio 5.55, $P < .001$) and (primarily hemorrhagic) stroke (odds ratio 12.1, $P = .003$).[30,31] This increased risk of ICH has been corroborated in meta-analysis[32] and is a reason that catheter-based therapeutics have been considered as a means to directly target PE and thereby reduce total exposure of thrombolytics in the body. Ultimately, identifying patients with intermediate PE who may deteriorate is essential to optimally decide which patients require ST or other advanced intervention, and represents a fundamental ambition in the PE field.

PERCUTANEOUS TREATMENT OF ACUTE PULMONARY EMBOLISM

In theory, percutaneous treatment of PE offers a rapid, targeted decrease in clot burden which may hasten symptom resolution without the risk of major hemorrhage that comes with ST.[14] Various society and consortium guidelines provide recommendations on the use of percutaneous treatment of PE, including those from the AHA,[19] ESC,[21] American College of Chest Physicians,[26] and the pulmonary embolism response teams (PERT) Consortium.[1] Given the paucity of trial data on interventional therapies for PE, recommendations are based primarily on expert opinion and case series, and thus limited in strength to IIa and IIb.[14,18] In general, guidelines suggest these interventional therapies as an alternative to ST in patients who have progressive deterioration or are at risk for cardiopulmonary instability despite initial anticoagulation. This includes patients with acute high-risk PE who have contraindications to ST or ongoing instability despite ST, patients with acute intermediate-high-risk PEs who are likely at elevated risk for progressive hypotension, and patients with thrombus-in-transit.[1,14,19,21,26] Interventional therapies may be considered in the highest risk normotensive patients to prevent right ventricular or hemodynamic failure and who may die before ST may take effect, or to hasten symptom resolution, theoretically offering the advantages of ST while posing a lower risk of ICH.[14,20]

If patients are not already intubated, catheter-directed treatment of PE may be provided using local anesthesia with central vascular access obtained via the femoral or internal jugular veins. Access may be limited by concurrent clot burden in the lower extremities or central veins. Image-guided vascular access with careful attention to sheath and catheter selection and manipulation is critical given concomitant therapeutic anticoagulation and possible thrombolytic therapy. Preprocedurally, consideration should be given to the planned deployment of vascular closure devices depending on the size of sheaths and experience of the operators, to reduce morbidity and bleeding from access site complications.

Catheter-directed therapies may be used to decrease PE clot burden via local infusion of thrombolysis, or mechanical and embolectomy strategies, or combinations of these approaches.

Catheter-Directed Thrombolysis

Catheter-directed thrombolysis (CDL) involves infusion of thrombolytics directly into the PA using a catheter that has been navigated through the venous system to the site of embolization. As with ST, CDL may be contraindicated in patients with significant bleeding risks. Compared with ST, lower doses of lytic agents required for CDL may reduce bleeding complication risks (typically <25% of systemic dose, though optimal dosing and duration of therapy is an area of active investigation). An additional theoretic benefit of CDL over ST is the avoidance of shunting of lytic agents to unobstructed PA segments which have lower resistance and are thus likely to receive more blood flow; however, *in vivo* flow studies show rapid washout of drug administered adjacent to PE, suggesting a need for direct intrathrombic injection.[33]

Although there are several case series of CDL, there is limited randomized data comparing this with ST.[14,20] Among patients with propensity-matched hospitalized PE in representative US cohort 2004 to 2014, there were equal 1.9% rates of ICH between ST versus CDL, though increased all-cause bleeding (15.9% vs 8.7%, $P < .001$) but reduced in-hospital mortality in CDL (6.5% vs 10.0%, $P = .02$).[34] However, given the heterogeneity of existing studies comparing ST and CDL, randomized data will be needed to rigorously compare bleeding rates between these modalities.[20]

Ultrasound-assisted thrombolysis

Ultrasound-assisted thrombolysis (USAT) was developed as a technology to improve the efficacy of CDL. USAT applies high-frequency ultrasound to fragment clots and ultimately potentiate thrombolytic agents. Specific ultrasound frequencies cause reversible disaggregation of fibrin polymers, allowing for faster, higher affinity binding of thrombolytics.[35] ULTIMA showed a 23% reduction in right ventricular (RV) to left ventricular (LV) diameter ratio at 24 hours in patients with intermediate-risk PE randomized to USAT (mean tPA dose 20.8 mg in the 87% patients who underwent bilateral USAT), versus anticoagulation, which showed a <3% reduction ($P < .001$).[36] FDA approval for the most commonly used device–EkoSonic Endovascular System (EKOS Corporation, Bothell, WA)—was obtained based on data from the single-arm, multicenter SEATTLE-II study which enrolled 150 patients with massive (20%) or submassive (80%) PE and demonstrated 37% reduced RV:LV 48 hours after USAT (mean tPA dose 23.7 mg).[37] Patients with higher baseline RV:LV, higher PA pressure, and radiographic indices of PA obstruction accrued more benefit from USAT, though treatment effects were attenuated with comorbid obesity, tobacco use, hepatic or renal insufficiency, or higher presenting heart rate.[38] OPTALYSE PE studied shorter thrombolytic durations and doses in USAT, and found comparable efficacy with regimens as short as 2 hours with 4 mg tPA.[39]

Evidence for USAT is primarily single-arm investigations with surrogate endpoints and additional investigations include:[40]

- HI-PEITHO, multicenter trial randomizing 406 patients with intermediate-high-risk PE to USAT versus anticoagulation to assess a primary clinical composite endpoint including PE-related death (https://clinicaltrials.gov/ct2/show/NCT04790370).
- KNOCKOUT PE, 1500 patient retrospective and prospective registry of intermediate-high and high-risk PE t0 examine outcomes including all-cause mortality, recurrent VTE, and pulmonary hypertension (https://clinicaltrials.gov/ct2/show/NCT03426124).

Catheter-Directed Embolectomy

Therapies for catheter-directed embolectomy (CDE) leverage several endovascular techniques to mechanically disrupt or extract *en bloc* emboli from the PA. Some techniques combine thrombus disruption and aspiration in the same catheter. Others augment mechanical treatment with directed administration of lytic therapy. Possible complications from catheter therapies include PA perforation and cardiac arrest. The former can lead to pericardial tamponade which may be fatal even with timely drainage, noting that the patient may have been exposed previously to systemic anticoagulation or thrombolytics. Mechanical thrombolysis can also lead to hemoglobinuria and hemodynamic changes (due to the release of adenosine and other vasoactive substances). Outcome data with CDE therapies for PE management have thus far been limited by sample size, heterogeneity of approaches and populations, and inconsistencies in comparison groups.

Mechanical fragmentation

Catheter-directed mechanical treatment may be performed by simple thrombus fragmentation using balloon angioplasty, passage of a guide wire, or rotation of a pigtail catheter-directed inside PE.[14,20] Without concurrent clot fragment aspiration, distal embolization occurs, though the theory for effect is increasing the overall surface area of perfused pulmonary vasculature, thereby decreasing pulmonary vascular resistance and RV afterload.[41–43] Modern embolectomy techniques have superseded this approach.

Rheolytic thrombectomy

Rheolytic thrombectomy mechanically disrupts clot by injecting high pressurized saline, creating a local Venturi effect, and then aspirating thrombus fragments through a more proximal port. Rheolytic thrombectomy can be combined with CDL, achieving success rates near 90% in this configuration, although most data come from uncontrolled case series.[44,45] Notable complications include hemoptysis, bradycardia, hypotension, and hemodynamic collapse.[46,47] Shear-induced release of vasoactive substances such as bradykinin and adenosine from platelets is believed to contribute to bradycardia and hypotension.[46] Due to adverse reported events, there is an FDA black box warning for use rheolytic therapies in the PA, including AngioJet (Boston Scientific, Minneapolis, MN), and this modality would be rarely considered (contraindications to ST, no other CDL or CDE device available).

Mechanical embolectomy

Suction embolectomy was first described by Greenfield in 1969. In cases where clot fragment cannot pass through the catheter, sustained suction is applied to keep thrombus attached to the catheter tip while it is withdrawn through the venotomy. Reported success with aspiration techniques (based on angiographic evidence of thrombus removal and decreased PA pressures) approaches 100% when used in conjunction with thrombolysis approaches.[48–50] In general, the caliber and relative inflexibility of large-bore catheters needed for successful aspiration prevent applicability to pulmonary embolectomy.[14,51] The AngioVac cannula (Angiodynamics, Latham, NY) aspirates intravascular material *en bloc* through a 22 French suction catheter using a venovenous bypass system. A filter located between the inflow and outflow cannulae traps solid material before returning blood to the patient. Various centers report experience extracting right heart thrombus-in-transit, with some application to the PA.[14,52–54]

The FlowTriever aspiration device (Inari Medical, Irvine, CA) was the first to receive FDA clearance for the catheter-directed mechanical management of PE (2018), based on the single-arm FLARE trial showing a reduction in RV:LV ratio in intermediate-high-risk PE; it was approved for treating thrombus-in-transit (2021).[55–57] FlowTriever is a 20 French catheter that allows for aspiration and also clot disruption, using 3 self-expanding nitinol discs which may be deployed within the clot and then retracted into the catheter along with disrupted and entrapped thrombus[52]; however, in practice, the disks may not be used as commonly, in favor of the aspiration functionality.[20] The smaller-bore Indigo aspiration catheter (Penumbra, Alameda, CA) is a 6- to 8-French device that ostensibly may be more navigable in the PA tree, but may have less capacity for larger clots; newer versions feature larger calibers and technology to target suction directly to clots. Indigo aspiration improved RV:LV ratio in intermediate-risk PE in the single-arm EXTRACT-PE trial.[58] Rates of major bleeding (hemoptysis, access site), PA injury (guidewire proration and distal PA perforation), and clinical deterioration were each reported less than 2%. Both FlowTriever and Indigo devices reported about 25% reduction in primary RV:LV endpoint, and both reduced PA systolic pressure by about 10%. Ongoing investigations of FlowTriever include:

- FLAME (FlowTriever for Acute Massive Pulmonary Embolism), high-risk PE, prospective observational cohort to assess all-cause mortality, deterioration, and need for rescue intervention (https://clinicaltrials.gov/ct2/show/NCT04795167)
- FLASH (FlowTriever All-Comer Registry for Patient Safety and Hemodynamics), real-world registry of intermediate-risk PE to assess device-related events and device-related death (https://clinicaltrials.gov/ct2/show/NCT03761173)
- PEERLESS, the first randomized trial comparing CDE (FlowTriever) versus CDL in intermediate-high-risk PE, assessing a win-ratio composite endpoint, encompassing all-cause mortality, ICH, deterioration, or treatment escalation (https://clinicaltrials.gov/ct2/show/NCT05111613)

SURGICAL TECHNIQUES FOR ACUTE PULMONARY EMBOLISM

Emergency surgical pulmonary embolectomy (SPE) may be considered for some patients with acute high-risk PE. Operative candidacy varies by center, surgeon, and specific clinical situation and comorbidities.[59] SPE is either excluded from most major society guidelines for the management of acute PE or recommended only as salvage therapy whereby other treatment options have failed or are contraindicated.[20,21] This is undoubtedly driven by historical data suggesting excessive mortality rates for patients undergoing SPE.[6,52,60] This philosophy is steadily changing as new data emerge, suggesting excellent contemporary outcomes with SPE, particularly when considered upfront, outside of the salvage indication.[21,61]

The SPEAR (Surgical Pulmonary Embolectomy as Routine therapy) consortium reported 214 SPE operations, of which 82% represented non–high-risk PE, and reported 11.7% in-hospital mortality (23.7% in high-risk patients, 9.1% in nonhigh risk patients).[61] In-hospital mortality in patients who did not require preoperative CPR was 8.6%, compared with 32.1% if preoperative CPR was required. A retrospective single-center review comparing SPE to veno-arterial (VA) ECMO for the treatment of high-risk PE (32 and 27 patients in the 2 groups, respectively) suggested a trend toward higher mortality in the VA-ECMO group (14.9% vs 6.3%)[62] although a bias toward ECMO rather than upfront SPE for patients with uncertain neurologic status after CPR may contribute. Notably, no mortalities in this analysis were from RV failure, suggesting the success in rescuing the RV. Outcomes that highlight the relative safety and efficacy of SPE when performed at expert centers have stimulated interest in the surgical community in incorporating SPE into the routine treatment algorithm for high-risk PE.[21,62–69]

Preparation for SPE includes invasive arterial monitoring, central venous access, and transesophageal echocardiography. A PA catheter may be used, but will generally be parked in the superior vena cava given distal clot burden. A single-lumen endotracheal tube is adequate in most settings. It is important to recognize the risk of cardiac arrest at the time of anesthesia induction depending on the degree of RV strain and cardiopulmonary dysfunction: peri-intubation sedation may blunt catecholamine surges on which the patient is dependent and reduce venous return in an already preload-dependent RV, and initiation of mechanical ventilation may increase pulmonary vascular resistance and further impair venous return. Accordingly, it is imperative that the surgical team be present at anesthesia induction and ready to rapidly initiate cardiopulmonary bypass.

Standard SPE approach is via midline sternotomy with the initiation of cardiopulmonary bypass via the aorta and dual vena cava for augmented venous drainage.[52] The aorta is then clamped, the heart arrested, and an incision made on the anterior main PA, starting 1.5 cm distal to the pulmonic valve, and extending to the proximal left PA.[70] With this exposure, clot is removed from the main, right, and left PAs using suction and forceps. Additional maneuvers for improved exposure and clot extraction include making a second incision in the right PA exposed between aorta and superior vena cava,[52] gentle compression of the lung to dislodge small distal clots (except if the patient received antecedent ST), and clot extraction from the segmental arteries using a small videoscope.[70,71] Other loci of thrombus-in-transit can be addressed surgically, including right heart thrombi and impending paradoxic embolism of PE, for which SPE is considered first-line therapy.[9,72] Before PA closure, the catheter in the superior vena-cava is advanced into the right PA under direct vision. When weaning from cardiopulmonary bypass, hemodynamics and echocardiographic assessment of RV function is carefully monitored. Diligent hemostasis before chest closure is of utmost importance given the need for postoperative therapeutic anticoagulation.

MECHANICAL CIRCULATORY SUPPORT OPTIONS

MCS with ECMO or other RV assist devices (RVAD) may be options in high-risk PE with refractory shock, cardiac arrest, or contraindications to ST, but who are not appropriate candidates for immediate intervention or surgery.[1] The goal of MCS is to sustain the systemic circulation and decompress the RV, while endogenous and anticoagulation-facilitated clot lysis occurs. MCS allows a period of end-organ recovery following arrest in patients with PE before proceeding with intervention, as well as periprocedural interventional support.

VA-ECMO is becoming a more common modality in treating highest risk catastrophic PE.[73,74] While the risk of mortality in cardiac arrest related to PE approaches 100%, meta-analysis suggests that ECMO is associated with approximately 60% survival to hospital discharge[75] Multiple single-center retrospective studies of ECMO in PE cohorts defined by cardiac arrest and/or cardiogenic shock on presentation are published; these vary in specific populations and the specific interventional PE therapy coupled with ECMO, however, report in-hospital survival rates 50% to 70%.[76–79]

The University of Maryland has extensively published on their experience with an initial VA-ECMO strategy in high- and catastrophic-risk PE. ECMO is continued until neurologic status is clarified, end-organ function is optimized, or 5 days of systemic anticoagulation have elapsed. At that time, ECMO decannulation is undertaken if the RV has recovered, or SPE performed if there is persistent RV dysfunction, with resultant greater than 95% hospital and 1-year survival.[77,80,81]

RVAD represent another evolving MCS option for high-risk PE, though only retrospective data and small series are reported.[52,82,83] Unlike VA-ECMO, some RVAD like a percutaneous axial pump (Impella-RP, Abiomed, Danvers, MA) are not able to provide oxygenation and ventilation support to the patient. Other RVADs like paracorporeal pumps with dual-lumen catheters for right atrium-PA bypass do allow the introduction of an oxygenator.

CONTROVERSIES AND THE ROLE OF PULMONARY EMBOLISM RESPONSE TEAMS

Limited comparative effective data on interventional therapies for PE leave gaps and available guideline statements provide recommendations, but are far from definitive.[1,14,16,18,19,21,26,52] This is especially manifest in the setting of ongoing or anticipated hemodynamic instability whereby clinicians have a host of ostensibly equivalent interventional strategies, and this is compounded by limited guidance to enable selection from the various modalities available for CDL or CDE (**Table 1**).

Enter the PERT–which, like other models of Heart teams,[18] leverages the collective expertise of multidisciplinary physicians. PERT physicians often include cardiac imaging, cardiac surgery, interventional cardiology and vascular medicine, interventional radiology, pulmonary and critical care, emergency medicine, and others.[1,14,16,18] PERT melds the Heart team concept with principles of rapid response teams to expressly assist clinicians in diagnosis, prognosis, and designing individualized management plans.[1,18] A robust multidisciplinary PERT can consider multiple options, reducing specialty-specific biases, and instead focusing on available options applied to individual patient factors that affect procedure-specific considerations.[1,18,52]

Though data demonstrating improved patient outcomes with PERT programs are only starting to emerge, many centers have implemented PERTs, focusing on interdisciplinary collaboration and streamlining processes of care for complex PE.[1,14,16,18,84,85]

SUMMARY AND FUTURE DIRECTIONS

Treatment of PE continues to evolve at a time when relatively novel interventional therapies are undergoing continuous implementation. Therapeutic anticoagulation is the mainstay in low-risk PE, but there is much less clarity and data to guide optimal treatment of more severe presentations, a fact that is reflected in the strength of guideline recommendations.

- Catastrophic-risk PE requires immediate hemodynamic support and interventions, including the consideration of MCS.
- ST is an option for patients presenting with acute high-risk PE and selected patients with acute intermediate-high PE. Many patients with high-risk PE have contraindications to ST, and this modality is underused due to fear of ICH, meriting consideration of an interventional therapy (see **Table 1**). Interventional and surgical treatment options are also available for the failure of ST, or for patients who may need more expeditious treatment efficacy.
- Thrombus-in-transit often requires CDE or SPE.
- Patients with intermediate-high-risk should have an individualized benefit-risk assessment, accounting for patient-specific preferences and bleeding risk. In general, the clinician treating PE should be flexible and continually reassess the patient, contemplating a role for interventions beyond anticoagulation for adverse hemodynamic or respiratory trajectory.[20,86]

In the absence of robust comparative effectiveness, data to help clinicians choose among interventional, surgical, and MCS options, PERTs including clinicians from various disciplines furnish patients with PE with expedient and thoughtful treatment plans that account for features of each individual case and expertise available at each center. Institutional expertise, and team and system familiarity with interventions are essential; institutions and operators should seek to master a portfolio of techniques, as low institutional volume is associated with higher mortality.[61,87] The volume-expertise relationship underlies the need for regional and national hub-and-spoke models for the care of PE, with protocols in place for expeditious, safe transfers.[88]

Table 1
Comparison of various interventional options for the management of pulmonary embolism

Modality	Specialists	Key Features and Considerations	Type of PE Addressed	Time to Initiation	Clinical Evidence Base
Therapeutic Anticoagulation	Any Clinician	• Inexpensive and easy to use • Some treatment failures • May take time to effect	All	Minutes	Prospective randomized trials
Systemic Thrombolysis	Any Clinician	• Rapid initiation of reperfusion • No special equipment • No special access requirements • Hemorrhage risk	Intermediate-high and high risk	Minutes	Prospective randomized trials
Catheter-Directed Thrombolysis	Interventional Cardiologist	• Vascular access and specialist required • Some bleeding risk, though lower thrombolytic exposures vs systemic administration	Intermediate-high and high risk; can address proximal or distal PE	Minutes to Hours	Small case series
Ultrasound-Assisted Thrombolysis	Interventional Cardiologist	• Vascular access and specialist required • Specialized equipment • Some bleeding risk, though lower thrombolytic exposures vs systemic administration	Intermediate-high and high risk; can address proximal or distal PE	Minutes to Hours	Single-arm trials and/or surrogate outcomes

Catheter-Directed Embolectomy	Interventional Cardiologist	• Vascular access and specialist required • Specialized equipment • Large bore vascular access • Limited access to distal disease (especially in pulmonary artery) • Intraprocedure and access complications	Intermediate-high and high risk; thrombus-in-transit, may or may not access proximal PE	Minutes to Hours	Case series
Surgical Pulmonary Embolectomy	Cardiac Surgeon	• Specialist required • Specialized equipment • Permits comprehensive proximal embolectomy • Comorbidity of sternotomy, cardiopulmonary bypass	Intermediate-high and high risk; proximal PA clot, or thrombus-in-transit	Minutes to Hours	Case series
Mechanical Circulatory Support	Cardiac Surgeon, Interventional Cardiologist, Critical Care	• Vascular access and specialist required • Supportive measure but does not directly treat PE. • However supports organ function and systemic perfusion during the critical initial phase, thus provides bridge to decision and bridge to intervention	High-risk	Minutes	Case series

Abbreviations: PA, pulmonary artery, PE, pulmonary embolism.

If recent technological innovations are any indication, the future of PE management will likely include the incorporation of more interventional therapies and MCS. However, our patients are owed rigorous clinical investigations so that this field uses data-driven therapies proven safe, efficacious, and cost-effective. Practically, it is unlikely that large or randomized trials will be feasible in highest risk PE gave lower incidence and atypical protocols that would be needed to enroll and randomize patients (cf community consents, randomization by center); registries are likely to be helpful to probe short-term high-risk mortality. The all-cause mortality rate in contemporary intermediate-high-risk PE was less than 2% in PEITHO,[30] so powering trials to show a benefit on mortality in intermediate-high-risk PE would be difficult. Accordingly, other endpoints including patient-centric outcomes may be needed such as cardiopulmonary functional assessment, relief of dyspnea, and quality-of-life.[20,40]

Until there is clarity about patient subgroups that derive maximal benefit from interventions, PERTs represent the contemporary mechanism to assess comparative benefits of various approaches.[1,14,16,18,52]

CLINICS CARE POINTS

- Maintain a high index of suspicion for the diagnosis of PE. Appropriate risk stratification based on society guidelines is a critical step in optimizing management for patients with PE.
- Therapeutic anticoagulation is the foundation of PE management and should be initiated early in most cases of acute PE. Therapy may be initiated before definitive diagnosis if the index of suspicion is sufficient.
- In patients with acute high-risk PE without contraindication to thrombolysis, ST should be considered.
- In patients with acute high-risk PE with have contraindications to ST, who fail ST, or who have higher risk features interventional approaches should be considered including CDL, CDE, and SPE.
- Consider MCS in patients with acute high-risk PE who present with cardiopulmonary collapse, intractable hypotension, or failure of ST.
- Reperfusion and debulking therapy are not first-line in intermediate-high-risk PE; however, frequent reassessments are required. With the manifestation of higher risk features or concern for clinical deterioration, ST (in the absence of contraindications), or CDL, CDE, or SPE should be considered.
- Thrombus-in-transit often requires the consideration of CDE of SPE, though ST has been reported.
- Comparative trials to investigate interventional options are being conducted.
- In the absence of high-level comparative effectiveness data among interventional treatment options for PE, multi-disciplinary PERTs should be considered as part of decision-making pathways for patients with acute intermediate or high-risk PE. Institutions should create a PERT to streamline processes of care and coordinate multidisciplinary care, and attention is needed to develop institutional expertise and volume in interventional techniques.

DISCLOSURE

The authors have nothing to disclose.

REFERENCES

1. Rivera-Lebron B, McDaniel M, Ahrar K, et al. Diagnosis, treatment and follow up of acute pulmonary embolism: consensus practice from the PERT consortium. Clin Appl Thromb Hemost 2019;25. 1076029619853037.
2. Mahan CE, Borrego ME, Woersching AL, et al. Venous thromboembolism: annualised United States models for total, hospital-acquired and preventable costs utilising long-term attack rates. Thromb Haemost 2012;108:291–302.
3. Goldhaber SZ, Bounameaux H. Pulmonary embolism and deep vein thrombosis. Lancet 2012;379:P1835–46.
4. Kniffin WD, Baron JA, Barrett J, et al. The epidemiology of diagnosed pulmonary embolism and deep venous thrombosis in the elderly. Arch Intern Med 1994;154: 861–6.
5. Carson JL, Kelley MA, Duff A, et al. The clinical course of pulmonary embolism. N Engl J Med 1992;326:1240–5.
6. Stein PD, Matta F. Case fatality rate with pulmonary embolectomy for acute pulmonary embolism. Am J Med 2012;125:471–7.
7. Kucher N, Rossi E, De Rosa M, et al. Massive pulmonary embolism. Circulation 2006;113:577–82.
8. Gupta R, Ammari Z, Dasa O, et al. Long-term mortality after massive, submassive, and low-risk pulmonary embolism. Vasc Med 2020;25:141–9.
9. Kabrhel C, Rempell JS, Avery LL, et al. Case records of the Massachusetts general hospital. Case 29-2014. A 60-year-old woman with syncope. N Engl J Med 2014;371:1143–50.
10. Anderson FA, Spencer FA. Risk factors for venous thromboembolism. Circulation 2003;107(SUPPL. 23):9–16.
11. Hariharan P, Dudzinski DM, Rosovsky R, et al. Relation among clot burden, right-sided heart strain, and adverse events after acute pulmonary embolism. Am J Cardiol 2016;118:1568–73.
12. Lynhe MD, Kline JA, Nielsen-Kudsk JE, et al. Pulmonary vasodilation in acute pulmonary embolism – a systematic review. Pulm Circ 2020;10. 2045894019899775.
13. Turetz M, Sideris AT, Friedman OA, et al. Epidemiology, pathophysiology, and natural history of pulmonary embolism. Semin Intervent Radiol 2018;35:92–8.
14. Dudzinski DM, Giri J, Rosenfield K. Interventional treatment of pulmonary embolism. Circ Cardiovasc Interv 2017;10:e004345.
15. Dalen JE, Banas JS, Brooks HL, et al. Resolution rate of acute pulmonary embolism in man. N Engl J Med 1969;280:1194–9.
16. Reza N, Dudzinski DM. Pulmonary embolism response teams. Curr Treat Options Cardiovasc Med 2015;17:387.
17. Todoran TM, Giri J, Barnes GD, et al. Treatment of submassive and massive pulmonary embolism: a clinical practice survey from the second annual meeting of the Pulmonary Embolism Response Team Consortium. J Thromb Thrombolysis 2018;46:39–49.
18. Dudzinski DM, Piazza G. Multidisciplinary pulmonary embolism response teams. Circulation 2016;133:98–103.
19. Jaff MR, McMurtry MS, Archer SL, et al. Management of massive and submassive pulmonary embolism, iliofemoral deep vein thrombosis, and chronic thromboembolic pulmonary hypertension: A scientific statement from the american heart association. Circulation 2011;123:1788–830.

20. Giri J, Sista AK, Weinberg I, et al. Interventional therapies for acute pulmonary embolism: Current status and principles for the development of novel evidence. Circulation 2019;140:E774–801.

21. Konstantinides SV, Meyer G, Becattini C, et al. 2019 ESC Guidelines for the diagnosis and management of acute pulmonary embolism developed in collaboration with the European Respiratory Society (ERS)The Task Force for the diagnosis and management of acute pulmonary embolism of the European Society of Cardiology (ESC). Eur Heart J 2020;41(4):543–603.

22. Kürkciyan I, Meron G, Sterz F, et al. Pulmonary embolism as cause of cardiac arrest: presentation and outcome. Arch Intern Med 2000;160:1529–35.

23. Boulafendis D, Bastounis E, Panayiotopoulos YP, et al. Pulmonary embolectomy (Answered and unanswered questions). Int Angiol 1991;10:187–94.

24. Ventetuolo CE, Klinger JR. Management of acute right ventricular failure in the intensive care unit. Ann Am Thorac Soc 2014;11:811–22.

25. Konstam MA, Kiernan MS, Bernstein D, et al. Evaluation and management of right-sided heart failure: a scientific statement from the American Heart Association. Circulation 2018;137:e578–622.

26. Stevens SM, Woller SC, Kreuziger LB, et al. Antithrombotic therapy for VTE Disease: second update of the CHEST guideline and expert panel report. Chest 2021;160:e545–608.

27. Khan F, Rahman A, Carrier M, et al. Long term risk of symptomatic recurrent venous thromboembolism after discontinuation of anticoagulant treatment for first unprovoked venous thromboembolism event: systematic review and meta-analysis. BMJ 2019;366:l4363.

28. Wan S, Quinlan DJ, Agnelli G, et al. Thrombolysis compared with heparin for the initial treatment of pulmonary embolism: a meta-analysis of the randomized controlled trials. Circulation 2004;110:744–9.

29. Wang C, Zhai Z, Yang Y, et al. Efficacy and safety of low dose recombinant tissue-type plasminogen activator for the treatment of acute pulmonary thromboembolism: a randomized, multicenter, controlled trial. Chest 2010;137:254–62.

30. Meyer G, Vicaut E, Danays T, et al. Fibrinolysis for patients with intermediate-risk pulmonary embolism. N Engl J Med 2014;370:1402–11.

31. Goldhaber SZ. Thrombolytic therapy for patients with pulmonary embolism who are hemodynamically stable but have right ventricular dysfunction: Pro. Arch Intern Med 2005;165:2197–205.

32. Chatterjee S, Chakraborty A, Weinberg I, et al. Thrombolysis for pulmonary embolism and risk of all-cause mortality, major bleeding, and intracranial hemorrhage: a meta-analysis. JAMA 2014;311:2414–21.

33. Schmitz-Rode T, Kilbinger M, Gunther RW. Simulated flow pattern in massive pulmonary embolism: significance for selective intrapulmonary thrombolysis. Cardiovasc Intervent Radiol 1998;21:199–204.

34. Geller BJ, Adusumalli S, Pugliese SC, et al. Outcomes of catheter-directed versus systemic thrombolysis for the treatment of pulmonary embolism: a real-world analysis of national administrative claims. Vasc Med 2020;25:334–40.

35. Siddiqi F, Odrljin TM, Fay PJ, et al. Binding of tissue-plasminogen activator to fibrin: effect of ultrasound. Blood 1998;91:2019–25.

36. Kucher N, Boekstegers P, Müller OJ, et al. Randomized, controlled trial of ultrasound-assisted catheter-directed thrombolysis for acute intermediate-risk pulmonary embolism. Circulation 2014;129:479–86.

37. Piazza G, Hohlfedler B, Jaff MR, et al. A prospective, single-arm, multicenter trial of ultrasound-facilitated, catheter-directed, low-dose fibrinolysis for acute

massive and submassive pulmonary embolism: the SEATTLE II study. JACC Cardiovasc Interv 2015;8:1382–92.

38. Sardar P, Piazza G, Goldhaber SZ, et al. Predictors of treatment response following ultrasound-facilitated catheter-directed thrombolysis for submassive and massive pulmonary embolism. Circ Cardiovasc Interv 2020;13:e008747.

39. Tapson VF, Sterling K, Jones N, et al. A randomized trial of the optimum duration of acoustic pulse thrombolysis procedure in acute intermediate-risk pulmonary embolism: the OPTALYSE PE trial. JACC Cardiovasc Interv 2018;11:1401–10.

40. Aggarwal V, Giri J, Nallamothu BK. Catheter-based therapies in acute pulmonary embolism: the good, the bad, and the ugly. Circ Cardiovasc Interv 2020;13: e009353.

41. Schmitz-Rode T, Janssens U, Duda SH, et al. Fragmentation of massive pulmonary embolism using a pigtail rotation catheter. Chest 1998;114:1427–36.

42. Murphy Jm, Mulvihill N, Mulcahy D, et al. Percutaneous catheter and guidewire fragmentation with local administration of recombinant tissue plasminogen activator as a treatment for massive pulmonary embolism. Eur Radiol 1999;9:959–64.

43. Fava M, Loyola S. Applications of percutaneous mechanical thrombectomy in pulmonary embolism. Tech Vasc Interv Radiol 2003;6:53–8.

44. Siablis D, Karnabatidis D, Katsanos K, et al. AngioJet rheolytic thrombectomy versus local intrapulmonary thrombolysis in massive pulmonary embolism: a retrospective data analysis. J Endovasc Ther 2005;12:206–14.

45. Fava M, Loyola S, Huete I. Massive pulmonary embolism: treatment with the hydrolyser thrombectomy catheter. J Vasc Interv Radiol 2000;11:1159–64.

46. Zhu DWX. The potential mechanisms of bradyarrhythmias associated with AngioJet thrombectomy. J Invasive Cardiol 2008;20(SUPPL. A):2A–4A.

47. Lin PH, Okada T, Steinberg JL, et al. Rheolytic pharmacomechanical thrombectomy in experimental chronic deep vein thrombosis: effect of L-arginine on thrombogenicity and endothelial vasomotor function. World J Surg 2007;31:664–75.

48. Moore JH, Koolpe HA, Carabasi RA, et al. Transvenous catheter pulmonary embolectomy. Arch Surg 1985;120:1372–5.

49. Hiramatsu S, Ogihara A, Kitano Y, et al. Clinical outcome of catheter fragmentation and aspiration therapy in patients with acute pulmonary embolism. J Cardiol 1999;34:71–8.

50. Heberlein WE, Meek ME, Saleh O, et al. New generation aspiration catheter: feasibility in the treatment of pulmonary embolism. World J Radiol 2013;5:430–5.

51. Behrens G, Bjarnason H. Venous thromboembolic disease: the use of the aspiration thrombectomy device AngioVac. Semin Intervent Radiol 2015;32:374–8.

52. Jaber WA, Fong PP, Weisz G, et al. Acute pulmonary embolism with an emphasis on an interventional approach. J Am Coll Cardiol 2016;67:991–1002.

53. Donaldson CW, Baker JN, Narayan RL, et al. Thrombectomy using suction filtration and veno-venous bypass: single center experience with a novel device. Catheter Cardiovasc Interv 2015;86:E81–7.

54. Al-Hakim R, Park J, Bansal A, et al. Early experience with angiovac aspiration in the pulmonary arteries. J Vasc Interv Radiol 2016;27:P730–4.

55. Bishay VL, Adenikinju O, Todd R. FlowTriever retrieval system for the treatment of pulmonary embolism: overview of its safety and efficacy. Expert Rev Med Devices 2021;18(11):1039–48. PMID. 34530650.

56. Tu T, Toma C, Tapson VF, et al. A prospective, single-arm, multicenter trial of catheter-directed mechanical thrombectomy for intermediate-risk acute pulmonary embolism: the FLARE study. JACC Cardiovasc Interv 2019;12:859–69.

57. Letter from Gregory O'Connell, Assistant Director DHT2C: Division of Coronary and Peripheral Intervention Devices, Food and Drug Administration, to Inari Medical, Inc., April 30, 2021. Available at: https://www.accessdata.fda.gov/cdrh_docs/pdf21/K211013.pdf. Accessed March 22, 2022.

58. Sista AK, Horowitz JM, Tapson VF, et al. Indigo aspiration system for treatment of pulmonary embolism: results of the EXTRACT-PE trial. JACC Cardiovasc Interv 2021;14:319–29.

59. Iaccarino A, Frati G, Schirone L, et al. Surgical embolectomy for acute massive pulmonary embolism: state of the art. J Thorac Dis 2018;10:5154–61.

60. Gulba DC, Schmid C, Borst HB, et al. Medical compared with surgical treatment for massive pulmonary embolism. Lancet 1994;343:576–7.

61. Keeling WB, Sundt T, Leacche M, et al. Outcomes after surgical pulmonary embolectomy for acute pulmonary embolus: a multi-institutional study. Ann Thorac Surg 2016;102:1498–502.

62. Choi JH, O'Malley TJ, Maynes EJ, et al. Surgical pulmonary embolectomy outcomes for acute pulmonary embolism. Ann Thorac Surg 2020;110:1072–80.

63. Goldberg JB, Spevack DM, Ahsan S, et al. Comparison of Surgical Embolectomy and Veno-arterial Extracorporeal Membrane Oxygenation for Massive Pulmonary Embolism. Semin Thorac Cardiovasc Surg 2021;Jun 19:S1043-0679(21)00292-6. https://doi.org/10.1053/j.semtcvs.2021.06.011. PMID 34157383.

64. Neely RC, Byrne JG, Gosev I, et al. Surgical embolectomy for acute massive and submassive pulmonary embolism in a series of 115 patients. Ann Thorac Surg 2015;100:1245–52.

65. Pasrija C, Kronfli A, Rouse M, et al. Outcomes after surgical pulmonary embolectomy for acute submassive and massive pulmonary embolism: A single-center experience. J Thorac Cardiovasc Surg 2018;155:1095–106.

66. Goldberg JB, Spevack DM, Ahsan S, et al. Survival and right ventricular function after surgical management of acute pulmonary embolism. JACC 2020;76:903–11.

67. Goldhaber SZ. ECMO and surgical embolectomy: two potent tools to manage high-risk pulmonary embolism. JACC 2020;76:912–5.

68. Goldhaber SZ. Surgical pulmonary embolectomy: the resurrection of an almost discarded operation. Tex Heart Inst J 2013;40:5–8.

69. Carrel T. Commentary: surgical embolectomy for massive pulmonary embolism revisited: a contemporary tribute to trendelenburg procedure. Semin Thorac Cardiovasc Surg 2021;2021 Jul 15:S1043-0679(21)00320-8. https://doi.org/10.1053/j.semtcvs.2021.07.008. PMID 34274433.

70. He C, Von Segesser, Kappetein PA, et al. Acute pulmonary embolectomy. Eur J Card Surg 2013;43:1087–95.

71. Pawale A, Seetharam K, Oswald E, et al. Video assistance for surgical pulmonary embolectomy. Eur J Card Surg 2017;52:989–90.

72. Nakamura K, Alba GA, Scheske JA, et al. A 57-year-old man with insidious dyspnea and nonpleuritic chest and back pain. Chest 2016;150:e41–7.

73. Elbadawai A, Mentias A, Elgendy Y, et al. National trends and outcomes for extracorporeal membrane oxygenation use in high-risk pulmonary embolism. Vasc Med 2019;24:230–3.

74. Kaso ER, Pan JA, Salerno M, et al. Venoarterial extracorporeal membrane oxygenation for acute massive pulmonary embolism: a meta-analysis and call to action. J Cardiovasc Transl Res 2021;(2021 Jul 19:1–10). https://doi.org/10.1007/s12265-021-10158-0. PMID 34282541.

75. Scott JH, Gordon M, Vender R, et al. Venoarterial extracorporeal membrane oxygenation in massive pulmonary embolism-related cardiac arrest: a systematic review. Crit Care Med 2021;49:760–9.
76. Gulani S, Das Gupta J, Osofsky R, et al. Venoarterial extracorporeal membrane oxygenation is an effective management strategy for massive pulmonary embolism patients. J Vasc Surg Venous Lymphat Disord 2021;9(2):307–14.
77. Ghoreshi M, DiChiacchio L, Pasrija C, et al. Predictors of recovery in patients supported with venoarterial extracorporeal membrane oxygenation for acute massive pulmonary embolism. Ann Thorac Surg 2020;110:70–5.
78. Chen YY, Chen YC, Wu CC, et al. Clinical course and outcome of patients with acute pulmonary embolism rescued by veno-arterial extracorporeal membrane oxygenation: a retrospective review of 21 cases. J Card Surg 2002;15:295.
79. Al-Bawardy R, Rosenfield K, Borges J, et al. Extracorporeal membrane oxygenation in acute massive pulmonary embolism: a case series and review of the literature. Perfusion 2019;34:22–8.
80. Pasrija C, Kronfli A, George P, et al. Utilization of veno-arterial extracorporeal membrane oxygenation for massive pulmonary embolism. Ann Thorac Surg 2018;105:498–504.
81. Pasrija C, Shah A, George P, et al. Triage and optimization: a new paradigm in the treatment of massive pulmonary embolism. J Thorac Cardiovasc Surg 2018;156: P672–81.
82. Bhalia A, Attaran R. Mechanical circulatory support to treat pulmonary embolism: venoarterial extracorporeal membrane oxygenation and right ventricular assist device. Tex Heart Inst J 2020;47:202–6.
83. Elder M, Blank N, Kaki A, et al. Mechanical circulatory support for acute right ventricular failure in the setting of pulmonary embolism. J Interv Cardiol 2018;34: 518–24.
84. Kabrhel C, Rosovsky R, Channick R, et al. A multidisciplinary pulmonary embolism response team: initial 30-month experience with a novel approach to delivery of care to patients with submassive and massive pulmonary embolism. Chest 2016;150:384–93.
85. Carroll BJ, Beyer SE, Mehegan T, et al. Changes in care for acute pulmonary embolism through a multidisciplinary pulmonary embolism response team. Am J Med 2020;133:1313–21.
86. Singh M, Shafi I, Rali P, et al. Contemporary catheter-based treatment options for management of acute pulmonary embolism. Curr Treat Options Cardiovasc Med 2021;23:44.
87. Jung RG, Simard T, Hibbert B, et al. Association of annual volume and in-hospital outcomes of catheter-directed thrombolysis for pulmonary embolism. Catheter Cardiovasc Interv 2022;99(2):440–6. PMID 35083846.
88. Rali P, Sacher D, Rivera-Lebron B, et al. Interhospital transfer of patients with acute pulmonary embolism: challenges and opportunities. Chest 2021;160: 1844–52.

Management of Coronary Artery Disease

Eric Francis Sulava, MD[a], Jeffery Chad Johnson, MD[b],*

KEYWORDS

- Coronary artery bypass grafting (CABG) • Heart team • Hybrid revascularization
- Minimally invasive CABG

KEY POINTS

- Surgical revascularization coronary artery bypass grafting (CABG) continues to be the preferred treatment of most patients with multivessel and left main coronary artery disease (CAD).
- The heart team approach is recommended when evaluating patients with CAD who may be candidates for surgical revascularization; this ensures the patient is considered individually and all factors are taken into account to develop the best, tailored treatment strategy.
- Use of arterial conduits, when available and appropriate, is preferred to venous grafts with internal thoracic artery conduits being superior to radial artery conduits.
- Minimally invasive and hybrid surgical/percutaneous revascularization strategies are being used more often and present additional options for some patients.
- Off-pump CABG presents an alternative revascularization treatment of some patients who are not good candidates for traditional CABG due to technical considerations (eg, heavily calcified aorta that cannot be cross-clamped).

BACKGROUND

Heart disease is the number one cause of death in the United States and is responsible for more than 650,000 deaths annually. Coronary heart disease results in more than 800,000 myocardial infarctions per year and is responsible for 13% of all deaths.[1] Although there has been a recent decrease in both the overall number and rate of deaths in recent years, it remains a significant economic and health burden. Moreover, with the population aging it is likely to remain a significant cause of death and morbidity.

[a] Department of Emergency Medicine, Naval Medical Readiness & Training Center Portsmouth, 620 John Paul Jones Circle, Portsmouth, VA 23708, USA; [b] Department of Surgery, Division of Cardiothoracic Surgery, Naval Medical Readiness & Training Center Portsmouth, 620 John Paul Jones Circle, Portsmouth, VA 23708, USA
* Corresponding author.
E-mail address: jchadjohnson@gmail.com

Surg Clin N Am 102 (2022) 449–464
https://doi.org/10.1016/j.suc.2022.01.005
0039-6109/22/Published by Elsevier Inc.

Surgical therapy for ischemic heart disease was first performed in the 1960s and coronary artery bypass grafting (CABG) techniques have been continually refined since that time.[2,3] In the 1970s, percutaneous coronary intervention (PCI) was introduced and has advanced from angioplasty, to the deployment of bare metal stents, and to modern drug eluting stents.[4–6] These 2 procedures comprise the mainstays of procedural treatment of coronary artery disease (CAD) today. A comprehensive examination the of medical, percutaneous, and surgical treatment of CAD in all settings is extremely far reaching. For this reason, this review outlines the surgical management of CAD, primarily in the stable setting. Patient presentation, evaluation, surgical indications, and surgical treatment are also examined.

PATIENT EVALUATION AND OVERVIEW

CAD is a pathologic process that leads to inadequate blood supply to the myocardium secondary to atherosclerotic plaque accumulation in the epicardial coronary arteries. This chronic and progressive disease can have dynamic and seemingly unpredictable transitions. There are long, clinically silent periods of plaque accumulation that lead to acute decompensation following plaque rupture. This widespread variation of clinical presentation can be conveniently organized into the disease classification of acute coronary syndrome (ACS) or stable ischemic heart disease (SIHD).[7]

ACS is defined as an abrupt reduction in coronary blood flow or a mismatch in myocardial oxygen supply and demand.[8] The 3 presentations of ACS are unstable angina, acute non-ST elevation myocardial infarction, and acute ST elevation myocardial infarction.[9] SIHD, also referred to as chronic coronary syndrome, encompasses stable anginal pain syndromes (chronic angina) and new-onset, low-risk chest pain. Differentiation will initially be largely history based, following a reassuring initial workup of nondiagnostic electrocardiogram (ECG), negative cardiac biomarkers, and exclusion of secondary causes of chest pain.[10]

DETERMINATION OF PRETEST RISK

Once the initial clinical evaluation suggests SIHD, the probability of SIHD must be determined before recommending further testing. When the probability is low, testing is usually not warranted because of the higher likelihood of a false-positive test. The same is true for high probability of SIHD, with noninvasive testing being unable to completely exclude underlying disease.

The 2012 American College of Cardiology Foundation (ACCF)/American Heart Association (AHA) Guidelines on SIHD reference combined tables based on data from the Coronary Artery Surgery Study (CASS), Diamond-Forrester model, and the Duke Databank for Cardiovascular Disease. These models determine pretest probability of SIHD by using multiple clinical and demographic factors. Intermediate ranges from 20% to 70% pretest probability of SIHD. There are limitations for these risk calculations, including risk overestimation for low-risk SIHD in patients, inappropriately excluding patients older than 70 years, and performing less well in the female population.[11]

APPROACH TO TESTING

Several factors influence the choice of additional diagnostic testing for patients with suspected CAD. In addition to calculating pretest probability, the clinician must consider the patient's ability to exercise, body habitus, cardiac medications, and resting ECG abnormalities that might affect interpretation of test results. Further testing is delineated by the method of stressing (exercise or pharmacologic) and the method to identify and measure ischemia (ECG, echocardiography, PET, single-photon emission computed tomography [SPECT], or MRI).[10] Functional, or stress testing, to detect inducible ischemia has been the "gold standard" and is the most common noninvasive test used to diagnose SIHD.

EXERCISE VERSUS PHARMACOLOGIC TESTING

In the testing environment, induced ischemia depends on the severity of stress imposed and the severity of the pathologic flow disturbance. Submaximal exercise or incomplete pharmacologic vasodilation can fail to produce ischemia, and therefore coronary stenoses less than 70% are often undetected by functional testing.[11] Exercise testing is generally preferred because it often can provide a higher physiologic stress than would be achieved by pharmacologic testing, while eliciting the prognostic indicator of exercise capacity.[11,12]

TESTING MODALITIES
Exercise Electrocardiography

The exercise ECG has been the cornerstone of diagnostic testing of patients with SIHD for several decades, although recent research calls its utility into question. The 2012 ACCF/AHA Guidelines on SIHD recommend starting with exercise ECG without imaging for intermediate-risk patients who can exercise and have an interpretable ECG.

There are limitations to this modality. Research has shown that exercise ECG has inferior performance compared with diagnostic imaging tests and has limited power to rule in/out obstructive CAD.[13] The addition of coronary computed tomography angiography (CCTA) or functional imaging clarifies the diagnosis, enables the targeting of preventive therapies and interventions, and potentially reduces the risk of myocardial infarction. The 2019 European Society of Cardiology (ESC) Guidelines for the Diagnosis and Management of Chronic Coronary Syndromes removed the recommendation for exercise ECG to be used as the initial test to establish a diagnosis of stable CAD.[7]

Functional Noninvasive Testing

Some cardiologists prefer to add imaging to the initial exercise evaluation. Noninvasive functional tests detect ischemia by wall motion abnormalities on stress cardiac magnetic resonance (CMR), stress echocardiography, or perfusion changes by SPECT or PET. These are highly accurate for the detection of high-grade, flow-limiting coronary stenosis when compared with coronary angiography and fractional flow reserve (FFR).[13] However, lower grade coronary atherosclerosis can remain undetected by functional testing.[7]

Stress Echocardiography

Echocardiography is a reliable noninvasive test that can detect evidence of myocardial ischemia or infarction. It can reveal new or worsening regional wall motion abnormalities (RWMA) and changes in global left ventricular (LV) function during or immediately following pharmacologically induced stress. Severe ischemia produces RWMA that can be visualized within seconds of coronary artery occlusion occurring before the onset of ECG changes or symptoms.[14,15] In several meta-analyses, the diagnostic sensitivity ranged from 70% to 85% for exercise and 85% to 90% for pharmacologic stress echocardiography, with specificity ranging from 77% to 89% and 79% to 90%, respectively.[16–18]

Nuclear Myocardial Perfusion Imaging

Nuclear myocardial perfusion imaging (MPI), using SPECT or PET, uses a radioactive tracer to identify myocardial tissue uptake using pharmacologic or exercise-induced stress. Sensitivity is similar between stress echocardiography and SPECT, with the caveat that SPECT provides better quality images in the obese population.[10] PET, which is less widely available, has increased sensitivity over traditional SPECT with values of 90% and 85%, respectively.[19] In the special population of patients with a known diagnosis of CAD, nuclear MPI and CMR have the ability to identify myocardium with reversible ischemia that may be amenable to revascularization.[11]

Stress Cardiac Magnetic Resonance

CMR has the ability to provide information on cardiac structure, function, and myocardial perfusion.[7,20] Unfortunately, CMR is more difficult to obtain, given the lack of widespread expertise, increased scan times, and compatibility issues with medical implants. CMR incorporates gadolinium contrast, which is contraindicated in patients with renal dysfunction. The 2012 ACCF/AHA Guideline on SIHD states that CMR is reasonable for patients with intermediate to high pretest probability of IHD who are incapable of moderate physical function and for patients with known SIHD who have an uninterpretable ECG. The 2019 ESC Guidelines also allow for CMR in patients with inconclusive echocardiographic testing.[7,11]

Coronary Computed Tomography Angiography

CCTA is a noninvasive alternative to stress testing that provides anatomic instead of functional information. This multislice imaging technique allows for noninvasive visualization of anatomic CAD with high-resolution images, similar to invasive coronary angiography. Its advantage over functional testing is the ability to identify nonobstructive CAD conditions.[10] Noting its tendency to overestimate the severity of coronary lesions in the presence of heavy coronary calcification, the strength of CCTA is its near-perfect negative predictive value.[11]

Coronary Angiography

Invasive coronary angiography (ICA) remains the "gold-standard" testing modality for the diagnosis of CAD. ICA defines coronary anatomy, the presence of coronary intraluminal obstruction, and the extent of coronary and collateral blood flow. ICA is recommended for initial testing only in patients who have survived sudden cardiac death, had a life-threatening ventricular arrythmia, or developed signs of heart failure. ICA is more routinely used for further diagnostic evaluation following a high-risk or inconclusive initial workup with noninvasive cardiac testing.[11]

The most commonly used nomenclature for defining coronary anatomy was developed for CASS. The extent of disease is defined as 1-vessel, 2-vessel, 3-vessel, or left main disease, with a significant stenosis being generally greater than 70% diameter occlusion. Unprotected left main CAD is considered significantly stenotic at greater than 50% diameter occlusion.[11] For lesions with intermediate severity stenoses, FFR can measure the pressure proximal and distal to stenotic lesions and determine proportional decrease of flow across a stenosis to assist in differentiation. Values less than 0.80 are associated with provocable ischemia and significant coronary artery stenosis.[11,21]

MEDICAL TREATMENT OPTIONS

Goals of SIHD treatment are to diminish disease progression, limit complications, and reduce ischemic symptoms. Medical providers must address risk modification and determine guideline-directed medical therapy (GDMT). Risk modification includes life-style changes such as dietary modification, weight reduction, smoking cessation, frequent exercise, and management of stress and depression. GDMT includes therapies that slow down the atherosclerotic disease, decrease future events of myocardial infarction, and attempts to eliminate angina. Medications used to decrease mortality include antiplatelet agents, β-blockers, renin-angiotensin-aldosterone blockers and lipid-lowering drugs. Medications for symptom control include nitrates, β-blockers, calcium channel blockers, and sodium channel blockers.[11] A summary of the ACCF/AHA approach to GDMT is included in **Table 1**. Medical therapy alone is inferior revascularization with regard to survival.

SURGICAL AND INTERVENTIONAL TREATMENT OPTIONS

The decision to treat CAD with PCI versus CABG is, from a procedural standpoint, one of the most critical decisions that can affect patient outcome. Timing and presentation will initially drive the choice of procedure. In patients with an acute presentation, restoration of coronary blood flow is the most important consideration. Such patients are typically treated with PCI initially to expeditiously restore myocardial blood flow, with CABG being reserved for salvage of failed intervention or those with unfavorable anatomy for PCI in such situations.

For patients with stable CAD a thoughtful, guidelines-based approach developed jointly by cardiologists and cardiac surgeons is followed. These guidelines were published by the ACC, AHA, the American Association for Thoracic Surgery, the Society of Thoracic Surgeons (STS), the Preventive Cardiovascular Nurses Association, and the Society for Cardiac Angiography and Interventions for the treatment of SIHD in 2014 and for CABG in 2011.[22,23] They were updated in 2016 to include dual antiplatelet therapy recommendations.[24] These guidelines provide an evidence-based framework to direct patient-tailored coronary revascularization strategies. Surgical management remains the best choice of treatment of patients with significant multivessel and unprotected left main CAD who are able to undergo CABG. Central concepts of the guidelines important for cardiac surgeons in the management of CAD are summarized in **Fig. 1**.

Heart Team Approach

Multidisciplinary evaluation of stable patients with cardiovascular disease, including significant CAD, allows for tailored evidence-based treatment of individual patients.[25] The heart team typically consists of an interventional cardiologist, a noninterventional cardiologist, and cardiac surgeon who review the patient's coronary disease pattern and complexity, technical feasibility of PCI and CABG, overall patient health and condition, STS risk estimate, and any other factors that might affect patient outcome. The recommendations of the heart team are discussed with the patient, and an informed treatment decision can then be made.

This approach can lead to a different recommended procedural treatment of CAD than that recommended by the original treating interventional cardiologist alone in up to 30% of multivessel CAD cases according to one retrospective study.[26] Although randomized controlled trial data are not currently available to assess impact on outcome, this approach nonetheless carries the highest level of recommendation (LOR 1) in the ACC/AHA guidelines.[22]

Table 1
Overview of guideline-directed medical therapy in stable ischemic heart disease

Modification		Intervention	Indication	Explanation
Lipid management	Moderate- to high-potency statin	Atorvastatin, 40–80 mg/d Rosuvastatin, 20–40 mg/d	With, or at high risk for, CVD. High potency for age <75 y, if tolerated. Moderate potency preferred for >75 y	LDL-C goal of ≤70 mg/dL
	Lipid-lowering medication	Ezetimibe, 10 mg	If lDL-C is not at goal with maximum statin therapy. Primary therapy for patients who cannot tolerate statins.	LDL-C goal of ≤70 mg/dL
	PCSK9 inhibitor	Evolucumab or alirocumab SQ	Not at goal with statin—ezetimibe combination therapy.	Not routinely used due to high cost and mode of delivery
Blood pressure management	SIHD goal of <130/80	β-Blocker (not atenolol), ACE inhibitors, or ARBs	First-line therapy for SIHD	β-blockers have additional benefit in patients with reduced EF following MI
		Dihydropyridine CCBs	Second-line therapy: BP not at goal and angina is present	With angina: β-blockers and CCB are preferred
		Dihydropyridine CCBs, thiazide diuretics, MRAs	Second-line therapy: BP not at goal and angina is absent	DM initial antihypertension treatment: combination of an ACE-I with a CCB or thiazide-/thiazide-like diuretic
Diabetes management	Goal HbA1c level of <7%	SGLT2 inhibitor or GLP-1 agonist	SGLT2 inhibitors have been shown to reduce cardiovascular events. GLP-1 agonist reduces ischemic events in patients with SIHD	SGLT2 inhibitors (empagliflozin, canagliflozin) increase loss of glucose through urinary tract. GLP-1 agonists (liraglutide, semaglutide) promote insulin secretion

Behavior modification	Physical activity	30–60 min of moderate aerobic activity on 5–7 d/wk	Patients with, or at risk for, CVD	Regular exercise reduces heart disease mortality, improves functional capacity, and can decrease angina
	Weight management	BMI ≤35 kg/m²		Risk of CVD, cardiovascular morbidity/mortality, is higher in overweight/obese patients
	Social historical factors	Tobacco and alcohol cessation		Smoking increases CVD mortality by 50%. Relationship between alcohol consumption and CVD, with probable harm beyond 2 drinks per day
Thrombotic risk management	Antiplatelet therapy	Aspirin, 75–162 mg/d	Used indefinitely (in the absence of contraindications) in patients with SIHD	Platelet aggregation is a key element of the thrombotic response to plaque disruption
		Clopidogrel, 75 mg/d	Can be used when aspirin is contraindicated	Can be used in patients with a history of GI bleeds

Abbreviations: ACEI, angiotensin-converting enzyme inhibitor; ARB, angiotensin-receptor blocker; BMI, body mass index; BP, blood pressure; CCB, calcium channel blocker; CVD, cardiovascular disease; DM, diabetes mellitus; EF, ejection fraction; GI, gastrointestinal; GLP-1, glucagon-like peptide 1; HbA1c, hemoglobin A1c; LDL-C, low-density lipoprotein cholesterol; MI, myocardial infarction; MRAs, mineralocorticoid receptor antagonists; PCSK9, proprotein convertase subtilisin/kexin type 9; SGLT2, sodium-glucose cotransporter-2; SIHD, stable ischemic heart disease.

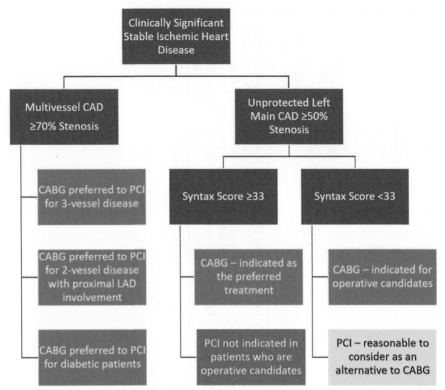

Fig. 1. Condensed summary of recommendations for surgical treatment of coronary artery disease and percutaneous treatment alternatives according to AHA/ACC/STS/AATS/PCNA/SCAI guidelines. Level of recommendation (LOR) is indicated by color: Green—LOR 1, yellow—LOR 2a/2b, red—LOR 3.

Unprotected Left Main Coronary Artery Disease

For patients with significant left main CAD, CABG is the preferred therapy to improve survival for patients who are surgical candidates. For patients with anatomically complex stenosis (SYNTAX score ≥33), CABG is superior to PCI for major adverse cardiac or cerebrovascular events (MACCE).[27] Patients with low to moderate anatomic complexity stenosis (SYNTAX score <33) and for whom the risk of adverse surgical outcomes is high, can be considered for PCI as an alternative to CABG without an increase in mortality.[28]

Multivessel Coronary Artery Disease

Patients with clinically significant multivessel CAD, defined as greater than or equal to 70% stenosis in 3 coronary arteries or in 2 coronary arteries with one being the proximal left anterior descending (LAD), should be considered for CABG as the preferred method of revascularization.[29] The left internal thoracic artery (LITA), if available, should be used to revascularize the LAD. Patients with significant stenoses in 2 coronary arteries with extensive ischemia, patients with mild to moderate LV dysfunction and multivessel CAD, and patients with isolated proximal LAD stenosis and extensive ischemia are also candidates to be considered for CABG to improve survival.[22]

Among patients with multivessel CAD, multiple arterial grafting is preferred to single arterial grafting and is associated with a lower all-cause mortality when compared with single arterial grafting CABG or PCI.[30,31]

Diabetic Patients

Patients with diabetes mellitus with clinically significant multivessel or unprotected left main CAD should preferentially receive CABG over PCI if they are suitable surgical candidates.[32] Multiple arterial grafting, including bilateral internal thoracic artery (BITA), can be considered with wound complication risk being mitigated to an acceptable level if ITA grafts are skeletonized.[33–35]

Conduit Selection

When planning surgical revascularization, it is critical to consider the type and amount of conduit available for use. The conduit type and source can affect long-term patency and clinical outcome. Likewise, when limited conduit is available, innovative configurations to achieve the most complete and highest quality revascularization should be considered. There is recent evidence to suggest that the use of multiple arterial grafting lowers all-cause mortality in multivessel and left main CAD, and liberal use of arterial grafts should be considered when available.[30] **Fig. 2** provides a summary of preferred conduits for use in CABG.

Internal thoracic artery

The right and left internal thoracic arteries are the best performing conduits over time, provided they are prepared appropriately and their target vessels are selected well. The LITA is the conduit of choice for the LAD. The right internal thoracic artery (RITA) can be used to revascularize the right coronary system, the distal circumflex coronary system, and the LAD. There is no difference in long-term patency between RITA and LITA grafts to equivalent targets, with both exhibiting greater than 90% patency at 10 years for appropriately chosen targets.[36] An important consideration when using the RITA to revascularize the right coronary circulation is to ensure there is a high-grade (>70%) stenosis proximal to the target when grafting the main RCA, use a free RITA graft, or use the RITA to graft more distal right coronary targets to

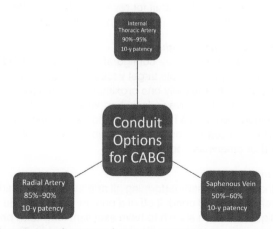

Fig. 2. Simplified summary of options for coronary revascularization conduits, including long-term patency rates for each.

prevent competitive flow and graft failure.[37,38] Both internal thoracic arteries can be prepared as in situ pedicled, skeletonized, or as free grafts.

There is an important caveat when preparing BITA grafts. The pedicled BITA technique is associated with a higher incidence of sternal wound complications than the skeletonized BITA technique. This effect may be magnified in the presence of diabetes and may affect single ITA grafting as well.[33–35] These are considerations that should be taken into account when considering a BITA technique in diabetic patients. Diabetic patients seem to benefit the most as a group from long-term mortality reduction when BITA revascularization is the chosen revascularization strategy. However, long-term mortality is similar between skeletonized and pedicled BITA grafts, although late MACCE may be higher among surgeons who perform the technique less often.[39]

Radial artery
The second most durable conduit available for use in CABG is the radial artery. Careful selection of eligible patients is required, including an Allen test to ensure adequate arterial circulation remains for the hand. The 10-year patency exceeds 85%, which is intermediate between ITA grafts and venous grafts.

Saphenous vein
The most commonly used conduit in CABG is the saphenous vein graft, typically in combination with the LITA. It is chosen for its ready availability, abundance, and caliber. However, these grafts are more prone to occlusion. The 1-month occlusion rate is greater than 10% and the 10-year patency rate is 50% to 60%.[40–42] Recent data on "no-touch" vein harvesting techniques seem to show a significant reduction in early occlusion and may improve long-term patency rates.[43]

Alternative conduits
Although surgical revascularization can usually be accomplished with the aforementioned conduit options, others have been described. These include the right gastroepiploic artery, lesser saphenous vein, and cryopreserved vein. These are not first-line or widely used options and are generally only entertained when none of other options are available.

Conduit Configurations

In addition to choosing the best conduit for revascularization, different configurations can be used to maximize the use of limited or preferable conduits.

Sequenced grafting of a single conduit
The most commonly used alternative configuration is a sequenced graft, wherein a single conduit is used to graft multiple target vessels. The advantage of this technique is that it reduces operative time (only one proximal anastomosis is required per graft) and enables a more complete revascularization when conduit availability is limited. Sequenced saphenous vein grafts have higher long-term patency than single grafts.[41] The disadvantage is that sequenced targets served by a single graft are jeopardized if inflow is occluded or otherwise compromised.

Composite conduit grafting
Another option that is used when performing all arterial or majority arterial revascularization is to branch one arterial conduit off of a primary arterial conduit as a composite graft. This technique has been shown to have excellent long-term patency when performed by surgeons experienced with this approach.[44,45] The disadvantage of branched grafting is that it is technically challenging with a learning curve and can

jeopardize multiple vascular territories; it is particularly devastating if such a complication were to affect an LITA graft to the LAD territory.

COMBINED THERAPY

Combining PCI with DES and CABG to achieve LITA to LAD grafting and effectively treat multivessel CAD has attracted great interest in recent years. The concept behind this hybrid approach is to achieve the most complete and high-quality revascularization possible when all targets may not be suitable for grafting. Likewise, this strategy opens the possibility to use minimally invasive CABG techniques for LITA to LAD grafting and to complete treatment of other significant stenoses with PCI.

One randomized controlled trial that compared hybrid CABG/PCI with CABG found no difference in mortality or MACCE at 5 years; however, this was not powered to definitively prove equivalence.[46] Other retrospective studies have likewise suggested no difference in outcome between these 2 treatment strategies.[47] For selected patients this option is reasonable to consider.

TREATMENT FAILURE AND COMPLICATIONS

Although CABG is considered the superior treatment option for multivessel and left main CAD in appropriately selected patients, treatment failure necessitating repeat revascularization does occur; this can often be addressed by PCI, although there is occasionally a role for redo CABG. Approximately 2% of contemporary CABG procedures in the United States are redo operations.[48]

Perioperative mortality is increased in redo CABG compared with primary CABG, although long-term survival is similar.[48,49] The procedure should be performed at centers with a higher volume of redo cardiac surgery. The usual indication for redo CABG is primary graft failure leading to LAD territory ischemia. If the LITA is available, it should be used in these situations; otherwise, the best available remaining conduit should be chosen for grafting. In non-LAD bypass situations, decisions are made on an individual case basis with the Heart Team.

Preoperative preparation for redo CABG should be thorough. In addition to the usual diagnostic studies that are obtained to define progressive or recurrent disease, adjunct studies should be obtained. At a minimum, a contrasted CT of the chest should be performed to assess patient anatomy as well as patency and location of prior grafts. Surgeons should also identify and confirm the presence of the conduit they plan to use for revascularization.

INNOVATIVE APPROACHES AND NEW DEVELOPMENTS

Innovative surgical approaches have been developed for surgical revascularization as well. Hybrid revascularization was discussed earlier, but minimally invasive and off-pump techniques expand the surgeon's armamentarium to treat CAD as well.

Off-Pump Coronary Artery Bypass Grafting

The ability to perform surgical revascularization without having to cannulate, cross-clamp, or place a patient on cardiopulmonary bypass is advantageous for select patients. Debate regarding equivalence or superiority of CABG versus off-pump CABG (OPCAB) is robust. Three large randomized controlled trials have been performed over the past 2 decades, all with 5-year follow-up.[50–54] The ROOBY trial found that OPCAB had a higher 5-year mortality and lower graft patency.[53] The CORNARY and GOPCABE trials showed no difference in MACCE or mortality between OPCAB and traditional CABG.[52,54]

Others have argued that high-volume surgeons at high-volume centers can achieve OPCAB outcomes comparable to traditional CABG.[55,56] An important takeaway for OPCAB techniques is that they can be appropriate for the treatment of certain subgroups of patients, such as those with aortic disease that prevents cross-clamp application.

Minimally Invasive Approaches

Minimally invasive direct coronary artery bypass (MIDCAB) refers to a variation of OPCAB that uses a technique typically involving a small thoracotomy and off-pump LITA to LAD bypass grafting. This procedure has been refined in recent years to use robotic technology and revascularization of additional territories is possible. The benefits of this approach include less pain, shorter length of stay, and less scarring. The technique is superior in outcome compared with PCI with regard to long-term mortality and need for revascularization.[57] MIDCAB can be combined with PCI in a hybrid approach to allow for complete revascularization with the benefit of an LITA to LAD graft as well.

EVALUATION OF OUTCOME AND LONG-TERM RECOMMENDATIONS

Patients are typically discharged from the care of their CT surgeon after a postoperative visit if there are no complications. They will, however, require cardiology/medical follow-up and testing as indicated. Optimal GDMT is very important in the postoperative setting for best results. Full recommendations can be found in the 2015 AHA statement on postoperative therapy.[58] When symptoms of progressive or recurrent CAD occur, diagnostic evaluation using coronary catheterization is usually indicated.

SUMMARY

Surgical management of CAD has been refined over almost 6 decades and is the standard of care for coronary revascularization among patients with multivessel or unprotected left main CAD. The goal of surgical therapy is complete revascularization, and using arterial conduits, specifically the LITA to LAD, is advocated. Minimally invasive, OPCAB, and hybrid procedures may benefit subsets of patients for whom traditional CABG is not advised or who have conditions that are more suited to these techniques. Optimizing long-term outcomes depends on diligent medical follow-up and adherence to optimal postoperative medical therapy.

CLINICS CARE POINTS

- Surgical treatment of coronary artery disease is most safely done in an elective setting; therefore, screening at-risk patients to identify them prior to acute presentation is critical.

- A learning curve exists for off-pump and multi-arterial grafting techniques; surgeons should achieve proficiency in these techniques before they employ them in practice in order to ensure the best possible outcomes.- Failure to initiate and maintain medical therapy after surgical intervention will result in inferior long-term outcomes; therefore, it is imperative to ensure postoperative medical therapy (i.e., beta blockers, statins, and aspirin) is prescribed and medical follow up is ensured.

DISCLOSURE

The authors have nothing to disclose.

REFERENCES

1. Underlying cause of death 1999-2019. Centers for Disease Control and Prevention, National Center for Health Statistics. Available at: http://wonder.cdc.gov/ucd-icd10.html. Accessed 31 August 2021.
2. Kolesov VI, Potashov LV. [Surgery of coronary arteries]. Eksp Khir Anesteziol 1965;10(2):3–8. Operatsii na venechnykh arteriiakh serdtsa.
3. Kolesov VI. [Initial experience in the treatment of stenocardia by the formation of coronary-systemic vascular anastomoses]. Kardiologiia 1967;7(4):20–5. Pervyi opyt lecheniia stenokardii nalozheniem venechno-sistemnykh sosudistykh soust'ev.
4. Gruntzig A. Transluminal dilatation of coronary-artery stenosis. Lancet 1978; 1(8058):263.
5. Sigwart U, Puel J, Mirkovitch V, et al. Intravascular stents to prevent occlusion and restenosis after transluminal angioplasty. N Engl J Med 1987;316(12):701–6.
6. Sousa JE, Costa MA, Abizaid A, et al. Lack of neointimal proliferation after implantation of sirolimus-coated stents in human coronary arteries: a quantitative coronary angiography and three-dimensional intravascular ultrasound study. Circulation 2001;103(2):192–5.
7. Knuuti J, Wijns W, Saraste A, et al. 2019 ESC Guidelines for the diagnosis and management of chronic coronary syndromes. Eur Heart J 2020;41(3):407–77.
8. Anderson JL, Morrow DA. Acute Myocardial Infarction. N Engl J Med 2017; 376(21):2053–64.
9. Amsterdam EA, Wenger NK, Brindis RG, et al. 2014 AHA/ACC Guideline for the Management of Patients with Non-ST-Elevation Acute Coronary Syndromes: a report of the American College of Cardiology/American Heart Association Task Force on Practice Guidelines. J Am Coll Cardiol 2014;64(24):e139–228.
10. Katz D, Gavin MC. Stable Ischemic Heart Disease. Ann Intern Med 2019;171(3): ITC17–32.
11. Fihn SD, Gardin JM, Abrams J, et al. 2012 ACCF/AHA/ACP/AATS/PCNA/SCAI/STS Guideline for the diagnosis and management of patients with stable ischemic heart disease: a report of the American College of Cardiology Foundation/American Heart Association Task Force on Practice Guidelines, and the American College of Physicians, American Association for Thoracic Surgery, Preventive Cardiovascular Nurses Association, Society for Cardiovascular Angiography and Interventions, and Society of Thoracic Surgeons. J Am Coll Cardiol 2012;60(24):e44–164.
12. Myers J, Prakash M, Froelicher V, et al. Exercise capacity and mortality among men referred for exercise testing. N Engl J Med 2002;346(11):793–801.
13. Knuuti J, Ballo H, Juarez-Orozco LE, et al. The performance of non-invasive tests to rule-in and rule-out significant coronary artery stenosis in patients with stable angina: a meta-analysis focused on post-test disease probability. Eur Heart J 2018;39(35):3322–30.
14. Wohlgelernter D, Cleman M, Highman HA, et al. Regional myocardial dysfunction during coronary angioplasty: evaluation by two-dimensional echocardiography and 12 lead electrocardiography. J Am Coll Cardiol 1986;7(6):1245–54.
15. Hauser AM, Gangadharan V, Ramos RG, et al. Sequence of mechanical, electrocardiographic and clinical effects of repeated coronary artery occlusion in human

beings: echocardiographic observations during coronary angioplasty. J Am Coll Cardiol 1985;5(2 Pt 1):193–7.

16. Fleischmann KE, Hunink MG, Kuntz KM, et al. Exercise echocardiography or exercise SPECT imaging? A meta-analysis of diagnostic test performance. JAMA 1998;280(10):913–20.

17. Imran MB, Palinkas A, Picano E. Head-to-head comparison of dipyridamole echocardiography and stress perfusion scintigraphy for the detection of coronary artery disease: a meta-analysis. Comparison between stress echo and scintigraphy. Int J Cardiovasc Imaging 2003;19(1):23–8.

18. Picano E, Molinaro S, Pasanisi E. The diagnostic accuracy of pharmacological stress echocardiography for the assessment of coronary artery disease: a meta-analysis. Cardiovasc Ultrasound 2008;6:30.

19. Mc Ardle BA, Dowsley TF, deKemp RA, et al. Does rubidium-82 PET have superior accuracy to SPECT perfusion imaging for the diagnosis of obstructive coronary disease?: A systematic review and meta-analysis. J Am Coll Cardiol 2012; 60(18):1828–37.

20. Tarantini G, Cacciavillani L, Corbetti F, et al. Duration of ischemia is a major determinant of transmurality and severe microvascular obstruction after primary angioplasty: a study performed with contrast-enhanced magnetic resonance. J Am Coll Cardiol 2005;46(7):1229–35.

21. Pijls NH, De Bruyne B, Peels K, et al. Measurement of fractional flow reserve to assess the functional severity of coronary-artery stenoses. N Engl J Med 1996; 334(26):1703–8.

22. Fihn SD, Blankenship JC, Alexander KP, et al. 2014 ACC/AHA/AATS/PCNA/SCAI/ STS focused update of the guideline for the diagnosis and management of patients with stable ischemic heart disease: a report of the American College of Cardiology/American Heart Association Task Force on Practice Guidelines, and the American Association for Thoracic Surgery, Preventive Cardiovascular Nurses Association, Society for Cardiovascular Angiography and Interventions, and Society of Thoracic Surgeons. J Am Coll Cardiol 2014;64(18):1929–49.

23. Hillis LD, Smith PK, Anderson JL, et al. 2011 ACCF/AHA Guideline for Coronary Artery Bypass Graft Surgery. A report of the American College of Cardiology Foundation/American Heart Association Task Force on Practice Guidelines. Developed in collaboration with the American Association for Thoracic Surgery, Society of Cardiovascular Anesthesiologists, and Society of Thoracic Surgeons. J Am Coll Cardiol 2011;58(24):e123–210.

24. Levine GN, Bates ER, Bittl JA, et al. 2016 ACC/AHA Guideline Focused Update on Duration of Dual Antiplatelet Therapy in Patients With Coronary Artery Disease: A Report of the American College of Cardiology/American Heart Association Task Force on Clinical Practice Guidelines. J Am Coll Cardiol 2016;68(10):1082–115.

25. Holmes DR Jr, Rich JB, Zoghbi WA, et al. The heart team of cardiovascular care. J Am Coll Cardiol 2013;61(9):903–7.

26. Tsang MB, Schwalm JD, Gandhi S, et al. Comparison of heart team vs interventional cardiologist recommendations for the treatment of patients with multivessel coronary artery disease. JAMA Netw Open 2020;3(8):e2012749.

27. Serruys PW, Morice MC, Kappetein AP, et al. Percutaneous coronary intervention versus coronary-artery bypass grafting for severe coronary artery disease. N Engl J Med 2009;360(10):961–72.

28. Stone GW, Sabik JF, Serruys PW, et al. Everolimus-Eluting Stents or Bypass Surgery for Left Main Coronary Artery Disease. N Engl J Med 2016;375(23):2223–35.

29. Head SJ, Milojevic M, Daemen J, et al. Mortality after coronary artery bypass grafting versus percutaneous coronary intervention with stenting for coronary artery disease: a pooled analysis of individual patient data. Lancet 2018; 391(10124):939–48.

30. Davierwala PM, Gao C, Thuijs D, et al. Single or multiple arterial bypass graft surgery vs. percutaneous coronary intervention in patients with three-vessel or left main coronary artery disease. Eur Heart J 2021. https://doi.org/10.1093/eurheartj/ehab537.

31. Rocha RV, Tam DY, Karkhanis R, et al. Multiple arterial grafting is associated with better outcomes for coronary artery bypass grafting patients. Circ 2018;138(19): 2081–90.

32. Esper RB, Farkouh ME, Ribeiro EE, et al. SYNTAX Score in patients with diabetes undergoing coronary revascularization in the FREEDOM trial. J Am Coll Cardiol 2018;72(23 Pt A):2826–37.

33. Peterson MD, Borger MA, Rao V, et al. Skeletonization of bilateral internal thoracic artery grafts lowers the risk of sternal infection in patients with diabetes. J Thorac Cardiovasc Surg 2003;126(5):1314–9.

34. Sa MP, Ferraz PE, Escobar RR, et al. Skeletonized versus pedicled internal thoracic artery and risk of sternal wound infection after coronary bypass surgery: meta-analysis and meta-regression of 4817 patients. Interact Cardiovasc Thorac Surg 2013;16(6):849–57.

35. Ding WJ, Ji Q, Shi YQ, et al. Incidence of deep sternal wound infection in diabetic patients undergoing off-pump skeletonized internal thoracic artery grafting. Cardiology 2016;133(2):111–8.

36. Tatoulis J, Buxton BF, Fuller JA. The right internal thoracic artery: the forgotten conduit–5,766 patients and 991 angiograms. Ann Thorac Surg 2011;92(1):9–15 [discussion 15-17].

37. Tatoulis J, Buxton BF, Fuller JA. Results of 1,454 free right internal thoracic artery-to-coronary artery grafts. Ann Thorac Surg 1997;64(5):1263–8 [discussion: 1268-1269].

38. Sabik JF 3rd, Stockins A, Nowicki ER, et al. Does location of the second internal thoracic artery graft influence outcome of coronary artery bypass grafting? Circulation 2008;118(14 Suppl):S210–5.

39. Gaudino M, Audisio K, Rahouma M, et al. Comparison of long-term clinical outcomes of skeletonized vs pedicled internal thoracic artery harvesting techniques in the arterial revascularization trial. JAMA Cardiol 2021. https://doi.org/10.1001/jamacardio.2021.3866.

40. Sabik JF 3rd, Lytle BW, Blackstone EH, et al. Comparison of saphenous vein and internal thoracic artery graft patency by coronary system. Ann Thorac Surg 2005; 79(2):544–51 [discussion: 544-551].

41. Vural KM, Sener E, Tasdemir O. Long-term patency of sequential and individual saphenous vein coronary bypass grafts. Eur J Cardiothorac Surg 2001;19(2): 140–4.

42. Goldman S, Zadina K, Moritz T, et al. Long-term patency of saphenous vein and left internal mammary artery grafts after coronary artery bypass surgery: results from a Department of Veterans Affairs Cooperative Study. J Am Coll Cardiol 2004;44(11):2149–56.

43. Tian M, Wang X, Sun H, et al. No-touch versus conventional vein harvesting techniques at 12 months after coronary artery bypass grafting surgery: multicenter randomized, controlled trial. Circulation 2021. https://doi.org/10.1161/CIRCULATIONAHA.121.055525.

44. Kim KB, Hwang HY, Hahn S, et al. A randomized comparison of the Saphenous Vein Versus Right Internal Thoracic Artery as a Y-Composite Graft (SAVE RITA) trial: one-year angiographic results and mid-term clinical outcomes. J Thorac Cardiovasc Surg 2014;148(3):901–7 [discussion: 907-908].

45. Kim MS, Hwang HY, Kim JS, et al. Saphenous vein versus right internal thoracic artery as a Y-composite graft: five-year angiographic and clinical results of a randomized trial. J Thorac Cardiovasc Surg 2018;156(4):1424–33.e1.

46. Ganyukov V, Kochergin N, Shilov A, et al. Randomized clinical trial of surgical vs. percutaneous vs. hybrid revascularization in multivessel coronary artery disease: residual myocardial ischemia and clinical outcomes at one year-hybrid coronary REvascularization Versus Stenting or Surgery (HREVS). J Interv Cardiol 2020; 2020:5458064. https://doi.org/10.1155/2020/5458064.

47. Basman C, Hemli JM, Kim MC, et al. Long-term survival in triple-vessel disease: Hybrid coronary revascularization compared to contemporary revascularization methods. J Card Surg 2020;35(10):2710–8.

48. Elbadawi A, Hamed M, Elgendy IY, et al. Outcomes of Reoperative Coronary Artery Bypass Graft Surgery in the United States. J Am Heart Assoc 2020;9(15): e016282.

49. Gallo M, Trivedi JR, Monreal G, et al. Risk factors and outcomes in redo coronary artery Bypass Grafting. Heart Lung Circ 2020;29(3):384–9.

50. Shroyer AL, Grover FL, Hattler B, et al. On-pump versus off-pump coronary-artery bypass surgery. N Engl J Med 2009;361(19):1827–37.

51. Lamy A, Devereaux PJ, Prabhakaran D, et al. Effects of off-pump and on-pump coronary-artery bypass grafting at 1 year. N Engl J Med 2013;368(13):1179–88.

52. Lamy A, Devereaux PJ, Prabhakaran D, et al. Five-year outcomes after off-pump or on-pump coronary-artery bypass grafting. N Engl J Med 2016;375(24): 2359–68.

53. Shroyer AL, Hattler B, Wagner TH, et al. Five-year outcomes after on-pump and off-pump coronary-artery bypass. N Engl J Med 2017;377(7):623–32.

54. Diegeler A, Borgermann J, Kappert U, et al. Five-Year Outcome After Off-Pump or On-Pump Coronary Artery Bypass Grafting in Elderly Patients. Circulation 2019; 139(16):1865–71.

55. Polomsky M, He X, O'Brien SM, et al. Outcomes of off-pump versus on-pump coronary artery bypass grafting: Impact of preoperative risk. J Thorac Cardiovasc Surg 2013;145(5):1193–8.

56. Taggart DP, Gaudino MF, Gerry S, et al. Ten-year outcomes after off-pump versus on-pump coronary artery bypass grafting: Insights from the Arterial Revascularization Trial. J Thorac Cardiovasc Surg 2021;162(2):591–9.e8.

57. Benedetto U, Raja SG, Soliman RF, et al. Minimally invasive direct coronary artery bypass improves late survival compared with drug-eluting stents in isolated proximal left anterior descending artery disease: a 10-year follow-up, single-center, propensity score analysis. J Thorac Cardiovasc Surg 2014;148(4):1316–22.

58. Kulik A, Ruel M, Jneid H, et al. Secondary prevention after coronary artery bypass graft surgery: a scientific statement from the American Heart Association. Circ 2015;131(10):927–64.

Evaluation and Treatment of Massive Hemoptysis

Beau Prey, MD[a],*, Andrew Francis, MD[a], James Williams, MD[a],
Bahirathan Krishnadasan, MD[b]

KEYWORDS

- Massive hemoptysis • Life-threatening hemoptysis • Bronchial artery • Embolization
- Bronchoscopy

KEY POINTS

- Massive hemoptysis is a life-threatening condition that requires immediate airway control from a multidisciplinary team.
- Patients with massive hemoptysis die from asphyxiation, not blood loss.
- Early management should include securing an airway for ventilation, followed by localization, and hemorrhage control.

INTRODUCTION
Background

Massive hemoptysis is a life-threatening airway hemorrhage with a historically poor prognosis. Conservative management alone has a mortality rate up to 75%.[1,2] As a result, emergent surgical management via an open thoracotomy was the primary method for localizing and controlling bleeding. This approach effectively reduced the mortality rates to less than 20% by the late 1970s.[2] Modern advancements in computed tomography (CT), bronchoscopy, and angiography/embolization have continued to reduce mortality through improved localization and hemorrhage control techniques. Bronchoscopy has become the most expeditious and effective method for acutely managing hemoptysis that is causing respiratory failure. Advancements in the capability of interventional radiology (IR) to identify and embolize the bleeding source have provided a minimally invasive, nonsurgical option for hemorrhage control.[3]

In addition, and perhaps critically, early activation of a multidisciplinary team to secure the airway and localize the source of bleeding is the most important immediate

[a] General Surgery Department, Madigan Army Medical Center, 9040 Jackson Avenue, Tacoma, WA 98431, USA; [b] Cardiothoracic Surgery, St. Joseph Medical Center, 1802 S. Yakima Avenue, Tacoma, WA 98405, USA
* Corresponding author.
E-mail address: bjprey@gmail.com

Surg Clin N Am 102 (2022) 465–481
https://doi.org/10.1016/j.suc.2021.11.002
0039-6109/22/Published by Elsevier Inc.
surgical.theclinics.com

action. Targeted blood product–based resuscitation, early correction of coagulopathies, and intensive care unit (ICU) management are also critical. Collectively, these techniques have reduced mortality rates to 13% to 17.8% over the past 50 years.[4–6]

Definition

Historically, the definition of massive hemoptysis has focused on the volume of blood lost per hour and per day. A common definition was 300 to 600 mL per 24 hours or 3 episodes of hemoptysis in 1 week,[7–11] but recommended values range widely in the literature, from 100 mL per 24 hours to 1000 mL per 24 hours or 100 mL/h[10,12–14] In one retrospective study of 1087 patients followed-up over a 14-year period, the average volume of blood loss in life-threatening hemoptysis was only 218 mL.[15] However, the diagnosis of massive hemoptysis should be made by assessing the patient, not measuring blood loss. More important than the specific rate or volume of expectorated blood loss (provided that can even be measured or accurately estimated) is the clinical effect the bleeding has on the patient. Patients with massive hemoptysis die from asphyxiation, not hemorrhagic shock; an understandable outcome given the mean total volume of the conducting airways in adults is only 150 mL.[16] This volume explains how a small amount of blood, if aspirated into the contralateral lung, can cause airway obstruction, respiratory failure, and death.

A better paradigm is to replace the term massive hemoptysis with life-threatening hemoptysis; if the patient develops respiratory failure, airway obstruction, or hypotension.[17] As with any life-threatening airway problem, identification and management must be prompt. Instead of attempts to quantify the volume or rate of blood loss, brisk hemoptysis should simply be recognized and its clinical effects assessed. In addition, providers must consider the patient's underlying physiologic reserve and comorbidities, as well as the capabilities and limitations of their personnel, facility, and equipment. Most patients with life-threatening hemoptysis have compromised lung function. A relatively small bleed may become life threatening simply due to patient factors or facility limitations.

Anatomy

The lungs are supplied by 2 vascular circulations, a low-pressure pulmonary arterial circuit (mean arterial pressure [MAP] 12–16 mm Hg), and a high-pressure bronchial arterial circuit (MAP 100 mm Hg). Life-threatening hemoptysis arises from the high-pressure bronchial arterial circuit in 90% of cases. The remaining 10% arise from the aorta (eg, aortobronchial fistula), nonbronchial systemic circulation (intercostals, coronaries, thoracic branches from the axillary and subclavian arteries, and the phrenic arteries), or the pulmonary vessels.[18–21] The pulmonary circuit is unlikely to cause life-threatening hemoptysis, as it interacts directly with the airway only at the level of the terminal bronchioles.[22,23] If, however, the main pulmonary artery or its proximal branches rupture, the volume of bleeding will be high and the patient's prognosis is poor.[7]

As stated previously, the bronchial arteries are responsible for most of the life-threatening hemoptysis. These arteries typically originate directly or indirectly from the aorta at the level of T3 to T8, most commonly from T5 to T6.[24] Bronchial arterial anatomy is highly variable, however, with up to 20% of patients having anomalous bronchial arteries arising from other systemic arteries. In 5% of patients, the bronchial artery branches into a spinal artery. As a result, embolization of the bronchial artery can cause spinal cord ischemia in 1.4% to 6.5% of cases.[25,26] These anatomic variations are critically important to consider when pursuing hemorrhage control.

Pathophysiology

Regardless of the location of the bleed, the pathophysiology involves derangements of the vasculature secondary to underlying lung disease. Chronic inflammation from infection or malignancy causes hypertrophy and tortuosity of the native bronchial arteries. Simultaneously, neovascularization, from the release of proangiogenic factors (eg, vascular endothelial growth factor and angiopoietin-1) leads to the development of new, thin-walled, fragile vessels.[27,28] These vascular derangements increase the probability of bleeding, especially from the high-pressure bronchial circuit. The exact pathophysiology causing these vascular derangements varies with each underlying cause. Suffice it to say, patients with the underlying causes discussed in the next section are more likely to develop hemoptysis.

Epidemiology

Life-threatening hemoptysis is uncommon. Only a small minority of patients at risk for hemoptysis will actually experience an episode of hemoptysis, which is likely to be limited to a single episode and to be non–life threatening. However, when life-threatening hemoptysis occurs, it invariably indicates a severe underlying disease.[29] In lung cancer, for example, 80% of patients will never develop hemoptysis, 19.4% of patients will develop non–life-threatening hemoptysis, and only 0.6% will develop life-threatening hemoptysis. Rarely does life-threatening hemoptysis present without warning signs, such as a sentinel bleed. Sentinel bleeding is reported in 80% of patients who develop malignancy-related life-threatening hemoptysis.[30–32] Any patient who reports symptoms consistent with a sentinel bleed should raise immediate concern.

Causes of life-threatening hemoptysis are provided in **Table 1**. The most common cause worldwide remains tuberculosis, with lung cancer being most prevalent in developed countries.[33,34] Pulmonary aspergillosis, bronchiectasis, necrotizing pneumonia, and cryptogenic (idiopathic) hemoptysis are the other most common causes. Identification of the cause of hemoptysis is important because the underlying derangements affect the patient's physiologic reserve, the probable location of the bleed, the probability of developing life-threatening hemorrhage, and the probability of recurrent hemorrhage. Recurrent hemoptysis is most often associated with cancer, aspergilloma, and bronchiectasis and tends to portend a higher mortality rate.[35]

Hemoptysis may also occur iatrogenically following clinical procedures such as transbronchial biopsies. Patient selection and preprocedure medical optimization are paramount.[3] Medications should be reconciled, anticoagulants should be held, and any coagulopathies should be reversed. Low-dose aspirin, however, has been shown to be safely continued for transbronchial lung biopsies.[36] Platelets should be generally maintained greater than 50,000 before a procedure. Other considerations, such as patient positioning and necessary equipment, should be confirmed before the procedure. For transbronchial biopsies specifically, some experts recommend routine use of bronchial blockers (or Fogarty balloons) to isolate procedural bleeding.[37] The procedure may also affect whether a rigid or flexible bronchoscope is used.[38]

Pulmonary artery (PA) rupture is a rare cause of massive hemoptysis, but is often lethal, and may be seen in the setting of tuberculosis or following the rupture of a Rasmussen aneurysm. The prevalence of these aneurysms ranges from 5% to 8% and is most often seen in geographic locations with a high prevalence of tuberculosis.[39] Pulmonary artery rupture may also be seen following procedural intervention.[3] For example, PA rupture may occur as a result of instrumentation of the pulmonary artery with a Swan-Ganz catheter.[40] The reported incidence of catheter-related rupture

Table 1 Causes of massive hemoptysis[3,7]	
Autoimmune	Diffuse Alveolar hemorrhage
	Goodpasture syndrome
	Granulomatous polyangiitis
	Microscopic polyangiitis
	Nodular polyangiitis
	Rheumatoid arthritis
	Systemic lupus erythematosus
	Systemic sclerosis
Cardiovascular	Aortic aneurysm
	Arteriovenous malformation
	Bronchial arterial fistula
	Congenital heart disease
	Congestive heart failure
	Mitral stenosis
	Pulmonary embolism/infarction
	Primary pulmonary hypertension
Iatrogenic	Aortobronchial fistula following aortic graft or other surgery
	Bevacizumab
	Endobronchial brachytherapy
	Erosion of airway stent
	Lung transplant
	Pulmonary artery rupture from right-sided heart catheterization
	Pulmonary injury from chest tube placement or thoracentesis
	Pulmonary vein stenosis after radio frequency ablation
	Thrombolytic therapy
	Tracheoinnominate artery fistula after tracheostomy
	Transbronchial lung biopsy/cryobiopsy
	Transthoracic needle aspiration
Infectious	Bronchiectasis (cystic fibrosis)
	Bacterial/viral bronchitis/pneumonia
	Flukes and parasites
	Invasive pulmonary fungal disease (aspergillosis, mycetomas)
	Lung abscess
	Necrotizing pneumonia
	Septic pulmonary embolism
Hematologic	Iatrogenic coagulopathies from anticoagulant and/or antiplatelet medications
	Platelet disease
	TTP
Miscellaneous	Idiopathic/cryptogenic (20%)
	Cocaine
	Foreign body aspiration
Pulmonary	Bronchiectasis (cystic fibrosis)
	Broncholithiasis
	Lymphangioleiomyomatosis
	Malignancy
	Pulmonary embolism/infarction
Trauma	Blunt or penetrating injuries
	Blast injuries
	Pseudohemoptysis

ranges between 0.03% and 0.2%, with mortality rates higher than 50%.[41] Catheter-related ruptures tend to be the result of balloon overdistention, with perforation by catheter tip being a less common cause.[42,43] A postmortem study found that the curvature of the PA catheter favored insertion into the right pulmonary arterial system, particularly the right lower and middle lobe branches, which could explain why roughly 70% of PA ruptures occur on the right side,[44] and this should be kept in mind during the initial management and treatment of hemoptysis in patients with a recent history of pulmonary artery instrumentation.[45]

DISCUSSION
Case Presentation

A 36-year-old female patient is transported by ambulance to the emergency department with reports of massive hemoptysis but no active hemorrhage. She has a history of histoplasmosis complicated by mediastinitis and development of a traction diverticulum. Two months before arrival, following appropriate treatment of the histoplasmosis, she underwent robotic resection of the diverticulum, which was complicated by a left bronchoesophageal fistula. The patient is now 1 month out from placement of an esophageal stent.

On presentation to the emergency department, she is stable without active hemorrhage or coagulopathy. She is admitted to the ICU with a plan for bronchoscopy, esophagogastroduodenoscopy, and esophageal stent repositioning/placement. Before the operation, she experiences a recurrent episode of hemoptysis, resulting in tachycardia and hypotension, but without respiratory distress. A blood transfusion is initiated and the patient responds appropriately, remaining hemodynamically stable with appropriate oxygenation in the ICU. She does not require intubation at this time. She proceeds urgently to the operating room and undergoes the procedures stated earlier with a multidisciplinary team including thoracic surgery and pulmonology. The location of the hemorrhage is presumed to be the known bronchoesophageal fistula. Bronchoscopy demonstrates active bleeding and granulation tissue at the fistula site, in the proximal bronchus intermedius; this is irrigated with ice cold normal saline with epinephrine followed by injection of tranexamic acid (TXA) into the fistula. The previous esophageal stent is repositioned proximally, and a second stent is placed through the gastroesophageal junction, overlapping the first stent. Significant clot is visualized in the patient's stomach during the procedure but there is no evidence of active hemorrhage. An air insufflation test with concomitant bronchoscopy demonstrates no further leak of air through the fistula site. A nasogastric tube is placed through the stents. Given the concern for a possible aortoenteric esophageal fistula, postprocedurally, she is taken to the ICU and IR is consulted.

Shortly after arrival in the ICU, she again develops large-volume hemoptysis with associated respiratory distress. The Massive Transfusion Protocol (MTP) is initiated. She goes into cardiac arrest, with return of pulses after 2 rounds of advanced cardiac life support. She is not placed in the lateral decubitus position due to the need for cardiopulmonary resuscitation. Her hemodynamics improve with continued resuscitation, and she is transferred urgently to IR for embolization of presumed bronchial artery bleed. Catheterization of the bronchial artery demonstrates immediate extravasation into the esophagus and subsequent communication with the trachea. An aortoenteric tracheal fistula is visualized on angiography. Vascular surgery is consulted. The patient is successfully treated with coil embolization of the left bronchial artery by IR followed by endovascular placement of a thoracic covered endograft with vascular surgery (**Figs. 1** and **2**). Following surgery, she remained intubated and sedated and was transferred to the ICU, in stable condition, with on-going targeted blood product–based resuscitation to reverse coagulopathies.

Although this patient is a unique case with a rare cause of life-threatening hemoptysis, her case illustrates several key points in the management of these patients:

- Her airway was frequently reassessed, aggressively maintained, and remained a priority throughout.
- Despite the fact that she was no longer actively bleeding at presentation, the suspicion for recurrent bleeding was high based on her history, and she was appropriately placed in the ICU.

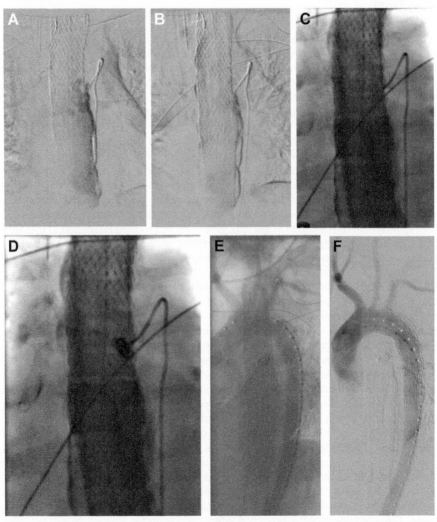

Fig. 1. (*A*) Initial angiogram showing contrast extravasation. Note the previously placed esophageal stent. (*B*) Angiogram showing contrast extravasation into the proximal bronchus and trachea. The catheter is positioned in the aorta with its tip at the level of the known fistula, demonstrating communication between the aorta and the airways. (*C*) Pre-bronchial artery embolization. (*D*) Postbronchial artery embolization. (*E*) Pre-TEVAR employment. Note contrast in the respiratory tree. (*F*) Post-TEVAR deployment.

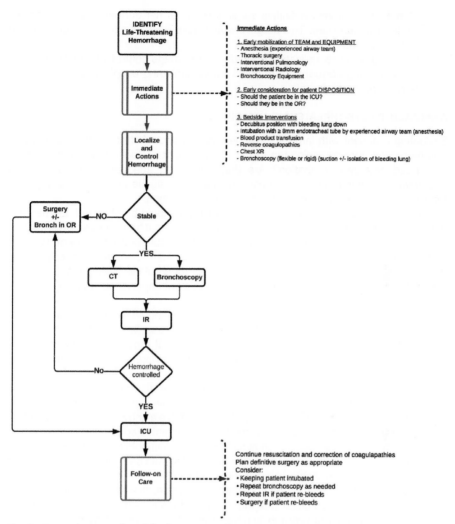

Fig. 2. General approach to life-threatening hemoptysis. Initial evaluation

- Bronchoscopy was used to localize and temporize her hemorrhage. This occurred in the operating room with an experienced airway team (anesthesia).
- The patient remained intubated in the immediate postoperative period, given the likelihood of recurrent hemorrhage and the need for reintubation and transport to IR. Leaving the patient intubated also facilitates additional bronchoscopies as needed.
- A multidisciplinary team was involved in her care from the beginning.
- A prompt and effective blood product resuscitation was initiated, allowing the patient to be stabilized and safely transported to IR for nonsurgical efforts at hemorrhage control.
- Bronchial artery embolization (BAE) was used successfully as a minimally invasive hemorrhage control technique, allowing the patient to avoid an emergent surgery. Although not discussed in the aforementioned scenario, the patient

ultimately underwent definitive surgical repair of her aortoesophageal tracheal fistula at a later date. This surgery would have been significantly more difficult and dangerous in the acute setting.

- This case also saw utilization of unique hemorrhage control interventions, given the underlying aortoenteric tracheal fistula, including esophageal stents and a thoracic aortic endograft.

APPROACH TO LIFE-THREATENING HEMOPTYSIS

Evaluating a patient with large-volume hemoptysis should start similarly to that of a trauma patient, by addressing the ABCs. Is the patient protecting their airway, or do they need emergent intubation? Are they ventilating adequately? Do they have adequate intravenous access? These questions should be answered rapidly, and resuscitation should begin with blood product transfusion.

When permitted, a thorough history and physical should be obtained. Elements in the questioning and examination should be able to rule out hemoptysis from epistaxis or hematemesis. Clues as to the underlying cause should become evident, whether that be previous infectious symptoms, recent airway instrumentation, underlying pulmonary disease or malignancy, or risk factors for tuberculosis. Medications, particularly anticoagulants and antiplatelets, are of significant importance, as they may be a source of reversible bleeding risk.

Laboratory assessment: initial laboratory evaluation should include type and cross-matching of blood products, complete blood counts, coagulation panel, liver and kidney function, and arterial blood gas. These results will provide critical information, including possible clues as to reversible causes of bleeding, such as coagulopathies, thrombocytopenia, or uremic platelet dysfunction.

Imaging modalities: more important than determining the cause of life-threatening hemoptysis is distinguishing the side from which the bleeding is originating. In some instances, this may be obvious, as the patient may have a known lung lesion or recent instrumentation that has precipitated the bleeding event. Regardless of whether the location is known or unknown, the first radiologic study should be a chest radiograph. Although this study has limited sensitivity (46%),[46] it should be implemented early, as it is quick and readily available in most circumstances. If the hemorrhage has been temporized, and the patient is hemodynamically stable, they should proceed to the CT scanner for dedicated chest imaging. A CT angiogram of the chest is a more sensitive tool than a chest radiograph to determine both the site and cause of bleeding, with a success rate of 70% and 77%, respectively.[1]

Imaging studies are great in the appropriate clinical setting, but the ideal diagnostic tool for massive hemoptysis is bronchoscopy. Bronchoscopy is readily available, can be performed at the bedside, aids with intubation efforts, localizes bleeding in about 50% to 93% of cases depending on rate of hemorrhage, and provides opportunity for various therapeutic options.[34,47,48] Bronchoscopy is discussed in greater detail later on in this article.

MANAGEMENT

The immediate priority should always be airway control in these patients. Intubation is usually required in life-threatening hemoptysis and ideally is performed by a trained anesthesiologist, preferably with a large-bore (≥8 mm) endotracheal tube. The large bore provides an adequate working channel for ongoing therapeutic interventions. Once the airway is protected, and the side of bleeding has been determined, the bleeding lung needs to be isolated to allow for ongoing ventilation. Placing the patient in the decubitus position, with the bleeding lung in the dependent position, allows ventilation of the unaffected side. This position prevents spillage of blood over the carina into the nonbleeding lung. The bronchus of the bleeding lung should ideally be occluded with a bronchial blocker or Fogarty balloon, resulting in a tamponade effect and preventing contamination of the contralateral lung. In the absence of these tools, the mainstem bronchus of the nonbleeding lung can be selectively intubated, thus allowing ongoing ventilation and potential occlusion of the opposite bronchus with the bronchial cuff. This method of intubation does not allow for intervention via fiberoptic bronchoscopy but is a temporizing measure that allows for ongoing ventilation while awaiting further treatment.

Dual-lumen endotracheal tubes seem as an attractive option, as they are frequently used in thoracic surgery for single lung ventilation. However, dual-lumen tubes should not be used in the setting of massive hemoptysis, as the lumens are too narrow to allow for therapeutic interventions. Instead, endotracheal tubes with an internal diameter of at least 8 mm are preferred, as they can accommodate a standard flexible bronchoscope.[49]

Once the airway has been secured, resuscitative efforts can attempt to replace blood loss and correct any coagulopathies. If the patient is hemodynamically stable, they can proceed to the CT scanner in order to localize the bleed or proceed to more definitive treatment options.

Bronchoscopy: bronchoscopy is an effective tool in the management of massive hemoptysis, as it serves a plethora of roles, from localization of bleeding, assisting with intubation, removal of blood from the airway, as well as a variety of therapeutic interventions.

Bronchoscope selection: whether the patient is stable with a slow bleed, or in extremis, flexible bronchoscopy is a quick and reliable tool that can be implemented at bedside in the emergency department, ICU, or operating room.

Although flexible bronchoscopy is convenient, and relatively easy to use, it has limited suction capabilities, and the visual field can be blurred or occluded quite easily. Rigid bronchoscopy, although technically more challenging, provides several benefits over flexible bronchoscopy. The rigid bronchoscope allows for more rigorous suction, while also facilitating ongoing ventilation of the healthy lung.[50] The larger working channel of the rigid bronchoscope makes clot evacuation and visualization easier and allows for concomitant use of other instrumentation, including flexible bronchoscope, bronchial blockers, and thermal ablation instruments. With the correct technical expertise, a rigid bronchoscope is the preferred endobronchial device in massive hemoptysis.

Endobronchial adjuncts: a commonly implemented tool in the setting of life-threatening hemoptysis is a bronchial blocker. These are inflatable balloons at the end of a catheter that can be placed to occlude a selected portion of the airway. Bronchial blockers serve 2 primary roles. First, they limit bleeding in a fixed volume, providing back pressure to assist with tamponade on the vessel, and thus contributing to hemostasis. Second, it contains the bleeding to one location, thus preserving the contralateral lung for ventilation.

Instillation of ice-cold saline is often used, with the thought that it promotes vasoconstriction at the affected site. There have been several small studies looking at the effectiveness of ice-cold saline in massive hemoptysis. One small series looked at 12 patients with massive hemoptysis (defined by expectoration of 600 mL of blood in 24 hours) who were treated with ice cold (4°C) saline lavage. All 12 patients stopped bleeding with this effort. Of those 12, 5 rebled during their same admission, but hemostasis was obtained in all of those with repeat lavage. The major side effect noted from this treatment is bradycardia. Ultimately, ice-cold saline lavages are a quick and readily available option for combatting life-threatening hemoptysis.[51]

Similar to cold saline lavage, endobronchial administration of epinephrine also causes vasoconstriction, although its efficacy in life-threatening hemoptysis is debated. Opponents of endobronchial epinephrine believe profuse hemorrhage will wash away epinephrine from the area of interest before it has the opportunity to work. Complications associated with endobronchial epinephrine include coronary vasospasm and arrhythmia.[52] For these reasons, epinephrine should be used cautiously in the patient with underlying coronary artery disease.[53]

TXA is an antifibrinolytic that has been studied extensively in patients with hemorrhagic trauma and is useful in the management life-threatening hemoptysis.[54] Both intravenous and nebulized TXA have been shown to be effective in decreasing bleeding and the need for further intervention in hemoptysis.[55,56]

There are also several thermoablative options to consider. Argon plasma coagulation, electrocautery, and neodymium-doped yttrium aluminum garnet laser, all have utility for hemostasis in the setting of large airway disease, particularly malignancy.[57] Importantly, these should not be used if the patient is requiring greater than 0.40 fraction of inspired oxygen (Fio_2) due to the risk of airway fire.[58,59]

Lastly, multiple other medications and endobronchial adjuncts have been proved useful for managing life-threatening hemoptysis. Various surgical hemostatic agents, including oxidized regenerated cellulose (Surgicel), gelatin-thrombin matrix (Floseal), silicone spigots (Endobronchial Watanabe Spigot), polymer surgical sealant (Coseal), and airway stents have all demonstrated utility to some degree in the setting of life-threatening hemoptysis.[60–63]

ENDOVASCULAR TREATMENTS

Bronchial artery embolization: following airway securement and stabilization, most of the patients with massive hemoptysis will require definitive treatment. First described in 1973, BAE has become the first-line, nonsurgical treatment of hemoptysis.[64] Following percutaneous access, typically via the femoral artery, an arteriogram is used to identify the bronchial arteries or nonbronchial systemic collaterals. Although it is rare to visualize active extravasation on angiography, there are other angiographic signs to identify culprit vessels for embolization, listed in **Box 1**.[9,65] Once identified, embolizing agents such as gelatin sponge, polyvinyl alcohol, N-butyl cyanoacrylate, metallic coils, and microspheres can be used intravascularly to occlude the vessel.[66]

A 2017 systematic review of 22 articles on BAE from 1976 to 2016 found that the immediate success rate, defined as complete cessation of hemoptysis, varied from 70% to 99%.[66] However, recurrence rates are high, with up to 57.5% of patients experiencing recurrent hemoptysis following initial embolization.[66] The mean time to

---

Box 1
Angiographic signs that suggest source of bleeding

1. Hypertrophy/enlarged (>3 mm in diameter) tortuous bronchial arteries with parenchymal hypervascularity and parenchymal staining

2. Bronchial artery aneurysms

3. Bronchial artery to pulmonary vein shunting

4. Bronchial artery to pulmonary artery shunting

5. Active extravasation

Table 2
Comparison of modern interventions for life-threatening hemoptysis

	Chest Radiograph	Computed Tomography	Flexible Bronchoscopy	Rigid Bronchoscopy	Angiography Bronchial Artery Embolization	Surgery
Portable/rapid (available at bedside)	++++	0	++	+	0	0
Simple to employ (technically, logistically)	++++	+++	++	+	0	0
Diagnostic (able to localize bleeding)	+	++++	++	++	+++	++
Diagnostic (able to identify cause)	0	++++	++	++	+	++++
Therapeutic (airway control)	0	0	++++	++++	0	0
Therapeutic (hemorrhage control)	0	0	++	+++	++++	++++
Appropriate for UNSTABLE patient	+	0	++	++	+	++++

hemoptysis recurrence is typically between 6 months and 1 year. Reasons for early recurrence include inadequate or incomplete embolization, whereas late recurrences are attributed to recanalization of embolized vessels, neovascularization, and underlying disease progression. BAE may be repeated to manage recurrent episodes of hemoptysis. Hemoptysis recurrence rates are higher in patients with aspergillomas, active tuberculosis, and underlying lung malignancy.[66] In such cases, BAE is often at best a temporary measure before surgical resection if the patient is a surgical candidate.[67] However, there are data to suggest that patients who are recurrence free for 36 months are unlikely to experience recurrent hemoptysis following successful initial BAE.[68] Despite advancements in embolization technology, recurrence rates remain unchanged over the past 40 years.[66]

Overall major complications from BAE including neurologic complications from in-advertent spinal artery embolization, bronchial-esophageal fistula, and gastrointestinal tract necrosis were low, occurring in less than 6.6% of patients.[66] The most common complications following BAE include transient chest/back pain and dysphagia occurring in up to 34.5% and 30% of patients, respectively.[66,69]

Surgical treatments: historically surgery was the only option available to manage massive hemoptysis but was associated with high morbidity and mortality. However, with improvements in imaging modalities, bronchoscopy, and interventional radiology, surgery is no longer the recommended first-line treatment in most of the cases. Unlike BAE, surgery offers a definitive cure if the offending portion of tissue can be safely excised.

With advances in surgical technique, including laparoscopic and robotic-assisted surgery, and improvements in postoperative care there has been renewed interest in surgery for management of massive hemoptysis. Recent studies examining the timing and role of surgery for managing massive hemoptysis have demonstrated lower mortality and complication rates if surgery can be delayed until after bleeding is controlled through other means.[70–72] In a retrospective review of 111 patients who underwent surgical lung resection for massive hemoptysis Andréjak and colleagues noted that fewer patients underwent pneumonectomy (17% vs 23%) if surgery was performed after bleeding was controlled.[70] Likewise, postoperative complications, including the need for mechanical ventilation, blood product transfusion, need for pressors, bronchopleural fistula, pneumonia, and hospital-acquired infection, were also reduced from 71% to 28% in the delayed surgical group.[70] The investigators also noted that both emergency surgery and pneumonectomy independently predicted complications including mortality.[70] Ideally, every effort should be made to control bleeding before surgery, as both mortality and morbidity increase with emergent surgical resection.[70–72] However, there are still circumstances where surgery is indicated for first-line therapy including pulmonary artery rupture, complex arteriovenous malformations, or refractory hemoptysis in the setting of benign lung disease and chest wall trauma.[73–75] In addition, surgery remains an option if hemorrhage control cannot be obtained through other less invasive means.

SUMMARY

Massive hemoptysis is more appropriately defined as life-threatening hemoptysis that causes airway obstruction, respiratory failure, and/or hypotension. Patients with this condition die from asphyxiation, not hemorrhagic shock. Any patient who presents with life-threatening hemoptysis requires immediate treatment to secure the airway and stabilize the patient. Early activation and coordinated response from a multidisciplinary team is critical. Once the airway is secure and appropriate resuscitation is initiated, priorities are to localize the source of the bleeding and gain hemorrhage control. Nonsurgical control of hemorrhage is superior to surgery in the acute situation. Most of these patients will require ICU level care.

Immediate actions to stabilize the patient and secure the airway include placement of the patient in the decubitus position with bleeding lung down, intubation with greater than or equal to 8 mm endotracheal tube, blood product transfusion and reversal of coagulopathies, bronchoscopy (to aid in securing the airway via suction, isolation of the bleeding lung via bronchial blocker or placement of the endotracheal tube in the main stem bronchus, and application of hemostatic adjuncts), engagement of a multidisciplinary team (including ICU, interventional radiology, thoracic surgery, interventional pulmonology, anesthesiology), and placement of the patient in the ICU.

Diagnostic options include chest radiography, CT, and bronchoscopy. Chest radiography is a quick, bedside tool that may be able to identify the side of the bleed. Both CT and bronchoscopy are capable of localizing the source of the bleed, and the combination of the 2 is more effective than each alone. CT is also capable of providing insight into the underlying cause of the bleeding. Angiography is capable of localizing the bleed in the event, whereas CT and bronchoscopy were unable to do so. The ability of IR to localize the bleed in a timely manner is significantly aided by information gained via CT and bronchoscopy; therefore, if the patient is stable, CT should be obtained.

Treatment options include early bronchoscopy as described earlier and angiography followed by BAE. In the appropriate patient, this minimally invasive, nonsurgical option for hemorrhage control is superior to emergent surgery. However, for the patient in extremis, who is too unstable for IR, surgery is the best option.

Table 2 summarizes the capabilities and limitations of these interventions.

CLINICS CARE POINTS

- Patients with life-threatening hemoptysis:
  - Die from asphyxiation, not hemorrhagic shock.
  - Require immediate treatment to secure the airway and stabilize the patient.
  - Require early activation and coordinated response from a multidisciplinary team.
  - Once the airway is secure and appropriate resuscitation is initiated, priorities are to localize the source of the bleeding and gain hemorrhage control.
  - Nonsurgical control of hemorrhage is superior to surgery in the acute situation.
  - Require ICU level care.

- Immediate actions to stabilize the patient and secure the airway include:
  - Placement of the patient in the decubitus position with bleeding lung down.
  - Intubation with greater than or equal to 8 mm endotracheal tube.
  - Blood product transfusion and reversal of coagulopathies.
  - Bronchoscopy (to aid in securing the airway, isolation of the bleeding lung, placement of the endotracheal tube in the main stem bronchus, and application of hemostatic adjuncts).
  - Early engagement of a multidisciplinary team (including ICU, interventional radiology, thoracic surgery, interventional pulmonology, anesthesiology).

- Diagnostic options include chest radiography, CT, flexible or rigid bronchoscopy, and angiography. Diagnostic sensitivity and localization of the bleed improves when multiple modalities are used.

- Treatment options include early bronchoscopy as described earlier and angiography followed by BAE. In the appropriate patient, a minimally invasive, nonsurgical option for hemorrhage control is superior to emergent surgery. However, for the patient in extremis, who is too unstable for IR, surgery is the best option.

DISCLOSURE

The authors have nothing to disclose.

REFERENCES

1. Crocco JA, Rooney JJ, Fankushen DS, et al. Massive hemoptysis. Arch Intern Med 1968;121(6):495–8.
2. Garzon AA, Gourin A. Surgical management of massive hemoptysis. A ten-year experience. Ann Surg 1978;187(3):267–71.
3. Davidson K, Shojaee S. Managing massive hemoptysis. Chest 2020;157(1): 77–88.
4. Lee BR, Yu JY, Ban HJ, et al. Analysis of patients with hemoptysis in a tertiary referral hospital. Tuberc Respir Dis (Seoul) 2012;73(2):107–14.
5. Ong TH, Eng P. Massive hemoptysis requiring intensive care. Intensive Care Med 2003;29(2):317–20.
6. Reechaipichitkul W, Latong S. Etiology and treatment outcomes of massive hemoptysis. Southeast Asian J Trop Med Public Health 2005;36(2):474–80.
7. Jin F, Li Q, Bai C, et al. Chinese expert recommendation for diagnosis and treatment of massive hemoptysis. Respiration 2020;99:83–92.
8. Burke CT, Mauro MA. Bronchial artery embolization. Semin Intervent Radiol 2004; 21(1):43–8.
9. Kalva SP. Bronchial artery embolization. Tech Vasc Interv Radiol 2009;12(2): 130–8.
10. Corey R, Hla KM. Major and massive hemoptysis: reassessment of conservative management. Am J Med Sci 1987;294(5):301–9.
11. Noë GD, Jaffé SM, Molan MP. CT and CT angiography in massive haemoptysis with emphasis on pre-embolization assessment. Clin Radiol 2011;66(9):869–75.
12. Amirana M, Frater R, Tirschwell P, et al. An aggressive surgical approach to significant hemoptysis in patients with pulmonary tuberculosis. Am Rev Respir Dis 1968;97(2):187–92.
13. Hirshberg B, Biran I, Glazer M, et al. Hemoptysis: etiology, evaluation, and outcome in a tertiary referral hospital. Chest 1997;112(2):440–4.
14. Knott-Craig CJ, Oostuizen JG, Rossouw G, et al. Management and prognosis of massive hemoptysis. Recent experience with 120 patients. J Thorac Cardiovasc Surg 1993;105(3):394–7.
15. Fartoukh M, Khoshnood B, Parrot A, et al. Early prediction of in-hospital mortality of patients with hemoptysis: an approach to defining severe hemoptysis. Respiration 2012;83:106–14.
16. Patwa A, Shah A. Anatomy and physiology of respiratory system relevant to anaesthesia. Indian J Anaesth 2015;59(9):533–41.
17. Ibrahim WH. Massive haemoptysis: the definition should be revised. Eur Respir J 2008;32(4):1131–2.
18. Remy J, Remy-Jardin M, Voisin C. Endovascular management of bronchial bleeding. In: Butler J, editor. The bronchial circulation. New York: Dekker; 1992. p. 667–723.
19. Khalil A, Parrot A, Nedelcu C, et al. Severe hemoptysis of pulmonary arterial origin: signs and role of multidetector row CT. Chest 2008;133:212–9.
20. Sakr L, Dutau H. Massive hemoptysis: an update on the role of bronchoscopy in diagnosis and management. Respiration 2010;80:38–58.

21. Uflacker R, Kaemmerer A, Picon PD, et al. Bronchial artery embolization in the management of hemoptysis: Technical aspects and long-term results. Radiology 1985;157:637–44.

22. Cahill BC, Ingbar DH. Massive hemoptysis. Assessment and management. Clin Chest Med 1994;15:147–67.

23. Deffebach ME, Charan NB, Lakshminarayan S, et al. The bronchial circulation: small, but a vital attribute to the lung. Am Rev Respir Dis 1987;135:463–81.

24. Roberts AC. Bronchial artery embolization therapy. J Thorac Imaging 1990;5: 60–72.

25. Cauldwell EW, Sickert RG, Lininger RE, et al. The bronchial arteries: an anatomic study of 150 human cadavers. Surg Gynecol Obstet 1948;86:395–412.

26. Yoon YC, Lee KS, Jeong YJ, et al. Hemoptysis: bronchial and nonbronchial systemic arteries at 16- detector row CT. Radiology 2005;234(1):292–8.

27. McDonald DM. Angiogenesis and remodeling of airway vasculature in chronic inflammation. Am J Respir Crit Care Med 2001;164(10 Pt 2):S39–45.

28. Kathuria H, Hollingsworth HM, Vilvendhan R, et al. Management of life-threatening hemoptysis. J Intensive Care 2020;8:23.

29. Hurt K, Bilton D. Haemoptysis: diagnosis and treatment. Acute Med 2012;11(1): 39–45.

30. Kvale PA, Selecky PA, Prakash UB. American College of Chest Physicians, Palliative care in lung cancer: ACCP evidence-based clinical practice guidelines (2nd edition). Chest 2007;132(3):368S–403S.

31. Arooj P, Bredin E, Henry MT, et al. Bronchoscopy in the investigation of outpatients with hemoptysis at a lung cancer clinic. Respir Med 2018;139:1–5.

32. Miller RR, McGregor DH. Hemorrhage from carcinoma of the lung. Cancer 1980; 46(1):200–5.

33. Dweik RA, Stoller JK. Role of bronchoscopy in massive hemoptysis. Clin Chest Med 1999;20(1):89–105.

34. Mondoni M, Carlucci P, Job S, et al. Observational, multicentre study on the epidemiology of haemoptysis. Eur Respir J 2018;51(1):1701813.

35. Mal H, Rullon I, Mellot F, et al. Immediate and long-term results of bronchial artery embolization for life-threatening hemoptysis. Chest 1999;115(4):996–1001.

36. Ernst A, Eberhardt R, Wahidi M, et al. Effect of routine clopidogrel use on bleeding complications after transbronchial biopsy in humans. Chest 2006; 129(3):734–7.

37. Hetzel J, Maldonado F, Ravaglia C, et al. Transbronchial cryobiopsies for the diagnosis of diffuse parenchymal lung diseases: expert statement from the cryobiopsy working group on safety and utility and a call for standardization of the procedure. Respiration 2018;95(3):188–200.

38. Ravaglia C, Bonifazi M, Wells AU, et al. Safety and diagnostic yield of transbronchial lung cryobiopsy in diffuse parenchymal lung diseases: a comparative study versus video-assisted thoracoscopic lung biopsy and a systematic review of the literature. Respiration 2016;91(3):215–27.

39. Syed M, Irby J. Airway management of ruptured pulmonary artery Rasmussen aneurysm and massive hemoptysis. BMC Res Notes 2015;8:346.

40. Singh AK, Gupta V, Rani B, et al. Rasmussen aneurysm. J Assoc Physicians India 2017;65:101–2.

41. Kearney TJ, Shabot MM. Pulmonary artery rupture associated with Swan-Ganz catheter. Chest 1995;108:1349–52.

42. Boyd KD, Thomas SJ, Gold J, et al. A prospective study of complications of pulmonary artery catheterizations in 500 consecutive patients. Chest 1983;84:245–9.

43. Chun GM, Ellestad MH. Perforation of the pulmonary artery by a Swan-Ganz catheter. N Engl J Med 1971;284:1041–2.

44. Sirivella S, Gielchinsky I, Parsonnet V. Management of catheter-induced pulmonary artery perforation: a rare complication in cardiovascular operations. Ann Thorac Surg 2001;72:2056–9.

45. Karak P, Dimick R, Hamrick KM, et al. Immediate trans-catheter embolization of Swan-Ganz catheter-induced pulmonary artery pseudoaneurysm. Chest 1997; 111:1450–2.

46. Revel MP, Fournier LS, Hennebique AS, et al. Can CT replace bronchoscopy in the detection of the site and cause of bleeding in patients with large or massive hemoptysis? Am J Roentgenol 2002;179(5):1217–24.

47. Hsiao EI, Kirsch CM, Kagawa FT, et al. Utility of fiberoptic bronchoscopy before bronchial artery embolization for massive hemoptysis. Am J Roentgenol 2001; 177:861–7.

48. Hirshberg B, Biran I, Glazer M, et al. Hemoptysis: etiology, evaluation, and outcome in a tertiary referral hospital. Chest 1997;112:440–4.

49. Campos JH. An update on bronchial blockers during lung separation techniques in adults. Anesth Analg 2003;97(5):1266–74.

50. Colchen A, Fischler M. Emergency interventional bronchoscopies. Rev Pneumol Cin 2011;67(4):209–13.

51. Conlan AA, Hurwitz SS. Management of massive hemoptysis with rigid bronchoscope and cold saline lavage. Thorax 1980;35(12):901–4.

52. Khoo KL, Lee P, Meta AC. Endobronchial epinephrine: confusion is in the air. Am J Respir Crit Care Med 2013;187(10):1137–8.

53. Steinfort DP, Herth FJ, Eberhardt R, et al. Potentially fatal arrhythmia complicating endobronchial epinephrine for control of iatrogenic bleeding. Am J Respir Crit Care Med 2012;185(9):1028–30.

54. CRASH-2 trial collaborators. Effects of tranexamic acid on death, vascular occlusive events, and blood transfusion in trauma patients with significant haemorrhage (CRASH-2): a randomised, placebo-controlled trial. Lancet 2010; 376(9734):23–32.

55. Bellam BL, Dhibar DP, Suri V, et al. Efficacy of tranexamic acid in haemoptysis: a randomized, controlled pilot study. Pulm Pharmacol Ther 2016;40:80–3.

56. Wand O, Guber E, Guber A, et al. Inhaled tranexamic acid for hemoptysis treatment: A randomized controlled trial. Chest 2018;154(6):1379–84.

57. Han CC, Prasetyo D, Wright GM. Endobronchial palliation using Nd:YAG laser is associated with improved survival when combined with multimodal adjuvant treatments. J Thorac Oncol 2007;2(1):59–64.

58. Morice RC, Ece T, Ece F, et al. Endobronchial argon plasma coagulation for treatment of hemoptysis and neoplastic airway obstruction. Chest 2001;119(3):781–7.

59. Dalar L, Sokucu SN, Ozdemir C, et al. Endobronchial argon plasma coagulation for treatment of Dieulafoy disease. Respir Care 2015;60(1):e11–3.

60. Valipour A, Kreuzer A, Koller H, et al. Bronchoscopy-guided topical hemostatic tamponade therapy for the management of life-threatening hemoptysis. Chest 2005;127(6):2113–8.

61. Peralta AR, Chawla M, Lee RP. Novel bronchoscopic management of airway bleeding with absorbable gelatin and thrombin slurry. J Bronchology Interv Pulmonol 2018;25(3):204–11.

62. Morikawa S, Okamura T, Minezawa T, et al. A simple method of bronchial occlusion with silicone spigots (Endobronchial Watanabe Spigot; EWS®) using a curette. Ther Adv Respir Dis 2016;10(6):518–24.

63. Lee SA, Kim DH, Jeon GS. Covered bronchial stent insertion to manage airway obstruction with hemoptysis caused by lung cancer. Korean J Radiol 2012; 13(4):515–20.

64. Rémy J, Voisin C, Dupuis C, et al. Treatment of hemoptysis by embolization of the systemic circulation. Ann Radiol (Paris) 1974;17(1):5–16.

65. Zhang JS, Cui ZP, Wang MQ, et al. Bronchial arteriography and transcatheter embolization in the management of hemoptysis. Cardiovasc Intervent Radiol 1994;17(5):276–9.

66. Panda A, Bhalla AS, Goyal A. Bronchial artery embolization in hemoptysis: a systematic review. Diagn Interv Radiol 2017;23(4):307–17.

67. Alexander GR. A retrospective review comparing the treatment outcomes of emergency lung resection for massive haemoptysis with and without preoperative bronchial artery embolization. Eur J Cardiothorac Surg 2014;45(2):251–5.

68. Fruchter O, Schneer S, Rusanov V, et al. Bronchial artery embolization for massive hemoptysis: long-term follow-up. Asian Cardiovasc Thorac Ann 2015; 23(1):55–60.

69. Stoll JF, Bettmann MA. Bronchial artery embolization to control hemoptysis: a review. Cardiovasc Intervent Radiol 1988;11(5):263–9.

70. Andréjak C, Parrot A, Bazelly B, et al. Surgical lung resection for severe hemoptysis. Ann Thorac Surg 2009;88(5):1556–65.

71. Shigemura N, Wan IY, Yu SC, et al. Multidisciplinary management of life-threatening massive hemoptysis: a 10-year experience. Ann Thorac Surg 2009; 87(3):849–53.

72. Pekçolaklar A, Çitak N, Aksoy Y, et al. Surgery for life-threatening massive hemoptysis; does the time of performed surgery and the timing of surgery affect the rates of complication and mortality? Indian J Surg 2021.

73. Fleisher AG, Tyers GF, Manning GT, et al. Management of massive hemoptysis secondary to catheter-induced perforation of the pulmonary artery during cardiopulmonary bypass. Chest 1989;95(6):1340–1.

74. Yun JS, Song SY, Na KJ, et al. Surgery for hemoptysis in patients with benign lung disease. J Thorac Dis 2018;10(6):3532–8.

75. Shepherd HM, Kotkar K, Bhalla S, et al. Emergent lung resection for massive hemoptysis from bronchial malformation. Ann Thorac Surg 2021;112(6):e423–6.

Minimally Invasive and Sublobar Resections for Lung Cancer

Caroline M. Godfrey, MD[a], Hannah N. Marmor, MD[c],
Eric S. Lambright, MD[c], Eric L. Grogan, MD, MPH[b,c],*

KEYWORDS

- Segmentectomy • Sublobar resection • Lung cancer • Minimally-invasive • VATS

KEY POINTS

- VATS segmentectomy has demonstrated superior preserved pulmonary function when compared with VATS lobectomy.
- Segmentectomy for ground-glass opacity nodules or part-solid nodules has shown oncologic equivalence to lobectomy.
- Emerging data suggest that anatomic segmentectomy may be at least oncologically equivalent to lobectomy in the treatment of stage IA peripheral NSCLC nodules less than or equal to 2 cm.
- As anatomic variations are common, the surgeon must be familiar with possible anatomic variants when performing VATS segmentectomy; when available, 3D-CT is a helpful tool to delineate bronchovascular anatomy in preoperative planning of segmentectomy.

BACKGROUND

Lung cancer is the second most common cancer worldwide with 11% of cancer diagnoses. Lung cancer remains the leading cause of global cancer-related death with 1.8 million deaths in 2020.[1] Stage I and stage II non–small cell lung cancer (NSCLC) have traditionally been treated with lobectomy, although practice patterns and guidelines have also included treating peripheral NSCLC with segmentectomy to preserve additional lung volume in selected cases. Current National Comprehensive Cancer Network (NCCN) guidelines recommend segmentectomy over lobectomy only for patients with poor pulmonary reserve or for peripheral nodules less than or equal to 2 cm

[a] Department of Thoracic Surgery, Vanderbilt University Medical Center, 1161 21st Avenue South, D-4311 MCN, Nashville, TN 37232, USA; [b] Section of Thoracic Surgery, Tennessee Valley VA Healthcare System, 1310 24th Ave S. Nashville, TN, 37212, USA; [c] Department of Thoracic Surgery, Vanderbilt University Medical Center, 609 Oxford House, 1313 21st Avenue South, Nashville, TN 37232, USA
* Corresponding author. Department of Thoracic Surgery, Vanderbilt University Medical Center, 609 Oxford House, 1161 21st Avenue South, Nashville, TN 37232.
E-mail address: Eric.grogan@vumc.org

Surg Clin N Am 102 (2022) 483–492
https://doi.org/10.1016/j.suc.2022.01.006
0039-6109/22/Published by Elsevier Inc.
surgical.theclinics.com

with adenocarcinoma in situ histology, greater than 50% ground-glass opacity (GGO) on computed tomography (CT), or radiologic doubling time greater than or equal to 400 days.[2] Recent retrospective and ongoing prospective trials suggest that segmental resection may be oncologically equivalent to lobectomy for the treatment of small, solid peripheral nodules.[3] Segmentectomy is also indicated for numerous nonmalignant conditions including ones that affect the lung tissue bilaterally, such as bronchiectasis, when a lung-sparing technique would be superior.[4]

This article reviews current controversies around sublobar resections including potential pulmonary functional benefits, oncologic outcomes, and appropriate applications of segmentectomy. We also discuss surgical management of ground-glass nodules, minimally invasive outcomes, and the surgical approach to common segmental resections.

Controversies

Preservation of lung function with segmentectomy

Although a greater amount of lung tissue is preserved after segmentectomy compared with lobectomy, it is crucial to determine whether this translates to preserved pulmonary function. Early comparative studies of open procedures demonstrated minimal to no improvement in residual lung function with segmentectomy when compared with lobectomy.[5] These results are thought to be due to the compensatory volume expansion of the remaining lobe after lobectomy. Ueda and colleagues[6] demonstrated that both the ipsilateral and contralateral functional lung volume had a greater increase following lobectomy when compared with segmentectomy, further contributing to this theory.

More recent studies have shown potential benefits in residual lung function supporting minimally invasive segmentectomy over lobectomy. Tane and colleagues[7] demonstrated that video-assisted thoracoscopic segmentectomy resulted in significantly preserved forced expiratory volume in 1 second (FEV_1) when compared with lobectomy (91.9% postoperative/preoperative FEV_1 when compared with 81.7%) in a group of matched patients. Kim and colleagues[8] found that patients with NSCLC undergoing video-assisted thoracoscopic surgery (VATS) sublobar resection demonstrated greater preserved pulmonary function at 3 and 12 months postoperatively when compared with those undergoing VATS lobectomy. As more minimally invasive lung cancer resections are being performed, the benefits of preserving lung function in segmentectomy have been clarified, making anatomic segmentectomy a more attractive option in appropriate clinical scenarios.

Oncologic outcomes of segmentectomy versus lobectomy

For years, lobectomy was considered the only oncologically acceptable resection for NSCLC except for octogenarian patients or patients without the pulmonary reserve to qualify for a lobectomy. This recommendation largely followed the data from the 1995 randomized controlled trial conducted by the Lung Cancer Study Group comparing lobectomy versus sublobar resection (including wedge resection and segmentectomy) for T1N0 NSCLC. This study demonstrated a 75% increase in recurrence rates ($P = 0.02$) and 30% increase in overall death rate ($P = 0.08$) for the sublobar resection group.[5] Patients with lung cancer were included with lesions discovered on plain chest radiographs alone and included nodules measuring 3 cm or less in all dimensions on posteroanterior and lateral chest radiographs, although no difference was observed in cancer death rates or locoregional recurrence among tumors less than 3, 9, or 27 cm^3.[5] As imaging technology has advanced, we are now able to detect smaller and part-solid nodules that may have more favorable histology and be more amenable to limited resection.[9]

Multiple retrospective studies have been unable to demonstrate oncologic equivalence between lobectomy and sublobar resections for T1N0 NSCLC (**Table 1**).[3,5,10–14]

Table 1
Summary of studies comparing overall survival and recurrence rate of NSCLC after segmentectomy versus lobectomy

Study	Year	Number of Patients	Prospective vs Retrospective	NSCLC Stage	Overall Survival: Lobectomy vs Sublobar	Recurrence Rate: Lobectomy vs Sublobar
JCOG0802	Ongoing	1106	Prospective	IA	Improved with segmentectomy	—
Landreneau et al[3]	2014	1192	Retrospective	I	No difference	No difference
Subramanian et al[10]	2018	650	Retrospective	IA	Similar	Decreased recurrence rate with lobectomy
Dai et al[11]	2016	15,760	Retrospective	T1aN0	Improved with lobectomy	—
Khullar et al[12]	2015	2961	Retrospective	T1aN0	Improved with lobectomy[a]	—
Jeon et al[13]	2014	164	Retrospective	IA	—	Decreased recurrence and local recurrence with lobectomy
Ginsberg and Rubinstein[5]	1995	247	Prospective RCT	T1N0	Improved with lobectomy	Decreased recurrence with lobectomy
Read et al[14]	1990	244	Retrospective	T1N0	No difference	—

[a] No difference in overall survival between segmentectomy and lobectomy when controlling for negative margins and adequate lymphadenectomy.

Many of these studies, however, have grouped all sublobar resections together, including wedge resections, which could obscure the results of a true comparison of anatomic segmentectomy to lobectomy.

More recent data have indicated that segmentectomy may be an oncologically sound surgical approach for small, peripheral NSCLC (see **Table 1**). In 2014, Landreneau and colleagues[3] published a retrospective analysis using propensity score matching that demonstrated no significant differences between 5-year survival (54% vs 60% respectively, $P = .258$) and 5-year freedom from recurrence (70% vs 71% respectively, $P = .467$) for segmentectomy when compared with lobectomy for clinical stage I NSCLC. There are currently 2 ongoing randomized phase 3 trials comparing lobectomy with segmentectomy for peripheral nodules less than 2 cm (JCOG0802/WJOG4607L[15] and CALGB140503). Preliminary findings of the JCOG trial presented at the American Association for Thoracic Surgeons meeting in 2021 demonstrated a 5-year overall survival of 91.1% for the lobectomy group and 94.3% for the segmentectomy group. These results reached significance, demonstrating noninferiority and superiority of segmentectomy as surgical treatment of clinical stage IA peripheral NSCLC less than or equal to 2 cm.[15] These novel data represent a potential upcoming shift in the surgical treatment recommendations for early-stage peripheral small nodule NSCLC.

Ground-glass opacity nodules

The classification of GGO nodules has emerged with the increased sensitivity of CT imaging to detect subcentimeter and nonsolid nodules. In the eighth edition of the TNM staging for lung cancer, the T1 classification includes the use of nonsize descriptors not used in prior editions.[16] The new T1a(mi) classification includes minimally invasive adenocarcinoma. T1a additionally includes both the rare superficial spreading tumor in central airways and the subcentimeter tumors.

GGOs are defined radiologically as opacities on CT imaging that do not obscure underlying pulmonary anatomy such as bronchi or vasculature.[17] GGOs have less aggressive characteristics, which potentially make them amenable to oncologically sound sublobar resections. The 5-year overall survival has been reported as 100% for pure GGO nodules and 93.4% to 98.4% for part-solid nodules.[18] Tumor size has not been shown to have significance in overall survival in either pure radiographic GGO tumors or part-solid tumors.[18] Furthermore, there is a slow progression of pure GGOs to part-solid nodules. In a prospective study of GGOs, 5.4% of pure ground-glass nodules developed into part-solid nodules during the follow-up period (mean follow-up 4.3 years) and 19.8% of heterogeneous ground-glass nodules developed into part-solid nodules, with a mean period of development of 3.8 and 2.1 years, respectively.[19]

As data have emerged validating the indolent nature of lung nodules presenting as GGOs, studies have also investigated the oncologic equivalence of sublobar resections for stage IA GGO or part-GGO nodules. Tsutani and colleagues[20] demonstrated an equivalent recurrence-free survival in patients with GGO-dominant tumors who underwent lobectomy (93.7%), segmentectomy (92.9%), and wedge resection (100%), indicating oncologic equivalence of sublobar resections for this type of tumor.

The 2021 NCCN guidelines included segmentectomy as an acceptable surgical option for peripheral nodules less than or equal to 2 cm with greater than 50% GGO on CT.[2]

Non–Lung Cancer Indications for Segmentectomy

Segmentectomy is also used in numerous nonmalignant pathologies. Segmentectomy was initially developed as a surgical treatment of tuberculosis and bronchiectasis to maximize the preservation of lung tissue in these multisegment bilateral pulmonary diseases.[4] Numerous nonmalignant pathologies such as intralobar sequestration, pulmonary arteriovenous malformations, bronchiectasis, bronchial atresia, nontuberculous mycobacterial infection, aspergilloma, and inflammatory pseudotumors are treated with segmentectomy, although the inflammatory nature of these pathologies may limit the ability to technically perform segmentectomy.

Minimally Invasive Approach to Segmentectomy

Video-assisted thoracoscopic surgery segmentectomy

Historically, any surgery with intermittent use of a thoracoscope could be classified as VATS, even if it was performed through a thoracotomy.[9] VATS now refers primarily to minimally invasive surgery with visualization of the surgical field using a thoracoscope and without the use of rib spreading. With an increase in popularity as well as surgeon comfort and expertise, more complex operations including segmentectomy are performed thoracoscopically.

The VATS approach to segmentectomy has been shown to reduce length of hospital stay as well as cases of postoperative pneumonia and unplanned intubation and increase rates of home discharge compared with open segmentectomy.[21]

Robotic-assisted thoracoscopic surgery segmentectomy

As technology has continued to advance, interest in robotic approaches to commonly performed minimally invasive procedures has increased. When compared with VATS, robotic-assisted thoracoscopic surgery (RATS) has been demonstrated to have equivalent or superior surgical outcomes. A meta-analysis conducted by Liang and colleagues[22] demonstrated lower 30-day mortality with RATS segmentectomy/lobectomy when compared with VATS approach (0.7% vs 1.1%, respectively, $P = .045$) and lower conversion rates to open surgery (10.3% vs 11.9%, $P < .001$).

Preoperative Planning

The anatomic landmarks involved in segmentectomy are more complex than for lobectomy and can vary between patients. Surgeon familiarity with common anatomic variants is critical and may be aided by preoperative imaging to delineate patient-specific anatomy.

Use of Preoperative 3D Computed Tomography

Performing minimally invasive segmentectomies can present many technical challenges, including identifying patient-specific anatomy. Preoperative 3D-CT can be used to identify anatomic variants, plan the operative approach, and predict surgical margins in sublobar resections. Using high-resolution CT (HRCT), Horinouchi and colleagues[23] found that 35% of T1N0 NSCLC extended beyond a single segment. Preoperative use of HRCT/3D-CT would allow the surgeon to identify nodules for which segmentectomy would not achieve a 2-cm surgical margin and adjust the surgical plan accordingly.

Le Moal and colleagues[24] presented a case series of patients who underwent preoperative planning using 3D-CT before robot-assisted thoracoscopic segmentectomy. Individual patient anatomy was accurately represented by the preoperative reconstruction.[24] More than 95% of pulmonary arteries are correctly identified on 3D-CT.[25] Reconstructing a 3D representation of the patient's specific bronchovascular anatomy allows the surgeon to plan dissection of the vascular anatomy and determine which intersegmenteal veins should be used as landmarks to dissect the intersegmental planes.[25]

Patterns of Bronchovascular Anatomic Variation

Bronchovascular anatomy can vary widely from patient to patient, although a few patterns predominate, the frequency of which has been described by Shimizu and colleagues[25] based on their analysis of 3D-CT angiography and bronchography images. The bronchi are classified based on the degree of branching with the trifurcated type being most common, which was found in 44.1% of patients in this study.[25] The patterns of pulmonary arterial and venous anatomy vary based on the pulmonary lobe. The pulmonary arteries for the right upper lobe (RUL) generally fall into 4 patterns based on whether the trunks are inferior or superior and whether there is an ascending artery. In 71.9% of patients, the "truncus superior and posterior ascending artery" pattern is seen.[25] The pulmonary veins for the lower lobes tend to be incredibly diverse in anatomy, although the veins for the upper lobes tend to follow more predictable patterns. In the RUL, the pulmonary veins generally fall into 4 patterns based on the presence of central and anterior veins, the most common type being "anterior with central" type, which is seen in 54% of patients.[25]

Procedural Approach

Positioning and access port placement

The positioning and port placement for anatomic segmentectomy should be performed in the same manner as for the corresponding lobectomy.[26]

Selected segmentectomy procedural outline

A schematic representation of the subsegments of the lung as well as some of the most common major segmental resections can be found in **Fig. 1**. We have selected some of the most performed segmental resections to highlight. Each segmental resection ends with division of the segmental plane. Details of this portion of the procedure are included at the end of the section. In cases in which segmentectomy is performed for lung cancer, a mediastinal lymph node dissection is performed with the segmentectomy.

Superior segmentectomy. A superior segmentectomy involves resection of the S^6 (superior) segment of the left or the right lung. As the procedure is similar on both sides, it is described generally and can be applied to either laterality.[27]

- The inferior pulmonary ligament is taken down, and the dissection of the bronchovascular structures begins with exposure of the superior segmental branch of the inferior pulmonary vein.
- The superior segmental artery is then identified by dissecting along the anterior aspect of the lower pulmonary artery in the fissure.
- The superior segmental artery is then divided followed by division of the superior segmental branch of the inferior pulmonary vein.
- The superior segmental bronchus is then exposed and divided using a stapler.
- If access to the artery proves to be challenging from the fissure approach, the segment can also be approached from the posterior hilum. This process would involve initial dissection and ligation of the superior segmental vein, followed by the superior segmental bronchus and then the artery.

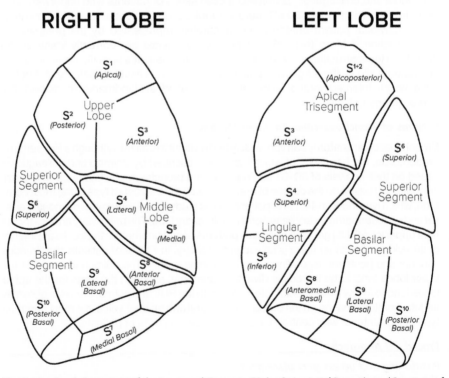

Fig. 1. Anatomic Segments of the Lung and Common Major Segmental Resections. (*Courtesy of Dominic Doyle.*)

- The segmental plane is then divided to free the segment. Methods for identification of the segmental plane are described in the following section.

Left apical trisegmentectomy. A left apical trisegmentectomy involves resection of the S^1 (apical), S^2 (posterior), and S^3 (anterior) segments of the left upper lobe; it is also referred to as a lingula-sparing left upper lobectomy because the lingula is the only portion of the left upper lobe preserved.

- Through the fissure or a posterior mediastinal approach, the posterior aspect of the pulmonary artery is identified and dissected to expose the apicoposterior and superior segmental branches. Taking care to preserve the superior segmental artery, the apicoposterior branches are divided
- Great care must be taken to preserve the lingular artery to complete a lingula-sparing operation. Awareness of anatomy including potential variants is critical because the lingular artery can takeoff proximally, running between the superior pulmonary vein and the bronchus or distally, arising from the basilar artery. A complete fissure can make identification of the lingular artery difficult.
- The apical branches of the pulmonary vein are then identified and divided, again ensuring preservation of the lingular branches. This maneuver allows further visualization of the anterior arterial branches, which can then be divided.
- The main pulmonary artery is identified, and the truncus anterior artery is dissected and divided.
- The bronchus is dissected, exposing the carina between the upper and lingular bronchus, and the apical bronchus is divided with a stapler. Before division, the lung is inflated to ensure that the lingular bronchus is intact.
- The segmental plane is then divided to free the segment. Methods for identification of the segmental plane are described in the following section.

Left lingular segmentectomy
- The lingular artery is identified within the fissure, dissected, and divided. Awareness of the anatomy, including potential variants, is critical because the lingular artery can takeoff proximally, near the anterior branches, running between the superior pulmonary vein and the bronchus. A complete fissure can make identification of the lingular artery difficult. One or two lingular arteries may be present and can also arise distally from the basilar artery when an incomplete inferior fissure is noted.
- Attention is then turned to the anterior hilum. The lung is then retracted posteriorly to expose the lingular vein, which is the inferiormost branch of the superior pulmonary vein. The lingular vein is then dissected and divided.
- The lingular bronchus is identified, dissected, and, after confirmation of preservation of the upper division bronchus, divided using a stapler.
- The segmental plane is then divided to free the segment. Methods for identification of the segmental plane are described in the following section.
- Alternatively, the left lingula can be approached from the anterior hilum by starting with the dissection of the lingular vein, followed by the bronchus, and finally the artery. In this approach, care must be taken when encircling the bronchus so as to minimize risk to the lingular branch of the pulmonary artery.

Delineation of segmental planes
One of the most challenging but critical technical aspects of a segmentectomy is the delineation and dissection of the segmental plane. Numerous methods of identifying this plane have been described in the literature including selective inflation/deflation of the segment, use of indocyanine green (ICG)/infrared, and use of the intersegmental veins to guide the dissection.

Selective inflation/deflation. Selectively inflating the affected segment can allow for accurate dissection along the plane demarcated by the inflation-deflation border; this can be achieved using several methods including jet ventilation or bronchus ligation with selective inflation of the affected segment. Jet ventilation does require another operator to manipulate the bronchoscope into the segmental bronchus to maintain isolated ventilation of the affected segment. In some circumstances, this may be too technically challenging to manipulate the bronchoscope at that level, and selective bronchial ligation with expansion of the selected segment may be preferred.[28] The utility of selective inflation/deflation is limited by collateral flow, which reduces the ability to isolate one segment.

Indocyanine green and infrared thoracoscopy. The use of infrared thoracoscopy, particularly in combination with injection of ICG, has been demonstrated as an effective alternative to selective inflation and allows for dissection of the intersegmental plane without inflation of the segment.[29] Both injection of ICG into the isolated segmental pulmonary artery and transbronchial injection into the segmental bronchus via bronchoscopy have been shown to effectively differentiate the affected segment from the surrounding lung parenchyma.[29] Transbronchial injection, when compared with segmental pulmonary arterial injection, of ICG has the advantage of being able to distinguish the lung parenchyma, not just the surface of the segmental lung tissue.[9] This method may be superior to selective inflation, particularly in patients with more significant collateral air flow, because this would diminish the effect of the selective inflation of the affected segment by also inflating some of the surrounding lung parenchyma.[29]

SUMMARY

The utility of segmentectomy and sublobar resections for lung cancer has long been a point of great debate. With the advent of minimally invasive techniques, segmentectomy has demonstrated improved preserved lung function when compared with lobectomy, prompting greater investigation of oncologic outcomes from the procedure. The pivotal 1995 Lung Cancer Study group prospective trial comparing sublobar resections with lobectomy demonstrated worse oncologic outcomes for sublobar resections, which since has been supported by multiple retrospective analyses. These studies have driven management guidelines including lobectomy for patients who could tolerate the procedure for solid-type NSCLC nodules. New data are emerging suggesting that anatomic segmentectomy could have oncologic equivalence, or even superiority, to lobectomy for patients with peripheral less yhan or equal to 2 cm NSCLC solid nodules. Although we await final reports of both ongoing prospective trials (JCOG0802/WJOG4607L[15] and CALGB140503), these new data represent a potential upcoming shift in surgical management of small, peripheral solid NSCLC and future increased use and relevance of the minimally invasive anatomic segmentectomy.

CLINICS CARE POINTS

- Minimally Invasive (MIS) sublobar resections have been demonstrated to preserve lung function when compared with MIS lobectomy and should be considered in the appropriate clinical scenario
- MIS approaches to pulmonary resections are associated with decreased length of hospital stay and decreased morbidity compared with open resections and should be considered among surgeons with the necessary expertise

- Sublobar resections have long been considered oncologically inferior to standard lobectomy for NSCLC, but recent retrospective and early prospective data support the oncologic equivalence, or even superiority, of anatomic segmentectomy when compared with lobectomy for stage IA peripheral NSCLC nodules less than or equal to 2 cm
- GGO-type and part-solid nodules are a marker of less aggressive phenotype and are amenable to sublobar resections for surgical treatment
- In performing anatomic segmentectomy, the surgeon must be aware of potential anatomic variants and can consider the use of 3D-CT for preoperative planning in settings where available
- Selective inflation/deflation of neighboring segments as well as ICG and infrared thoracoscopy can be helpful adjuncts for delineating the segmental plane during segmentectomy

DISCLOSURE

None of the authors have any conflicts of interest. Dr. Godfrey's time was supported by the Surgical Oncology Training Grant T32 (CA106183-18). Dr. Marmor's time was supported by the Surgical Oncology Training Grant T32 (CA106183-18). Dr. Grogan's time was supported by the Veteran's Administration, the Vanderbilt Department of Thoracic Surgery and the 5U01CA152662 grant.

REFERENCES

1. Sung H, Ferlay J, Siegel RL, et al. Global cancer statistics 2020: Globocan estimates of incidence and mortality worldwide for 36 cancers in 185 countries. CA: A Cancer J Clinicians 2021;71(3):209–49.
2. National Comprehensive Cancer Network. Non-small Cell Lung Cancer (Version 5.2021). Available at: https://www.nccn.org/professionals/physician_gls/pdf/nscl.pdf. Accessed August 10, 2021.
3. Landreneau RJ, Normolle DP, Christie NA, et al. Recurrence and survival outcomes after anatomic segmentectomy versus lobectomy for clinical stage I non–small-cell lung cancer: A propensity-matched analysis. J Clin Oncol 2014; 32(23):2449–55.
4. Churchill ED, Belsey R. Segmental pneumonectomy in bronchiectasis: the lingula segment of the left upper lobe. Ann Surg 1939;109(4):481–99.
5. Ginsberg RJ, Rubinstein LV. Randomized trial of lobectomy versus limited resection for T1 N0 non-small cell lung cancer. The Ann Thorac Surg 1995;60(3):615–23.
6. Ueda K, Tanaka T, Hayashi M, et al. Computed tomography-defined functional lung volume after segmentectomy versus lobectomy. Eur J Cardio-Thoracic Surg 2010;37(6):1433–7.
7. Tane S, Nishio W, Nishioka Y, et al. Evaluation of the residual lung function after thoracoscopic segmentectomy compared with lobectomy. Ann Thorac Surg 2019;108(5):1543–50.
8. Kim SJ, Lee YJ, Park JS, et al. Changes in pulmonary function in lung cancer patients after video-assisted thoracic surgery. Ann Thorac Surg 2015;99(1):210–7.
9. Nakazawa S, Shimizu K, Mogi A, et al. VATS segmentectomy: past, present, and future. Gen Thorac Cardiovasc Surg 2018;66(2):81–90. Epub 2017 Dec 18.
10. Subramanian M, McMurry T, Meyers BF, et al. Long-term results for clinical stage IA lung cancer: comparing lobectomy and sublobar resection. The Ann Thorac Surg 2018;106(2):375–81.

11. Dai C, Shen J, Ren Y, et al. Choice of surgical procedure for patients with non-small-cell lung cancer ≤ 1 cm or > 1 to 2 cm among lobectomy, segmentectomy, and wedge resection: a population-based study. J Clin Oncol 2016;34(26): 3175–82.

12. Khullar OV, Liu Y, Gillespie T, et al. Survival after sublobar resection versus lobectomy for clinical stage ia lung cancer: an analysis from the national cancer data base. J Thorac Oncol 2015;10(11):1625–33.

13. Jeon HW, Kim YD, Kim KS, et al. Sublobar resection versus lobectomy in solid-type, clinical stage IA, non-small cell lung cancer. World J Surg Oncol 2014;12:215.

14. Read RC, Yoder G, Schaeffer RC. Survival after conservative resection for T1 N0 M0 non-small cell lung cancer. Ann Thorac Surg 1990;49(3):391–400.

15. Asamura H, Okada M, Saji H, et al. Randomized trial of segmentectomy compared to lobectomy in small-sized peripheral non-small cell lung cancer. Abstract presented at: American Association for Thoracic Surgery 101st Annual Meeting; April 30th–May 2nd, 2021, Virtual.

16. Detterbeck FC, Boffa DJ, Kim AW, et al. The eighth edition lung cancer stage classification. Chest 2017;151(1):193–203.

17. Chen KN. The diagnosis and treatment of lung cancer presented as ground-glass nodule. Gen Thorac Cardiovasc Surg 2020;68(7):697–702.

18. Hattori A, Matsunaga T, Takamochi K, et al. neither maximum tumor size nor solid component size is prognostic in part-solid lung cancer: impact of tumor size should be applied exclusively to solid lung cancer. Ann Thorac Surg 2016; 102(2):407–15.

19. Kakinuma R, Noguchi M, Ashizawa K, et al. Natural history of pulmonary subsolid nodules: a prospective multicenter study. J Thorac Oncol 2016;11(7):1012–28.

20. Tsutani Y, Miyata Y, Nakayama H, et al. Appropriate sublobar resection choice for ground glass opacity-dominant clinical stage IA lung adenocarcinoma: wedge resection or segmentectomy. Chest 2014;145(1):66–71.

21. Sabra MJ, Alwatari Y, Bierema C, et al. Five-year experience with vats versus thoracotomy segmentectomy for lung tumor resection. Innovations (Phila). 2020; 15(4):346–54.

22. Liang H, Liang W, Zhao L, et al. Robotic versus video-assisted lobectomy/segmentectomy for lung cancer: a meta-analysis. Ann Surg 2018;268(2):254–9.

23. Horinouchi H, Nomori H, Nakayama T, et al. How many pathological T1N0M0 non-small cell lung cancers can be completely resected in one segment? Special reference to high-resolution computed tomography findings. Surg Today 2011; 41(8):1062–6.

24. Le Moal J, Peillon C, Dacher JN, et al. Three-dimensional computed tomography reconstruction for operative planning in robotic segmentectomy: a pilot study. J Thorac Dis 2018;10(1):196–201.

25. Shimizu K, Nakazawa S, Nagashima T, et al. 3D-CT anatomy for VATS segmentectomy. J Vis Surg 2017;3:88.

26. Yan TD. Surgical atlas of thoracoscopic lobectomy and segmentectomy. Ann Cardiothorac Surg 2014;3(2):183–91.

27. McKenna RJ, et al. Segmentectomy. In: Wang J., Ferguson M K, editors. Atlas of minimally invasive surgery for lung and esophageal cancer. S.I. Springer; 2017.

28. Oizumi H, Kato H, Endoh M, et al. Techniques to define segmental anatomy during segmentectomy. Ann Cardiothorac Surg 2014;3(2):170–5.

29. Misaki N, Chang SS, Gotoh M, et al. A novel method for determining adjacent lung segments with infrared thoracoscopy. J Thorac Cardiovasc Surg 2009; 138(3):613–8.

Chemo and Immuno-Therapeutic Options for Nonsmall Cell Lung Cancer Lung Cancer

Rafael Santana-Davila, MD

KEYWORDS

- Nonsmall cell lung cancer • Immune checkpoint inhibitors • Immunotherapy
- Chemoimmunotherapy

KEY POINTS

- Immunotherapy has dramatically changed the paradigm and outcome of patients with NSCLC.
- Immunotherapy is being used for the treatment of patients across stages of NSCLC.
- Further research is needed to accurately define those patients that can benefit the most from immunotherapy.

Immunotherapy through immune checkpoint inhibitors (ICI) has dramatically changed the treatment paradigm and outcome of patients with a variety of malignancies. In this review we will focus on nonsmall cell lung cancers (NSCLC). Here, treatment with PDL1 inhibitors was first approved in patients with metastatic disease after 1st line treatment with a platinum doublet after several trials demonstrated an improved outcome comparing ICI treatment versus the then current second-line treatment, docetaxel.[1,2] Subsequent studies focused on first-line treatment. Keynote-024 demonstrated the superiority of treatment with pembrolizumab versus chemotherapy in patients with NSCLC that had a PD-L1 expression on at least 50% of malignant cells and no sensitizing mutation of the epidermal growth factor receptor (EGFR) gene or translocation of the anaplastic lymphoma kinase (ALK) gene. Pembrolizumab treatment was associated with an increase in progression-free and overall survival median OS 30 vs 14.2 months (hazard ratio (HR): 0.63; 95% confidence interval (CI): 0.47–0.86) with fewer adverse events compared with platinum chemotherapy.[3] Keynote-042 was a similar study with the main difference that included patients with expression of pdl1 of 1% of greater.[4] This was also a positive study that demonstrated that the OS was significantly longer in the pembrolizumab group patients (16.7 vs 12.1 months,

Fred Hutch Cancer Research Center, University of Washington, Seattle Cancer Care Alliance, 825 Eastlake Avenue East, Seattle, WA 98109, USA
E-mail address: rafaelsd@uw.edu

Surg Clin N Am 102 (2022) 493–498
https://doi.org/10.1016/j.suc.2022.02.005
0039-6109/22/© 2022 Elsevier Inc. All rights reserved.

HR: 0.81, P = .001), for patients with PD-L1 $\geq$50% (20 vs 12.2 months, HR: 0.69, P = .0003), PD-L1 $\geq$20% (17.7 vs 13.0 months, HR: 0.77, P = .002), and PD-L1 $\geq$1% (16.7 vs 12.1 months, HR: 0.81, P = .001). It is important to note that these results were largely driven by patients who had a PDL1 of greater than 50%, this group constituted 47% of patients. In a prespecified exploratory analysis of patients with PD-L1 score 1% to 49%, the median OS was 13.4 months in the pembrolizumab group and 12.1 months in the chemotherapy group (HR: 0.92, 95% CI: 0.77–1.11). Similar results were found when using the PD-L1 inhibitor atezolizumab, IMpower110 was a phase 3 study that showed that treatment with atezolizumab resulted in a significantly longer overall survival than platinum-based chemotherapy among patients with NSCLC with high PD-L1 expression (20.2 months vs 13.1 months; hazard ratio for death, 0.59; P = .01).[5]

On another front, pembrolizumab was combined with chemotherapy in 2 separate trials depending on histology (nonsquamous and squamous). Both were double-blinded studies and both showed a benefit of combining ICI with chemotherapy followed by maintenance ICI and pemetrexed in nonsquamous histology where OS was 22.0 months in the pembrolizumab-combination group versus 10.7 months in the placebo-combination group (HR: 0.56; 95% CI: 0.45–0.70).[6] In patients with squamous histology maintenance was pembrolizumab alone, here median OS was 17.1 versus 11.6 months for the chemotherapy alone arm (HR: 0.71; 95% CI: 0.58–0.88). Similarly, the IMpower130 trial with enrolled patients with nonsquamous NSCLC atezolizumab and a platinum doublet chemotherapy showed a benefit when compared with chemotherapy alone median OS of 18.6 months versus 13.9 months in the chemotherapy alone arm (HR: 0.79; 95% CI: 0.64–0.98; P = .033).[7]

Combination immunotherapy has also been found to be effective in the treatment of metastatic NSCLC. The IMpower225 study was designed when a platinum doublet was the standard of care.[8] Here patients with NSCLC without EGFR or ALK abnormalities were divided according to PD-L1 Expression. Patients with greater than 1% PDL1 expression were randomized to receive nivolumab 3 mg/kg every 2 weeks plus ipilimumab 1 mg/kg every 6 weeks, nivolumab monotherapy 240 mg every 2 weeks, or platinum-doublet chemotherapy. Patients with less than 1% PD-L1 expression were randomized to receive nivolumab plus ipilimumab, nivolumab 360 mg every 3 weeks plus platinum-doublet chemotherapy, or platinum-doublet chemotherapy alone. The primary endpoint of the trial was overall survival with nivolumab plus ipilimumab as compared with chemotherapy in patients with a PD-L1 expression level of $\geq$1%. Median OS was 17.1 in the combination immunotherapy versus 14.9 with chemotherapy (HR: 0.76, 95% CI: 0.65–0.90). OS benefit was also observed in patients with a PD-L1 expression level of less than 1%, with a median duration of 17.2 months with nivolumab plus ipilimumab and 12.2 months with chemotherapy (HR: 0.64, 95% CI: 0.51–0.81). It is, however, unknown how would combination immunotherapy would compare to the current standard of chemoimmunotherapy. To complicate things further Checkmate 9LA was a study that compared combination immunotherapy with the same dosage and frequency as the checkmate 227 trial but with the addition of 2 cycles of histology appropriate chemotherapy versus chemotherapy alone. Median OS in the experimental group was 14.1 months versus 10.7 months in the control group (HR: 0·69, 96.71% CI: 0.55–0.87; P = .00065).

HOW TO CHOOSE WHAT REGIMEN IN THE METASTATIC SETTING?

Clearly, there has been substantial progress in the treatment of patients with metastatic lung cancer in the last 2 decades, median OS in most contemporary studies exceeds 1 year and there is hope that first-line studies will show long-term survivors in a fraction of patients although no studies are mature enough to give precise statistics.[9] With the availability of new treatments there is controversy as to which regimen is the right one for an individual patient who has no driver mutations. In my own practice for patients that have a PDL1 expression by the 22C3 pharmDx test of 50% or more and do not have a large burden of disease or evidence of rapid progression, pembrolizumab, cemiplimab, or atezolizumab alone is an appropriate consideration that reduces the incidence of side effects compared with using chemoimmunotherapy. Adding ipilimumab in this groups does not improve efficacy and only adds toxicity.[10] For patients with rapidly progressive disease, a large disease burden or in those who I'm concerned will not likely receive second-line therapy at that time of progression, I discuss using chemoimmunotherapy with pembrolizumab and a platinum doublet.

In patients with PD-L1 low tumors (0%–49%), the preferred standard is chemoimmunotherapy with pembrolizumab and a platinum doublet. Some patients (excluding those with negative expression of PD-L1) will want to avoid the toxicities of chemotherapy and prefer to receive immunotherapy alone, I tend to discourage this as there is evidence that this is approach is likely inferior, although it is an acceptable option for patients that want to avoid adverse events. For patients that want to avoid the specific adverse events of chemotherapy and the association of the cyclical patterns of these adverse events, in specific the episode of neutropenia and fatigue that come with chemotherapy, I discuss the use of combination immunotherapy with nivolumab and ipilimumab.

For patients had have received immunotherapy and have experience progressive disease there is no current role in rechallenging with immunotherapy outside of a clinical trial.

PATIENTS THAT PRESENT WITH EARLIER STAGE DISEASE

For patients with stage III disease or unresectable stage II disease.

The Pacific study was a randomized controlled trial for patients with stage III disease that was treated with chemotherapy and radiation. There were no requirements as to which chemotherapy to use during the radiation treatment and which is the optimal chemotherapy regimen is not known. Those patients that did not have progressive disease went on to be randomized to 12 months of durvalumab versus placebo. The median OS for durvalumab was 47.5 versus 29.1 months for the placebo arm (0.68; 95% CI: 0.53–0.87; $P = .00251$) with estimated 4-year OS rates of 49.6% versus 36.3% for durvalumab versus placebo.[11] In a post hoc analysis it was patients with PD-L1 expression of greater than 1% who appear to benefit the most (HR: 0.60, 95% CI: 0.43–0.84), although this was not an endpoint and therefore PD-L1 staining should not be used for decision making in this patient population. Patients treated with durvalumab experienced more grade 3 and 4 adverse events compared with those treated with placebo (31 vs 26%).[12] The most frequent cause of discontinuation for durvalumab was pneumonitis in 6.1% of cases versus 3.9% in the placebo group. Quality of life did not appear to be different from those treated with immunotherapy compared with placebo.[13]

USE IN PATIENTS WITH DISEASE AMENABLE TO RESECTION

The use of immunotherapy as part of multimodality therapy for patients with disease amenable for resection is a rapidly evolving field. As of the first quarter of 2022, the only approved modality is its use as adjuvant therapy after resection and adjuvant chemotherapy. This is based on a randomized open-label study whereby 1005 patients with resected NSCLC stage IB to IIIA were enrolled to receive atezolizumab of best supportive care (BSC) after adjuvant chemotherapy. The primary endpoint was disease-free survival and was assessed in a hierarchical pattern first in a subpopulation of stage II–IIIA patients whose tumors expressed PD-L1 on 1% of tumor cells. This constituted 476 patients of which 248 were randomized to atezolizumab. The 3-year DFS rates at 3 years were 60% in the atezolizumab group versus 48% in the control group, stratified HR of 0.66 (95% CI: 0.50–0.88), $P = .0039$. The next analysis included all patients with stage II to IIIA here 882 patients participated of which 442 received atezolizumab. The 3-year DFS rates were 56% in the atezolizumab group versus 49% in BSC arm, (median DFS 42.3 vs 35.3 months Stratified HR: 0.79 (95% CI: 0.64–0.96), $P = .020$). Subsequently came the analysis in the intention to treat population (all patients stages IB to IIIA), 507 patients received atezolizumab, the 3-year DFS was 58% in the atezolizumab group and 53% in the control group, stratified HR ratio: 0.81 (95% CI: 0.67–0.99), $P = 0.040$, this last analysis did not meet statistical significance and therefore nor further analysis was carried out. Furthermore, the survival data were immature with only 187 (19%) deaths. Adverse events occurred in 68% of patients in the treatment group, 11% were of grade 3 to 4 severity and there were 4 treatment-related deaths (myocarditis, interstitial lung disease, multiple organ dysfunction, and acute myeloid leukemia). Immune-mediated adverse events requiring systemic corticosteroid treatment occurred in 60 patients (12%) treated with atezolizumab and in 4 patients (1%) who received BSC, it is important to remember that when adverse events needs systemic steroids this are typically high doses and for several week durations while they are tapered. Atezolizumab was approved as an adjuvant treatment by the FDA in October of 2021.

Several other ICI are currently being evaluated in the adjuvant setting, pembrolizumab (NCT02504372), nivolumab (NCT02595944), and durvalumab (NCT04585477).

NEOADJUVANT TREATMENT

In patients that will be treated with surgical resection, neoadjuvant chemotherapy before surgery provides similar outcomes compared with surgical treatment after chemotherapy.[14,15] Several phase 2 studies have evaluated the role of single-agent ICI in this setting,[16] the largest of this trials is the LCMC3 trials which enrolled 191 patients that had stage IB-IIIB NSCLC, here patients received atezolizumab for 2 cycles, In patients without EGFR/ALK mutations who underwent surgery, the MPR rate was 20% (30/147; 95% CI: 14%–28%) and the pathologic complete response (pCR) rate was 7% (10/147; 95% CI: 3–12).[17] Chemoimmunotherapy has also been evaluated. CheckMate 816 was a randomized study whereby 358 patients were randomized to receive a platinum doublet or chemotherapy with nivolumab every 3 weeks for 3 cycles. Stage IIIA was present in 64% of cases. The primary endpoints were pCR and event-free survival (EFS). Surgery was performed in 83.2% in the experimental arm and 75.4% in the control, progressive disease was the most frequent reason for surgery cancellation. Patients treated with immunotherapy had a pCR rate of 24% compared with 2.2% in the control arm. A pCR benefit was independent of stage, histology, PDL1 expression, or tumor mutation burden.[18] There was no increase in the median duration of surgery or length of hospitalization arms. Adverse events were similar with 33.5% grade 3 to 4 events in the experimental arm and 36.9% in the control arm. Grade 3 to 4 surgery-related AEs were reported in 11% versus 15% of the chemoimmunotherapy versus chemo arms, respectively. Grade 5 surgery-related AEs were reported in 2 versus 0 pts in the chemoimmunotherapy versus chemo arms. A recent press release announced that the primary endpoint of EFS was positive. Other similar phase 3 trials are ongoing with durvalumab (NCT03800134), pembrolizumab (NCT03425643), atezolizumab (NCT03456063), and tislelizumab (NCT04379635). It is important to note that most of these trials do not have OS as their primary endpoint, most use a pCR as a surrogate. While pCR has been associated with an increase in cure rates[19,20] it has not been validated across different therapeutic classes of agents (immunotherapy vs chemotherapy) or across different histologies of NSCLC and therefore its validity as a proper surrogate of OS is debatable and prone to controversy.

SUMMARY AND FURTHER DIRECTIONS

It is clear that immunotherapy has changed the outcome of patients with NSCLC and the standard of care is rapidly changing as new clinical trials report new outcomes. Although PDL1 expression levels have emerged as the most important biomarker, it is far from perfect and an s better one that can correlate more accurately when immunotherapy alone can be given is desperately needed. It is important to remember that PDL1 is only one of the multitudes of immune checkpoints and is likely that malignant tumors rely on a variety of mechanisms to evade the immune system. As we understand the interaction between malignant cells and the immune system, new immunotherapies will be developed that will continue to change the paradigm of how NSCLC is treated.

CLINICS CARE POINTS

- Immunotherapy has proven to be a succesful treatment strategy for patient with NSCLC.
- Further investigation is establishing when to use immunotherapy alone versus chemo immunotherapy and whats is its role in the treatment of patients with curable disease.

DISCLOSURE

The author has received honoraria for serving as an advisor for AstraZeneca, Takeda Science Foundation, EMD Sorono, Mirati Therapeutics. The author receive research funding through my institution by Eli Lilly & Co, Genentech, Beyond Spring Pharmaceuticals, ISA Pharmaceuticals, Merck, Pfizer, BMS and ALX oncology.

REFERENCES

1. Herbst RS, Baas P, Kim DW, et al. Pembrolizumab versus docetaxel for previously treated, PD-L1-positive, advanced non-small-cell lung cancer (KEYNOTE-010): a randomised controlled trial. Lancet 2016;387:1540–50.
2. Borghaei H, Paz-Ares L, Horn L, et al. Nivolumab versus docetaxel in advanced nonsquamous non-small-cell lung cancer. N Engl J Med 2015;373:1627–39.
3. Reck M, Rodríguez-Abreu D, Robinson AG, et al. Updated analysis of KEYNOTE-024: pembrolizumab versus platinum-based chemotherapy for advanced non-small-cell lung cancer with PD-L1 tumor proportion score of 50% or greater. J Clin Oncol 2019;37:537–46.
4. Mok TSK, Wu YL, Kudaba I, et al. Pembrolizumab versus chemotherapy for previously untreated, PD-L1-expressing, locally advanced or metastatic non-small-cell lung cancer (KEYNOTE-042): a randomised, open-label, controlled, phase 3 trial. Lancet 2019;393:1819–30.

5. Herbst RS, Giaccone G, de Marinis F, et al. Atezolizumab for first-line treatment of PD-L1-selected patients with NSCLC. N Engl J Med 2020;383:1328–39.

6. Gadgeel S, Rodríguez-Abreu D, Speranza G, et al. Updated analysis from KEYNOTE-189: pembrolizumab or placebo plus pemetrexed and platinum for previously untreated metastatic nonsquamous non-small-cell lung cancer. J Clin Oncol 2020;38:1505–17.

7. West H, McCleod M, Hussein M, et al. Atezolizumab in combination with carboplatin plus nab-paclitaxel chemotherapy compared with chemotherapy alone as first-line treatment for metastatic non-squamous non-small-cell lung cancer (IMpower130): a multicentre, randomised, open-label, phase 3 trial. Lancet Oncol 2019;20:924–37.

8. Hellmann MD, Paz-Ares L, Bernabe Caro R, et al. Nivolumab plus ipilimumab in advanced non-small-cell lung cancer. N Engl J Med 2019;381:2020–31.

9. Friedlaender A, Liu SV, Addeo A. Tracking the tail. J Immunother Cancer 2020;8: e000971.

10. Boyer M, Şendur MAN, Rodríguez-Abreu D, et al. Pembrolizumab plus ipilimumab or placebo for metastatic non-small-cell lung cancer with PD-L1 tumor proportion score ≥ 50%: Randomized, double-blind phase III KEYNOTE-598 study. J Clin Oncol 2021;39:2327–38.

11. Faivre-Finn C, Vicente D, Kurata T, et al. Four-year survival with durvalumab after chemoradiotherapy in stage III NSCLC-an update from the PACIFIC trial. J Thorac Oncol 2021;16:860–7.

12. Antonia SJ, Villegas A, Daniel D, et al. Overall survival with durvalumab after chemoradiotherapy in stage III NSCLC. N Engl J Med 2018;379:2342–50.

13. Hui R, Özgüroğlu M, Villegas A, et al. Patient-reported outcomes with durvalumab after chemoradiotherapy in stage III, unresectable non-small-cell lung cancer (PACIFIC): a randomised, controlled, phase 3 study. Lancet Oncol 2019;20: 1670–80.

14. Felip E, Rosell R, Maestre JA, et al. Preoperative chemotherapy plus surgery versus surgery plus adjuvant chemotherapy versus surgery alone in early-stage non-small-cell lung cancer. J Clin Oncol 2010;28:3138–45.

15. NSCLC M-aCG. Preoperative chemotherapy for non-small-cell lung cancer: a systematic review and meta-analysis of individual participant data. Lancet 2014;383:1561–71.

16. Friedlaender A, Naidoo J, Banna GL, et al. Role and impact of immune checkpoint inhibitors in neoadjuvant treatment for NSCLC. Cancer Treat Rev 2022; 104:102350.

17. Kwiatkowski DJ, Rusch VW, Chaft JE, et al. Neoadjuvant atezolizumab in resectable non-small cell lung cancer (NSCLC): interim analysis and biomarker data from a multicenter study (LCMC3). J Clin Oncol 2019;37:8503.

18. Spicer J, Wang C, Tanaka F, et al. Surgical outcomes from the phase 3 CheckMate 816 trial: Nivolumab (NIVO) + platinum-doublet chemotherapy (chemo) vs chemo alone as neoadjuvant treatment for patients with resectable non-small cell lung cancer (NSCLC). J Clin Oncol 2021;39:8503.

19. Mouillet G, Monnet E, Milleron B, et al. Pathologic complete response to preoperative chemotherapy predicts cure in early-stage non-small-cell lung cancer: combined analysis of two IFCT randomized trials. J Thorac Oncol 2012;7:841–9.

20. Waser NA, Adam A, Schweikert B, et al. Pathologic response as early endpoint for survival following neoadjuvant therapy (NEO-AT) in resectable non-small cell lung cancer (rNSCLC): systematic literature review and meta-analysis. Ann Oncol 2020;31:S806.

Epidemiology of Coronary Artery Disease

John P. Duggan, MD[a], Alex S. Peters, MD[a], Gregory D. Trachiotis, MD[b,c], Jared L. Antevil, MD[d],*

KEYWORDS

- Coronary disease • Cardiovascular diseases • Myocardial infarction
- Coronary artery bypass • Percutaneous coronary intervention

KEY POINTS

- Although the mortality of coronary artery disease (CAD) has declined over recent decades, CAD remains the leading cause of death in the United States (US) and presents a significant economic burden.
- Epidemiologic studies have identified numerous strong risk factors for CAD. Some risk factors for the development of CAD are decreasing within the US population, including smoking, hypertension, dyslipidemia, and physical inactivity. Other risk factors, such as advanced age, diabetes, and obesity are increasing in prevalence.
- Therapies for CAD have evolved over time–the most significant historic advances were the development and refinement of coronary artery bypass grafting (CABG), percutaneous coronary intervention (PCI), and lipid-lowering medications.
- The contemporary optimal treatment of CAD relies on a multi-modality and multi-disciplinary approach, individualizing therapy for each patient based on the best available evidence.
- Despite the increasing prevalence of CAD nationwide, there has been a steady decline in the number of CABGs and PCIs performed in the US for the past decade. Patients with CABG are becoming increasingly older and with more comorbid conditions, although mortality associated with CABG has remained steady.

INTRODUCTION

Coronary artery disease (CAD) is presently the leading cause of death in the United States (US), as it has been since 1990 (**Fig. 1**).[1] The quantity of years of life lost due

a Department of Surgery, Walter Reed National Military Medical Center, 4494 Palmer Road North, Bethesda, MD 20814, USA; b Division of Cardiology, Cardiothoracic Surgery and Heart Center, Veterans Affairs Medical Center, 50 Irving Street Northwest, Washington, DC 20422, USA; c Department of Surgery, George Washington University Hospital, 2300 I Street NW, Washington, DC 20052, USA; d Division of Cardiothoracic Surgery, Veterans Affairs Medical Center, 50 Irving Street Northwest, Washington, DC 20422, USA
* Corresponding author.
E-mail address: jared.antevil@va.gov

Surg Clin N Am 102 (2022) 499–516
https://doi.org/10.1016/j.suc.2022.01.007
0039-6109/22/Published by Elsevier Inc.

surgical.theclinics.com

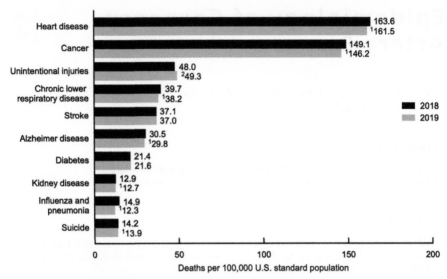

Fig. 1. Age-adjusted death rates for the 10 leading causes of death in the United States in 2018 and 2019. (*Reprinted from* Kochanek et al.[1]).

to premature mortality from CAD is greater than the sum of lung cancer, colon cancer, breast cancer, and prostate cancer (**Fig. 2**).[2] 10.9% of adults aged 45 or older and 17.0% of adults aged 65 or older are estimated to have CAD, and approximately 800,000 Americans suffer a myocardial infarction (MI) each year.[2] CAD is a major source of health care costs, estimated at $126.2 billion in 2010 and expected to increase to more than $177 billion by 2040.[3] Vast improvements in care have led to a steady decline in CAD deaths over the past several decades.[4]

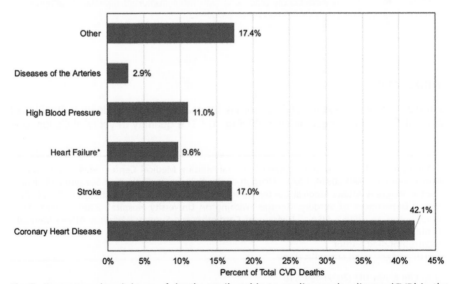

Fig. 2. Percentage breakdown of deaths attributable to cardiovascular disease (CVD) in the US in 2018. (*Reprinted from* Virani et al.[2]).

Our current understanding of the natural history and risk factors of CAD was largely informed by the investigators of the Framingham Heart Study. The Framingham Heart Study began in 1948 to identify characteristics that contribute to the development of cardiovascular disease (CVD). At the time CAD was responsible for more than 50% of deaths in the US and there was only a limited understanding of the natural history of CAD.[5] The investigators sought to enroll subjects with no known or apparent heart disease and follow this cohort over time to identify and determine risk factors for heart disease. The study initially enrolled 5209 residents of Framingham, Massachusetts, chosen because it was representative of the US population at the time and because of its proximity to Boston and Harvard Medical School.[5] To date, thousands of articles have been published based on Framingham data, and factors such as high blood pressure, cholesterol, diabetes, smoking, and obesity had been identified as risk factors for CAD.[5,6] The study currently includes the second and third generations of initial subjects and continues to produce relevant epidemiologic information about CVD.

EFFECT OF AGE

Age is a major risk factor for the development of atherosclerotic CVD and CAD,[7] partially because longer life allows for greater duration of exposure to other risk factors (**Fig. 3**).[8] In one study using Framingham data, age was more strongly associated with risk of a CVD event than any other factor among men, and second only to hypertension among women.[7]

US census data indicate that the overall US population is aging. The number of Americans older than 65 is projected to increase from 40 million to more than 80 million by 2040, driven largely by the prolonged life expectancy of "baby boomers." As age is a major risk factor for CAD, it is not surprising that the prevalence of CAD is expected to increase dramatically over this same time period, from 11.7 million to 17.3 million by 2040.[3]

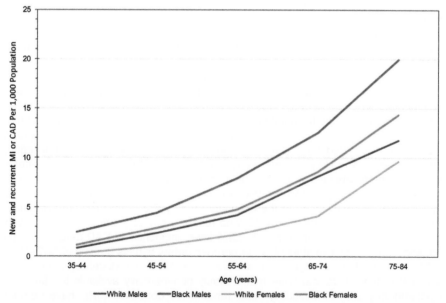

Fig. 3. Incidence of fatal CAD, by age in the US 2005 to 2014. (*Reprinted from* Virani et al.[2]).

EFFECT OF BLOOD PRESSURE

High blood pressure was identified as a risk factor for mortality by life insurance companies in the early 20th century shortly after the development of the sphygmomanometer. However, medical professionals at the time largely believed that elevated blood pressures were not harmful, instead arguing that elevated blood pressure was a necessary compensatory condition to permit perfusion in the setting of atherosclerosis.[9] This concept was challenged in 1961 when elevated blood pressure was identified as a risk factor for CVD in the early outcomes of the Framingham Heart Study.[6] This was followed by many additional randomized controlled trials, and by 1990 there was strong evidence supporting antihypertensive use.[9]

Presently, hypertension is known to be a major independent risk factor for CAD.[10] There is a strong progressive association between blood pressure and age-specific mortality from CAD, with one large meta-analysis noting a 20 mm Hg increase in systolic BP or 10 mm Hg increase in diastolic BP is associated with roughly twice the risk of death from CAD for patients aged 40 to 69.[11] In one study using Framingham data, blood pressure had the strongest association with CVD events in women and was second only to age as a risk factor for men.[7]

Blood pressure is a key feature of the American College of Cardiology (ACC)/American Heart Association (AHA) Heart Risk Calculator,[12] and blood pressure control is a core component of current AHA guidelines on the primary prevention of CVD.[13] The prevalence of hypertension in US adults is estimated at 32.4% or about 82 million adults. Among adults who self-report hypertension, about 76% use antihypertensive medications.[14] Expenditures related to hypertension were $79 billion in 2016.

EFFECT OF CHOLESTEROL

Elevated total cholesterol and elevated low-density lipoproteins (LDL) are strongly associated with increased risk of atherosclerotic CVD, while elevated high-density lipoprotein (HDL) cholesterol has been associated with a decreased risk of atherosclerotic CVD. These associations are quite strong, and both serum cholesterol and HDL are incorporated into the ACC/AHA Heart Risk Calculator.[10] Additionally, lipid control and statin treatment are key components of AHA guidelines on the primary prevention of CVD.[13]

The relationship between cholesterol and atherosclerosis was known several decades before the availability of large-scale epidemiologic data. Physicians in the early 20th century were aware of the increased incidence of MI in families with familial hypercholesterolemia, and the relationship between cholesterol and atherosclerosis had been convincingly demonstrated in histologic and animal studies. The Framingham Heart Study provided strong epidemiologic evidence supporting the connection, even in those with mildly elevated cholesterol,[6] and by 1960 the AHA was recommending dietary changes to reduce cholesterol intake.[15,16]

Evidence supporting medication used to lower cholesterol and lipid levels emerged in 1985 with the publication of the Coronary Primary Prevention Trial. In this study, middle-age men without known CAD who received cholestyramine achieved lower serum cholesterol and had a 20% to 25% lower incidence of CAD death, nonfatal MI, angina, new positive stress test, or coronary artery bypass grafting (CABG).[17]

Statin medications for hypercholesterolemia were first introduced by a Japanese scientist in the 1970s and were made widely commercially available in 1987.[18,19] Contemporary studies, including many randomized controlled trials, have demonstrated the efficacy of statin therapy in reducing dyslipidemia and the risk of CVD,

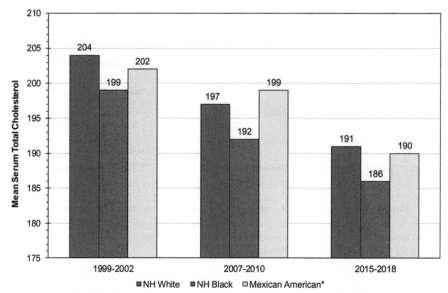

Fig. 4. Age-adjusted trends in mean serum total cholesterol among US adults by race and year. (*Reprinted from* Virani et al.[2]).

including CAD, and in reducing mortality from CAD.[20-23] Statin therapy has become a mainstay in the primary and secondary prevention of CAD.

Among US adults, mean serum total cholesterol, LDL, and triglycerides have declined over the past 20 years (**Fig. 4**).[2] The use of lipid-modifying agents has remained steady in the past decade in the US at around 40 million individuals,[18] though there have been increases in statin use among adults older than age 40.[19] Statin use and high-intensity statin use have been increasing among patients who have had an atherosclerotic CVD event, particular patients with CAD.[22] The development of generic statins have led to lower total cost, down from $17.2 billion in 2003 to $16.9 billion in 2013, and lower out-of-pocket cost, only $2 per 30-day period as of 2016 according to one estimate.[22]

While the propagation of statins and widespread reduction in dyslipidemia has been an encouraging trend over the past 2 decades, inequities in statin use among specific demographic groups have been a recent subject of interest. Multiple studies have shown lower use among younger adults, women, and some racial and ethnic minorities. These disparities are not fully explained by access to care or health insurance characteristics and remain the subject of research and policy efforts to ensure equitable care for all patients.[19]

EFFECT OF DIABETES MELLITUS

Diabetes mellitus was one of the first risk factors for CAD identified in the Framingham study[6] and continues to be a major contributor to the burden of CAD in the US and worldwide.[2] The Centers for Disease Control and Prevention (CDC) estimates 34.2 million Americans have diabetes, about 10% of the population, including 21.4% of those more than age 65. The number of youth and adolescents with diabetes is also at an all-time high – nearly one-quarter of a million Americans under age 20– and has doubled since 2003. An additional 88 million Americans are prediabetic (**Fig. 5**).[23]

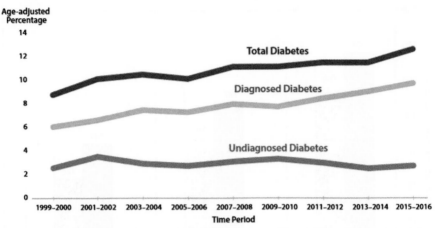

Fig. 5. Temporal trends in the prevalence of diabetes mellitus in the US. (*Reprinted from* Centers for Disease Control and Prevention.[23]).

CVD is the leading cause of morbidity and mortality in patients with diabetes.[24] Diabetics are almost twice as likely to die from CVD compared with patients without diabetes; much of this risk is related to CAD and MI.[24,25] In 2016, there were an estimated 1.7 million hospitalizations for CVD in diabetics, including 438,000 for CAD.[23] Diabetes is associated with many other CAD risk factors, including obesity, physical inactivity, tobacco use, hypertension, and hyperlipidemia.[23,26] Pathophysiologically, diabetes is associated with accelerated atherosclerosis leading to complex CAD[26–28] and greater atherosclerotic disease of the aorta,[29] diastolic dysfunction, and heart failure.[24] The association between diabetes and CAD is so profound that some studies suggest that patients with diabetes with no history of MI have the same risk of cardiovascular death as nondiabetic patients with prior MI.[30]

EFFECT OF TOBACCO USE
Smoking

Cigarette smoking became the most prevalent form of tobacco use during the early 20th century, peaking in 1964 at which time 40% of US adults regularly smoked cigarettes, including the majority (53%) of adult men. Even though much was known about the deleterious health effects of cigarette smoking, including its association with lung cancer, cigarette smoking was considered a perfectly acceptable practice in homes and public spaces.[31]

In the early 1960s, a presidentially directed comprehensive review of 7000 scientific articles by 150 experts convincingly demonstrated the increased risks of lung cancer, chronic bronchitis, emphysema, CAD, and mortality associated with smoking cigarettes. Importantly, this report gained widespread attention from the US public and media. Cigarette smoking was thus identified as a major public health concern, marking a major shift in American culture. Cigarette smoking began to decline after the publication of this report in 1964, a trend that has continued for over 5 decades (**Fig. 6**).[31,32]

With ongoing efforts by physicians and public health officials to educate the public and advocate for appropriate public policy, rates of cigarette smoking are at an all-time low among US adults. Despite these improvements, smoking has remained the leading cause of preventable disease, disability, and death in the US. As of 2018%,

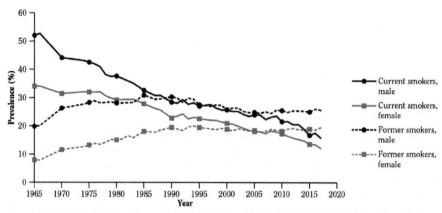

Fig. 6. Temporal trends in the prevalence of current and former smokers in the US. (*Reprinted from* U.S. Department of Health and Human Services, Centers for Disease Control and Prevention, National Center for Chronic Disease Prevention and Health Promotion, Office on Smoking and Health.[32]).

19.7% of US adults used any type of tobacco product, and 13.7% of US adults reported cigarette use every day or some days.[2,33]

While smoking has been linked to serious diseases of multiple organ systems, the most significant mechanism by which smoking causes death and disability is CAD. Exposure to tobacco smoke is associated with a relative risk of developing CAD between 1.4 and 6.3, depending on age and the tobacco dose.[34,35] Smokers have an increased relative risk of death from CAD of 2.50 in men and 2.86 in women.[36] Even exposure to second-hand smoke confers an increased risk of CAD.[35] Death from MI and CAD is lower among former smokers than current smokers, though quitting does not completely eliminate future risk.[32] While the pathophysiology is known to be multifactorial, the direct effects of nicotine–release of catecholamines stimulating increased heart rate and myocardial demand, endothelial dysfunction, lipid abnormalities, and insulin resistance are thought to be principally responsible.[34]

EFFECT OF SMOKELESS TOBACCO AND ELECTRONIC NICOTINE DELIVERY SYSTEMS

Smokeless tobacco products also contain high doses of nicotine and have been extensively studied. These products carry a significant risk of CAD (RR: 2.23); the effects of smoking plus use of smokeless tobacco have been shown to be multiplicative (smoking alone RR: 2.95, smoking plus smokeless RR 4.09).[37]

While smoking has steadily declined since 1964, the usage of electronic nicotine delivery systems, also known e-cigarettes or vaping, has increased dramatically in recent years and has become a $2 billion industry.[38] Presently e-cigarettes are the most common nicotine product among youth – 10.5% of middle school students and 27.5% of high school students reporting use within 30 days.[39] By comparison, cigarette use in the preceding 30 days among middle and high school students in the US was 2.3% and 5.8%, respectively, in 2019.[2,33]

As vaporized nicotine products are relatively new, there are scant epidemiologic data available to assess associated risks. The heterogeneity of chemicals contained within them is vast and difficult to study.[38] The strongest similarity between e-cigarettes and combustible cigarettes is nicotine, which is known to acutely cause catecholamine release, increased myocardial demand, and induce endothelial dysfunction, and is known to be addictive.[34,38] Given the staggeringly high proportion of youth and adolescents using e-cigarettes, and the known increased risk of future cigarette use, e-cigarettes may reverse the trend of decreased morbidity and mortality due to tobacco and nicotine use in the US that has been sustained since the Surgeon General's report in 1964.

EFFECT OF OBESITY

Obesity is defined as a body mass index (BMI) greater than 30. Body weight was identified as a risk factor for CVD early in the Framingham study and has been extensively studied since then.[33] The relationship between BMI and risk of death from CVD is not linear; studies have instead demonstrated a J-shaped curve with differences in risk starting to emerge around BMI 26.5 in men and 25 in women, with a steep inflection point and exponentially increasing risk beyond BMI 40.[40] In one study involving only women, obesity (BMI > 30) conferred a relative risk of 2.48 for the development of CAD, while severe obesity (BMI > 40) conferred a relative risk of more than 5. Weight gain during adulthood, even as little as 4 to 10 kg, was associated with increased risk. Increased levels of physical activity attenuated the negative effects of obesity but did not eliminate CAD risk.[41,42]

Despite a common misperception of adipose tissue as simply a storage repository for biologic fuel, adipose tissue is quite metabolically active and is known to secrete many cytokines and bioactive mediators that may lead to the progression of CAD. These have been noted to increase the risk of thrombotic disease including MI, cause dysregulation of lipid levels, induce insulin resistance, contribute to endothelial dysfunction, and accelerate atherosclerosis.[42]

Independent of BMI or the measured amount of subcutaneous fat, visceral fat mass has been shown to be a significant risk factor for CAD, hyperglycemia, hyperlipidemia, and hypertension,[40] and has been associated with severity of CAD measured angiographically.[43] This may be because visceral fat is more metabolically active than subcutaneous fat, secreting higher volumes of cytokines and bioactive mediators.[44]

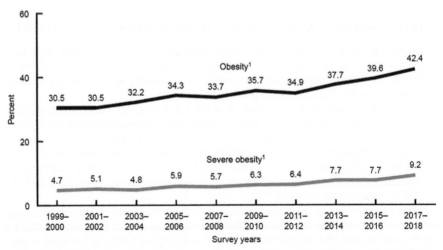

Fig. 7. Temporal trends in the prevalence of obesity (BMI > 30) and severe obesity (BMI > 40). (*Reprinted from* Virani et al.[2]).

The proportion of US adults who are at a healthy bodyweight has been declining for several decades, presently down to 27.7% of the population from 41.7% in 1988 to 1994. Over the same period of time, the proportion of US adults who are obese has nearly doubled from 22.8% to 38.6% (**Fig. 7**). The proportion of children aged 6 to 11 who are obese has increased from 11.3% to 17.9%, and the proportion of children aged 12 to 19 who are obese has increased from 10.5% to 20.6%.[4]

EFFECTS OF PHYSICAL INACTIVITY

Physical inactivity is often thought of as one component, along with nutrition, that contributes to the development of obesity. However, lack of exercise is a significant risk factor for the development of CAD independent of bodyweight. While it is true physical inactivity contributes to the development of obesity, and that the combination of the 2 confers a greater risk of CAD than either in isolation, the risk of developing CAD is elevated in patients with healthy bodyweight who are physically inactive, and the risk of CAD is lower in obese patient who exercise in comparison with those who do not.[41]

Physical activity and exercise can attenuate but not eliminate the deleterious effects of obesity.[42] Exercise is associated with lower incidence of CVD, lower mortality, and lower incidence of CVD risk factors including hypertension, obesity, and impaired blood glucose.[45] Enhanced activity of nitric oxide synthase and circulating progenitor cells at the endothelial level along with coronary angiogenesis have been postulated as the mechanisms by which regular physical activity and exercise may prevent or attenuate the development of CAD.[46]

Recent findings related to the levels of physical activity of average Americans are a mix of encouraging and discouraging trends. It has been encouraging to note that among adults, there has been a steadily increasing percentage of the population that is meeting US Health and Human Services (HHS) recommendations for exercise, a trend that has been ongoing since 2008 (**Fig. 8**). As of 2018, more than half of

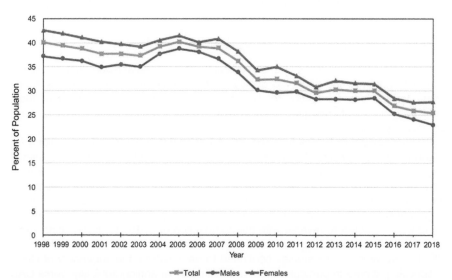

Fig. 8. Temporal trends in physical inactivity in US adults. (*Reprinted from* Virani et al.[2]).

American adults engaged in greater than 150 minutes per week of moderate physical activity or 75 minutes per week of vigorous physical activity, meeting the recommended activity recommendations. This measure has steadily increased from just more than 40% in 2008. Nearly one-quarter of US adults engage in no leisure-time physical activity, which was 36.3% in 2008 and has decreased steadily.[4,45]

However, over the same time-period inactivity among American youth has gotten much worse, with the number of children and adolescents meeting activity recommendations slowly dropping year over year since 2011. Less than one-quarter of US children and adolescents engage in 60 minutes of moderate physical activity per day as recommended by HHS with higher rates among males (30.9%) in comparison to females (15.4%).[47] These trends are likely contributing to the burdens of childhood obesity and diabetes among America's youth and may lead to more widespread CVD in the future.

HISTORY OF CORONARY ARTERY BYPASS GRAFTING

Attempts to surgically treat CAD during the early 20th century were largely unsuccessful. However, the 1960s saw many critical advancements in the care of CAD, including the development of coronary angiography[48] and the proliferation of safe and effective technology and techniques for cardiopulmonary bypass.[49] There were also many breakthroughs in surgical technique, including left internal mammary artery (LIMA) grafting to the left anterior descending artery (LAD)[50] as well as aortocoronary grafting using reversed saphenous vein. Initially used as a technique for revisions or as a "bail out" during coronary endarterectomy,[51] the use of saphenous vein as coronary grafting conduit was later broadly applied to revascularize other coronary vessels for patients whose anterior wall was revascularized with internal mammary arterial grafting.[52]

Once CABG was established as a safe and reproducible treatment option for patients with CAD, several randomized controlled trials were undertaken to determine which patients might benefit from surgical revascularization. These studies broadly demonstrated a survival advantage of CABG over medical therapy alone in many patient populations and ushered in an era of profound growth of surgical procedural volumes. These studies also laid the foundation for modern indications for CABG including left main disease and 3-vessel disease.

THERAPIES FOR CORONARY ARTERY DISEASE

The mainstay of treatment of CAD is medical therapy aimed at risk reduction, alleviation of symptoms, and improved quality of life. Elective revascularization is appropriate for patients for whom medical therapy does not adequately meet these objectives; urgent or emergent revascularization is indicated in the setting of an acute coronary syndrome.

Coronary angioplasty was first performed in a human in 1977 and was quickly followed by the development of bare-metal stents in the mid-1980s and drug-eluting stents in the late 1990s and early 2000s.[53] Many randomized controlled trials were undertaken to evaluate bare-metal stents versus CABG in patients in multi-vessel disease. These studies tended to demonstrate a long-term survival advantage or fewer major adverse cardiac and cerebrovascular events in patients with CABG.[54,55] This trend was expected to reverse with the comparison of CABG to drug-eluting stents in more recent randomized controlled trials, such as SYNTAX,[56] FREEDOM,[57] and BEST.[58] However, these studies continued to demonstrate the superiority of CABG in specific patients–in particular those with clinically or angiographically worse CAD. The feasibility of treating left main disease with percutaneous coronary intervention

(PCI) has recently been evaluated in 2 large randomized controlled trials, with some-what mixed results.[59,60]

When patients with complex CAD require revascularization, leading cardiology and cardiothoracic surgery societies recommend balanced, multidisciplinary decision-making with a "Heart Team" to determine whether CABG or PCI represents optimal therapy for an individual patient. At a minimum, the Heart Team consists of an inter-ventional cardiologist and a cardiac surgeon. Utilization of the Heart Team promotes patient autonomy via better informed consent, helps ensure the best evidence-based approach for each individual patient, reduces variability among providers and institu-tions, and may have a mortality benefit.[61,62]

RECENT TRENDS IN INVASIVE THERAPIES

According to the data from the Nationwide Inpatient Sample (NIS) database, 201,000 CABGs were performed in 2016, down from 337,000 in 2003. Data from the Society of Thoracic Surgeons (STS) database showed a similar decline throughout the early 2000s.[63,64] The NIS database reported that 440,000 PCIs were performed in 2016, down from 777,000 in 2003. Decreasing national CABG procedural volume has been the trend since the 1990s with the emergence of PCI as a less invasive alterna-tive. However, the decrease in PCI volume is a more recent development (**Fig. 9**). It has been suggested that the downtrend in all revascularization procedures has been due to a combination of improvements in medical therapy and the dissemination of data questioning the benefit of revascularization in stable CAD.[63]

CABG continues to be the most commonly performed procedure in cardiac surgery; approximately 85% of all cardiac surgeries are isolated CABG. The large majority of CABGs are performed with cardiopulmonary bypass; off-pump procedures declined steadily through the last decade and hit a nadir around 10% in 2013 to 2014, though there was a slight uptrend to around 13% in 2016.

SHIFTING DEMOGRAPHICS FOR PATIENTS WITH CORONARY ARTERY BYPASS GRAFTING

The indications for CABG, as well as the increasing age of the population and increasing prevalence of diabetes, obesity, and other comorbidities, have led to a

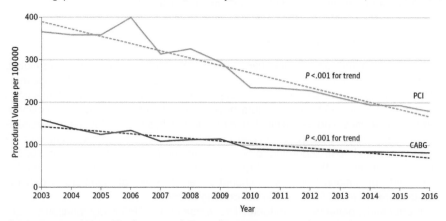

Fig. 9. Temporal Trend in the Annual Rate of Percutaneous and Surgical Coronary Revascu-larization per 100,000 US Adults. Dashed line indicates the mean trend and the solid line the year-to-year trend. (*Reprinted from* Alkhouli et al.[63]).

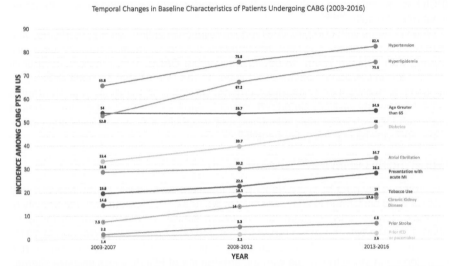

Fig. 10. Temporal changes in baseline characteristics of patients undergoing CABG (2003–2016). (*Data derived* from Alkhouli et al.[63]).

shifting demographic of patients undergoing CABG, with a trend toward patients with CABG being older and with more comorbidities than in the past. Data from the NIS database have demonstrated a 2-fold increase in the proportion of patients with CABG with chronic kidney disease between 2003 and 2016 and a 3-fold increase in patients with prior stroke. It is also becoming more common for CABG to be performed nonelectively, often for acute MI (**Fig. 10**). Despite these findings, the STS and NIS databases both demonstrate decreased absolute mortality for patients with CABG over time.[63–65] Similar recent trends have been noted within the Veterans Affairs health care system; patients have become more medically complex–older, higher average BMI, more diabetes, and more heart failure—and more angiographically complex (more left main disease, higher prevalence of previous PCI). Despite these changes, perioperative mortality has decreased over time.[66]

UNIQUE POPULATIONS–DIABETICS

The FREEDOM trial specifically investigated CABG versus PCI with drug-eluting stents in diabetics with multivessel disease and demonstrated reduced all-cause mortality, fewer major adverse cardiac and cerebrovascular events, and fewer MIs among patients undergoing CABG.[57] As data have accumulated regarding the efficacy of CABG for diabetics, and as the incidence of diabetes has risen in the general population, the proportion of patients with CABG who are diabetic has grown to an all-time high, up to about 50% according to one estimate, up from less than 40% in 2006.[64] Given projections for the continued growth of the prevalence of diabetes in the US and world populations,[67] surgeons should expect to see high numbers of patients with diabetes referred for CABG in the coming decades.

Unfortunately, patients with diabetes fare worse after CABG in comparison to non-diabetics, a disparity that has decreased with improvements in surgical technique, cardiac anesthesia, and cardiac critical care. Indeed, patients with diabetes have greater risks of perioperative complications such as stroke, renal failure, deep sternal

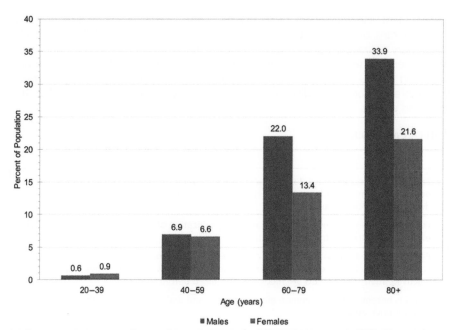

Fig. 11. Prevalence of CAD by age and sex in the US, 2015 to 2018. (*Reprinted from* Virani et al.[2]).

wound infection, and death within 30 days,[68] as well as worse all-cause mortality at 5 years.[69]

UNIQUE POPULATIONS–WOMEN

CAD and associated mortality are more common in men than in women (**Fig. 11**), and women who have CAD are more likely to have a nonobstructive pattern.[70] However, data from the STS database noted proportionately more women undergoing CABG over time throughout the 1990s (25.7% of all patients with CABG in 1990 vs 28.7% in 1999).[65] Women undergoing CABG tend to be older than their male counterparts and have more comorbid conditions at the time of operation, including obesity, diabetes, hypertension, chronic kidney disease, chronic lung disease, and concomitant valvular disease. Women are also more likely to present with ACS or cardiogenic shock,[62] although some data have indicated that women with ACS are less likely to undergo angiography and revascularization.[71] While long-term outcomes seem to be similar between men and women, periprocedural outcomes are worse for women, including mortality, prolonged ICU stay, and wound complications.[62]

SUMMARY

Although the mortality of CAD has declined over recent decades, CAD remains the leading cause of death in the US and presents a highly significant economic burden. Epidemiologic studies have identified numerous strong risk factors for CAD. Some risk factors for the development of CAD are decreasing within the US population, including smoking, hypertension, dyslipidemia, and physical inactivity. Other risk factors, such as advanced age, diabetes, and obesity are increasing in prevalence. Therapies for CAD have evolved over time–the most significant historic advances were the development and refinement of CABG, PCI, and lipid-lowering medications. The contemporary optimal treatment of CAD relies on a multi-modality and multi-disciplinary approach, individualizing therapy for each patient based on the best available evidence. There has been a steady decline in the number of CABGs and PCIs performed in the US for the past decade. Patients with CABG are becoming older and with more comorbid conditions, although mortality associated with CABG has remained steady.

CLINICS CARE POINTS

- Epidemiologic studies have demonstrated the increasing prevalence of CAD and increasing prevalence of many CAD risk factors. However, the number of CABGs and PCIs has decreased in recent years.
- For patients who may require revascularization, utilization of a "Heart Team" approach is an essential best practice to optimize patient outcomes.
- Patients referred for CABG will likely continue to be older, have more significant comorbid conditions, and have more angiographically complex lesions. It is imperative to ensure elective patients with CABG are medically optimized before surgery.
- CABG is becoming more common among women and diabetics, both of whom have worse perioperative outcomes.

DISCLOSURE

The authors have nothing to disclose.

REFERENCES

1. Kochanek KDXJ, Arias E. Mortality in the United States, 2019. NCHS data brief, no 395. Hyattsville, MD: National Center for Health Statistics; 2020.
2. Virani SS, Alonso A, Aparicio HJ, et al. Heart disease and stroke statistics-2021 update: a report from the american heart association. Circulation 2021;143(8): e254–743.
3. Odden MC, Coxson PG, Moran A, et al. The impact of the aging population on coronary heart disease in the United States. Am J Med 2011;124(9):827–33.e825.
4. Office of Disease Prevention and Health PromotionHealthy People 2020. Washington, DC: U.S. Department of Health and Human Services; 2021. Available at: https://www.healthypeople.gov/2020/data-search/. Accessed 01 August 2021.
5. Mahmood SS, Levy D, Vasan RS, et al. The framingham heart study and the epidemiology of cardiovascular disease: a historical perspective. Lancet 2014; 383(9921):999–1008.
6. Kannel WB, Dawber TR, Kagan A, et al. Factors of risk in the development of coronary heart disease–six year follow-up experience. The framingham study. Ann Intern Med 1961;55:33–50.
7. D'Agostino RB, Vasan RS, Pencina MJ, et al. General cardiovascular risk profile for use in primary care: the Framingham Heart Study. Circulation 2008;117(6): 743–53.
8. Lloyd-Jones DM, Leip EP, Larson MG, et al. Prediction of lifetime risk for cardiovascular disease by risk factor burden at 50 years of age. Circulation 2006; 113(6):791–8.

9. Kotchen TA. Historical trends and milestones in hypertension research: a model of the process of translational research. Hypertension 2011;58(4):522–38.

10. Goff DC Jr, Lloyd-Jones DM, Bennett G, et al. 2013 ACC/AHA guideline on the assessment of cardiovascular risk: a report of the American college of cardiology/american heart association task force on practice guidelines. J Am Coll Cardiol 2014;63(25 Pt B):2935–59.

11. Lewington S, Clarke R, Qizilbash N, et al. Age-specific relevance of usual blood pressure to vascular mortality: a meta-analysis of individual data for one million adults in 61 prospective studies. Lancet 2002;360(9349):1903–13.

12. Rosendorff C, Black HR, Cannon CP, et al. Treatment of hypertension in the prevention and management of ischemic heart disease: a scientific statement from the american heart association council for high blood pressure research and the councils on clinical cardiology and epidemiology and prevention. Circulation 2007;115(21):2761–88.

13. Arnett DK, Blumenthal RS, Albert MA, et al. 2019 ACC/AHA guideline on the primary prevention of cardiovascular disease: a report of the american college of cardiology/american heart association task force on clinical practice guidelines. Circulation 2019;140(11):e596–646.

14. Samanic CM, Barbour KE, Liu Y, et al. Prevalence of self-reported hypertension and antihypertensive medication use among adults - United States, 2017. MMWR Morb Mortal Wkly Rep 2020;69(14):393–8.

15. Hajar R. Statins: past and present. Heart Views 2011;12(3):121–7.

16. Endo A. A historical perspective on the discovery of statins. Proc Jpn Acad Ser B Phys Biol Sci 2010;86(5):484–93.

17. The lipid research clinics coronary primary prevention trial results. I. reduction in incidence of coronary heart disease. JAMA 1984;251(3):351–64.

18. Blais JE, Wei Y, Yap KKW, et al. Trends in lipid-modifying agent use in 83 countries. Atherosclerosis 2021;328:44–51.

19. Salami JA, Warraich H, Valero-Elizondo J, et al. National trends in statin use and expenditures in the US adult population from 2002 to 2013: insights from the medical expenditure panel survey. JAMA Cardiol 2017;2(1):56–65.

20. Randomised trial of cholesterol lowering in 4444 patients with coronary heart disease: the Scandinavian Simvastatin Survival Study. Lancet 1994;344(8934): 1383–9.

21. Grundy SM, Stone NJ, Bailey AL, et al. 2018 AHA/ACC/AACVPR/AAPA/ABC/ ACPM/ADA/AGS/APhA/ASPC/NLA/PCNA Guideline on the Management of Blood Cholesterol: A Report of the American College of Cardiology/American Heart Association Task Force on Clinical Practice Guidelines. *J Am Coll Cardiol* Jun 25 2019;73(24):e285–350. https://doi.org/10.1016/j.jacc.2018.11.003.

22. Yao X, Shah ND, Gersh BJ, et al. Assessment of trends in statin therapy for secondary prevention of atherosclerotic cardiovascular disease in US adults from 2007 to 2016. JAMA Netw Open 2020;3(11):e2025505.

23. Centers for Disease Control and Prevention. National diabetes statistics report, 2020. Centers for Disease Control and Prevention. Atlanta, GA: U.S. Dept of Health and Human Services; 2020.

24. Leon BM, Maddox TM. Diabetes and cardiovascular disease: epidemiology, biological mechanisms, treatment recommendations and future research. World J Diabetes 2015;6(13):1246–58.

25. Lee CD, Folsom AR, Pankow JS, et al. Cardiovascular events in diabetic and nondiabetic adults with or without history of myocardial infarction. Circulation 2004;109(7):855–60.

26. Kappetein AP, Head SJ, Morice MC, et al. Treatment of complex coronary artery disease in patients with diabetes: 5-year results comparing outcomes of bypass surgery and percutaneous coronary intervention in the SYNTAX trial. Eur J Cardiothorac Surg 2013;43(5):1006–13.

27. Nicholls SJ, Tuzcu EM, Kalidindi S, et al. Effect of diabetes on progression of coronary atherosclerosis and arterial remodeling: a pooled analysis of 5 intravascular ultrasound trials. J Am Coll Cardiol 2008;52(4):255–62.

28. Lester WM, Roberts WC. Diabetes mellitus for 25 years or more. Analysis of cardiovascular findings in seven patients studied at necropsy. Am J Med 1986;81(2): 275–9.

29. Iwakawa N, Tanaka A, Ishii H, et al. Impact of diabetes mellitus on the aortic wall changes as atherosclerosis progresses: aortic dilatation and calcification. J Atheroscler Thromb 2020;27(6):509–15.

30. Haffner SM, Lehto S, Rönnemaa T, et al. Mortality from coronary heart disease in subjects with type 2 diabetes and in nondiabetic subjects with and without prior myocardial infarction. N Engl J Med 1998;339(4):229–34.

31. U.S. Department of Health and Human Services. The health consequences of smoking: 50 Years of progress. A report of the surgeon general. Atlanta, GA: U.S. Department of Health and Human Services, Centers for Disease Control and Prevention,; 2014. National Center for Chronic Disease Prevention and Health Promotion, Office on Smoking and Health, 2014. Printed with corrections.

32. U.S. Department of Health and Human Services.. Smoking Cessation. A Report of the Surgeon General. Atlanta, GA: U.S. Department of Health and Human Services, Centers for Disease Control and Prevention, National Center for Chronic Disease Prevention and Health Promotion, Office on Smoking and Health; 2020.

33. Hubert HB, Feinleib M, McNamara PM, et al. Obesity as an independent risk factor for cardiovascular disease: a 26-year follow-up of participants in the Framingham Heart Study. Circulation 1983;67(5):968–77.

34. U.S. Department of Health and Human Services. How tobacco smoke causes disease: the biology and behavioral basis for smoking-attributable disease: a report of the surgeon general. Atlanta, GA: U.S. Department of Health and Human Services, Centers for Disease Control and Prevention, National Center for Chronic Disease Prevention and Health Promotion, Office on Smoking and Health; 2010.

35. Law MR, Morris JK, Wald NJ. Environmental tobacco smoke exposure and ischaemic heart disease: an evaluation of the evidence. BMJ 1997;315(7114): 973–80.

36. Thun MJ, Carter BD, Feskanich D, et al. 50-year trends in smoking-related mortality in the United States. N Engl J Med 2013;368(4):351–64.

37. Teo KK, Ounpuu S, Hawken S, et al. Tobacco use and risk of myocardial infarction in 52 countries in the INTERHEART study: a case-control study. Lancet 2006; 368(9536):647–58.

38. U.S. Department of Health and Human Services. E-Cigarette use among youth and young adults. A Report of the Surgeon General. Atlanta, GA: U.S. Department of Health and Human Services, Centers for Disease Control and Prevention, National Center for Chronic Disease Prevention and Health Promotion, Office on Smoking and Health; 2016.

39. Wang TW, Gentzke AS, Creamer MR, et al. Tobacco product use and associated factors among middle and high school students - United States, 2019. MMWR Surveill Summ 2019;68(12):1–22.

40. Calle EE, Thun MJ, Petrelli JM, et al. Body-mass index and mortality in a prospective cohort of U.S. adults. N Engl J Med 1999;341(15):1097–105.
41. Li TY, Rana JS, Manson JE, et al. Obesity as compared with physical activity in predicting risk of coronary heart disease in women. Circulation 2006;113(4): 499–506.
42. Van Gaal LF, Mertens IL, De Block CE. Mechanisms linking obesity with cardiovascular disease. Nature 2006;444(7121):875–80.
43. Zamboni M, Armellini F, Sheiban I, et al. Relation of body fat distribution in men and degree of coronary narrowings in coronary artery disease. Am J Cardiol 1992;70(13):1135–8.
44. Matsuzawa Y. The metabolic syndrome and adipocytokines. FEBS Lett 2006; 580(12):2917–21.
45. Piercy KL, Troiano RP, Ballard RM, et al. The Physical Activity Guidelines for Americans. JAMA 2018;320(19):2020–8.
46. Winzer EB, Woitek F, Linke A. Physical Activity in the Prevention and Treatment of Coronary Artery Disease. J Am Heart Assoc 2018;7(4).
47. Merlo CL, Jones SE, Michael SL, et al. Dietary and Physical activity behaviors among high school students - youth risk behavior survey, United States, 2019. MMWR Suppl 2020;69(1):64–76.
48. Sones FM Jr, Shirey EK. Cine coronary arteriography. Mod Concepts Cardiovasc Dis 1962;31:735–8.
49. Stoney WS. Evolution of cardiopulmonary bypass. Circulation 2009;119(21): 2844–53.
50. Kolessov VI. Mammary artery-coronary artery anastomosis as method of treatment for angina pectoris. J Thorac Cardiovasc Surg 1967;54(4):535–44.
51. Mueller RL, Rosengart TK, Isom OW. The history of surgery for ischemic heart disease. Ann Thorac Surg 1997;63(3):869–78.
52. Favaloro RG. Landmarks in the development of coronary artery bypass surgery. Circulation 1998;98(5):466–78.
53. Iqbal J, Gunn J, Serruys PW. Coronary stents: historical development, current status and future directions. Br Med Bull 2013;106:193–211.
54. Booth J, Clayton T, Pepper J, et al. Randomized, controlled trial of coronary artery bypass surgery versus percutaneous coronary intervention in patients with multivessel coronary artery disease: six-year follow-up from the Stent or Surgery Trial (SoS). Circulation 2008;118(4):381–8.
55. Daemen J, Boersma E, Flather M, et al. Long-term safety and efficacy of percutaneous coronary intervention with stenting and coronary artery bypass surgery for multivessel coronary artery disease: a meta-analysis with 5-year patient-level data from the ARTS, ERACI-II, MASS-II, and SoS trials. Circulation 2008; 118(11):1146–54.
56. Serruys PW, Morice MC, Kappetein AP, et al. Percutaneous coronary intervention versus coronary-artery bypass grafting for severe coronary artery disease. N Engl J Med 2009;360(10):961–72.
57. Farkouh ME, Domanski M, Sleeper LA, et al. Strategies for multivessel revascularization in patients with diabetes. N Engl J Med 2012;367(25):2375–84.
58. Park SJ, Ahn JM, Kim YH, et al. Trial of everolimus-eluting stents or bypass surgery for coronary disease. N Engl J Med 2015;372(13):1204–12.
59. Holm NR, Mäkikallio T, Lindsay MM, et al. Percutaneous coronary angioplasty versus coronary artery bypass grafting in the treatment of unprotected left main stenosis: updated 5-year outcomes from the randomised, non-inferiority NOBLE trial. Lancet 2020;395(10219):191–9.

60. Stone GW, Sabik JF, Serruys PW, et al. Everolimus-eluting stents or bypass surgery for left main coronary artery disease. N Engl J Med 2016;375(23):2223–35.

61. Neumann FJ, Sousa-Uva M, Ahlsson A, et al. 2018 ESC/EACTS guidelines on myocardial revascularization. Eur Heart J 2019;40(2):87–165.

62. Hillis LD, Smith PK, Anderson JL, et al. 2011 ACCF/AHA guideline for coronary artery bypass graft surgery: a report of the american college of cardiology foundation/american heart association task force on practice guidelines. Circulation 2011;124(23):e652–735.

63. Alkhouli M, Alqahtani F, Kalra A, et al. Trends in characteristics and outcomes of patients undergoing coronary revascularization in the United States, 2003-2016. JAMA Netw Open 2020;3(2):e1921326.

64. D'Agostino RS, Jacobs JP, Badhwar V, et al. The society of thoracic surgeons adult cardiac surgery database: 2018 update on outcomes and quality. Ann Thorac Surg 2018;105(1):15–23.

65. Ferguson TB Jr, Hammill BG, Peterson ED, et al. A decade of change–risk profiles and outcomes for isolated coronary artery bypass grafting procedures, 1990-1999: a report from the STS national database committee and the duke clinical research institute. society of thoracic surgeons. Ann Thorac Surg 2002;73(2):480–9 [discussion 489-490].

66. Cornwell LD, Omer S, Rosengart T, et al. Changes over time in risk profiles of patients who undergo coronary artery bypass graft surgery: the veterans affairs surgical quality improvement program (VASQIP). JAMA Surg 2015;150(4):308–15.

67. Bommer C, Sagalova V, Heesemann E, et al. Global economic burden of diabetes in adults: projections from 2015 to 2030. Diabetes Care 2018;41(5):963–70.

68. Shahian DM, O'Brien SM, Filardo G, et al. The society of thoracic surgeons 2008 cardiac surgery risk models: part 1–coronary artery bypass grafting surgery. Ann Thorac Surg 2009;88(1 Suppl):S2–22.

69. Alserius T, Hammar N, Nordqvist T, et al. Improved survival after coronary artery bypass grafting has not influenced the mortality disadvantage in patients with diabetes mellitus. J Thorac Cardiovasc Surg 2009;138(5):1115–22.

70. Brown JC, Gerhardt TE, Kwon E. Risk factors for coronary artery disease. StatPearls. Treasure Island (FL): StatPearls Publishing; 2021.

71. Anand SS, Xie CC, Mehta S, et al. Differences in the management and prognosis of women and men who suffer from acute coronary syndromes. J Am Coll Cardiol 2005;46(10):1845–51.

Epidemiology of Valvular Heart Disease

Alex S. Peters, MD[a], John P. Duggan, MD[a], Gregory D. Trachiotis, MD[b,c],
Jared L. Antevil, MD[d],*

KEYWORDS

- Heart valve diseases • Cardiovascular diseases • Aortic valve stenosis
- Mitral valve Insufficiency

KEY POINTS

- Although there are various pathologies of the 4 heart valves that are of clinical relevance, acquired diseases of the aortic and mitral valves are the most common cause of morbidity and mortality.
- Aortic stenosis (AS) is increasing in incidence in the United States (US), driven largely by an aging demographic, and is the most common indication for valve intervention.
- Aortic valve replacement is the only effective treatment of as, is increasingly accomplished via transcatheter techniques and has a dramatic mortality benefit.
- Mitral valve regurgitation (MR) is the most common form of valvular heart disease (VHD) in the US, whereby MR is most often the result of mitral valve prolapse; rheumatic heart disease (RHD) is a more common etiology of MR in underdeveloped countries.
- Interventions for MR in the US are increasing, with a trend toward valve repair over replacement, and increasing utilization of transcatheter techniques to treat MR.

INTRODUCTION

There are various pathologies of the 4 heart valves that are of clinical relevance. The etiologies of these conditions are numerous. Disorders of the heart valves can be categorized as congenital or acquired and by the effect on valve function, for instance, whether they cause stenosis or regurgitation. Of the deaths each year attributed to valvular heart disease (VHD), the most commonly involved valves are the aortic valve followed by the mitral valve, with deaths secondary to right-sided VHD being quite rare **(Fig. 1)**.[1] This article will focus primarily on aortic and mitral VHD, given their greater clinical impact.

[a] Department of Surgery, Walter Reed National Military Medical Center, 4494 Palmer Road North, Bethesda, MD 20814, USA; [b] Division of Cardiology, Cardiothoracic Surgery and Heart Center, Washington DC Veterans Affairs Medical Center, 50 Irving Street Northwest, Washington, DC 20422, USA; [c] Department of Surgery, George Washington University Hospital, 900 23rd St NW, Washington, DC 20037, USA; [d] Division of Cardiothoracic Surgery, Washington DC Veterans Affairs Medical Center, 50 Irving Street Northwest, Washington, DC 20422, USA
* Corresponding author.
E-mail address: jared.antevil@va.gov

Surg Clin N Am 102 (2022) 517–528
https://doi.org/10.1016/j.suc.2022.01.008
0039-6109/22/Published by Elsevier Inc.

surgical.theclinics.com

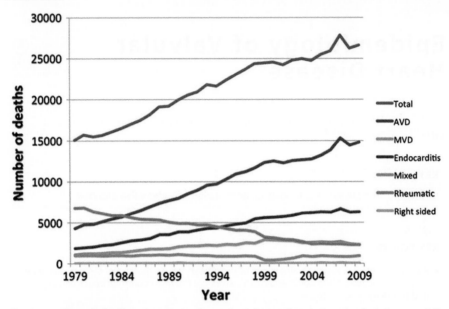

Fig. 1. Number of deaths per year in the United States due to heart valve disease. AVD, aortic valve disease. MVD, mitral valve disease. (Reproduced from Coffey et al.[1])

Aortic Valve Disease

Significance

In the United States (US), aortic valve disease (AVD) is the most common cause of mortality and reason for procedural intervention among the various types of VHD.[2,3] Data reported to the Centers for Disease Control showed that of the 24,192 deaths due to VHD in 2019, 16000 were secondary to AVD.[2] Mortality due to AVD steadily increased from the 1970s to the 2000s, with an annual increase of approximately 1.6%, which is likely driven by the aging population and the increased prevalence of degenerative AVD with aging.[1] Based on the estimates of population growth and assumption of stable mortality, the number of deaths attributed to VHD is expected to double by 2030, and will likely be driven by AVD.[1] AVD is also the most common indication for procedural intervention for VHD in the US. In 2017, the cumulative number of transcatheter aortic valve replacements (TAVR) and surgical aortic valve replacements (SAVR) was nearly 84,000, more than double the 30,000 procedures performed on the mitral valve that year.[3]

Aortic Stenosis

Aortic stenosis (AS) is a narrowing of the normal aortic valve area from various causes that leads to increased resistance to flow and increased flow rates across the valve. In 2020 the American College of Cardiology (ACC) and American Heart Association (AHA) published guidelines that defined 4 stages of AS based on the aortic valve velocity, valve area, pressure gradients, and symptoms. Broadly these stages range from "at risk of AS" based on congenital anomalies or aortic valve sclerosis to severe symptomatic AS.[4]

Etiology

The 3 principle causes of AS are a congenital bicuspid valve, calcification of a normal tri-leaflet valve, and rheumatic heart disease (RHD).

Congenital bicuspid valve: Bicuspid aortic valve (BAV) is the most common congenital cardiac defect and is present in 0.5% to 2% of the population, with a male predominance of roughly 3:1.[5] BAV anatomy is important clinically as it is a common cause of AS requiring procedural intervention, and because of its association with other anomalies, namely the dilation of the proximal ascending aorta.[5,6] From a series of 932 patients aged 26 to 91 undergoing isolated aortic valve replacement (AVR) the overall incidence of bicuspid anatomy was 49%, and another 4% had a unicuspid valve.[6] Thus, in patients requiring AVR roughly half have a congenitally abnormal valve. Importantly, the incidence of congenital abnormalities varies with age. All patients less than 50 years old had a congenitally abnormal valve, with 58% being bicuspid. In those 51 to 70 years old, two-thirds of patients undergoing AVR had a bicuspid valve and one-quarter had a tri-leaflet valve. Finally, in those greater than 70 years old a calcified tri-leaflet valve was present in 57% and a bicuspid valve in 40%.[6]

Calcific aortic valve disease: Calcific AVD, formerly known as senile or degenerative disease, is the most common cause of AS in adults.[7] Calcific AVD exists on a spectrum from aortic valve sclerosis, which is thickening and/or calcification without significant obstruction, to hemodynamically significant calcific AVD, referred to as AS.[8] The prevalence of aortic valve sclerosis and AS both increase with age. The prevalence of aortic valve sclerosis ranges from approximately 9% in patients 51 years old to 42% in those 81 years old.[9] The rate of progression of aortic valve sclerosis to hemodynamically significant AS is approximately 1.8% to 1.9% of patients per year.[8] The prevalence of AS in the general population in developed countries is 0.4% and 1.7% in those greater than 65.[10] For those greater than 75 the prevalence is estimated to be 3.4% of the population.[8]

Rheumatic heart disease: The third major cause of AS is RHD, which occurs after infection with *Streptococcus pyogenes* and the development of acute rheumatic fever. Molecular mimicry leads to valve inflammation which over time can cause fibrosis and fusion of the commissures, leading to stenosis, which is also often accompanied by regurgitation.[11] Low-income countries and low-income groups within high-income countries bear the majority of the burden of this disease. In New Zealand, Indigenous populations are significantly more affected by this disease entity than nonindigenous persons. Forty per 100,000 and 80 per 100,000 people of Maori and Pacific island origin, respectively, are affected by acute rheumatic fever, compared with 2.1 per 100,000 in non-Maori/Pacific persons.[11] The Global Burden of Disease (GBD) study estimates mortality and prevalence of many disease entities worldwide, including RHD. A review of the GBD study data from 1990 to 2015 estimated there were 9.2 deaths per 100,000 in 1990 and 4.8 deaths per 100,000 in 2015, a reduction of 47.8%.[12] In the same review, most of the cases in 1990 and 2015 (77% and 82%, respectively) occurred in endemic regions, with the highest numbers of deaths occurring in India, China, and Pakistan. The prevalence of RHD in 2015 was 444 per 100,000 in endemic regions and 3.4 per 100,000 in nonendemic regions.[12]

Aortic Regurgitation

In high-income countries calcific AVD, BVD, and aortic root dilation are the most common causes of aortic regurgitation (AR).[13] In low-income regions RHD is the leading cause of AR.[4] In 2 large studies in the US and the United Kingdom (UK) the prevalence of clinically significant AR ranged from 0.5% to 1.6% in the general population, and in those 75 years and older the prevalence was 2.0%.[9,10] Some degree of mild AR seems to be more common as 13% of men and 8.5% of women in the Framingham Offspring study had mild or greater AR.[14] The prevalence of moderate or greater AR in an African American cohort was the same as the general population in the US at 0.5%.[15] A slightly greater prevalence of moderate or greater AR was found in a cohort of 3500 Native Americans with a rate of 3.5%.[16] In Europe, the etiologies of AR were estimated in a multicenter study including 4900 patients. The most common etiology was degenerative at 50%, followed by congenital and rheumatic both at 15%, and endocarditis at 7%.[17]

Treatment of Aortic Valve Disease

Medical therapy and prognosis

For severe AS the only therapy with a demonstrated survival benefit is AVR.[7] In symptomatic patients with severe AS who are managed medically, the median survival is less than 2 years, and the mortality rate at 5 years seems to be between 80% and 90% (**Fig. 2**).[18,19] Presenting symptoms confer a difference in mortality with the average survival for patients with angina, syncope, and dyspnea being 5, 3, and 2 years, respectively.[20] Even for asymptomatic patients with severe stenosis AVR seems to be superior as demonstrated by a series of asymptomatic patients randomized to surgery versus "watchful waiting," which demonstrated a significantly higher mortality rate at 2 years in the watchful waiting group.[21]

Multiple studies have shown that survival after successful AVR for AS is equivalent to the general population. Patients more than the age of 65 who had AVR in the UK had postoperative survival equivalent to matched patients without AS at an interval of up to 8 years after AVR,[22] and a study in Iceland demonstrated equivalent survival at a median follow-up of 4.7 years.[23]

Medical management for AS has focused on the prevention of the progression of aortic valve sclerosis and mild to moderate AS to severe disease. Unfortunately, medical management alone has not been shown to prevent progression of AS or improve survival.[4,7] However, the ACC/AHA 2020 guidelines for the management of VHD recommended that patients with AS receive antihypertensive therapy and statin therapy

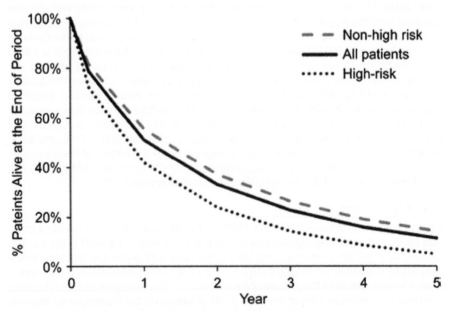

Fig. 2. Survival rates more than 5 years of all patients with symptomatic aortic stenosis and those at high- and non-high operative risk. (Reproduced from Clark et al.[19])

according to standard guidelines, as there is evidence to suggest that ischemic events in patients with AS are decreased with these medications.[4]

For patients with asymptomatic severe AR, the risk of developing symptoms, LV dysfunction, or death is strongly related to the degree of LV dilation.[24,25] In symptomatic patients, the mortality rate is approximately 6% per year for patients with New York Heart Association (NYHA) Class II symptoms and 24% per year for those with NYHA class III or IV symptoms.[26]

Recommended medical therapy for AR per the AHA/ACC 2020 guidelines includes the treatment of hypertension and heart failure according to standard guidelines, but it is not a substitute for AVR in patients who are candidates for surgery.[4] AVR is recommended for all symptomatic patients and for patients with asymptomatic severe AR and either depressed systolic function or a severely dilated LV.[4] The degree of symptoms and ventricular dysfunction predicts postoperative survival, with improved outcomes in those with milder symptoms and less dysfunction.[27–29]

Aortic valve replacement

Over the past 60 years, since the first SAVR in 1960, there has been a significant evolution of AVR. Initial valves consisted of a mechanical valve with a "valve-in-cage" design. Over time mechanical valves that more accurately mimicked the normal function and hemodynamics of the native aortic valve were developed. A major limitation of mechanical valves is the need for lifelong anticoagulation. Bioprosthetic valves were introduced in the late 1960s. These valves have the benefit of being less thrombogenic, thus eliminating the need for lifelong anticoagulation, but at the expense of limited durability.

The use of bioprosthetic valves has increased substantially in more recent years: in 1998 53.3% of implanted valves were bioprosthetic and in 2011 that percentage increased to 63.6%.[30] **Fig. 3** shows the change over time overall and stratified by patient age. Improved durability of bioprosthetic valves, the increased safety of reoperative valve surgery, and the possibility of "valve-in-valve" TAVR for degenerated bioprosthetic valves are likely driving the trend toward increased use of bioprosthetic valves.

Perhaps the greatest recent advancement in AVD has been the advent of TAVR in the early 2000s. Initially, this procedure was reserved for patients with AS with prohibitive surgical risk. Over the past 2 decades studies have demonstrated noninferiority of TAVR to SAVR for patients at intermediate risk for surgery, and more recently short-term data suggest equivalent results for low-risk patients with AS and a tri-leaflet aortic valve.[31] With expanding indications, TAVR overtook SAVR as the most common method for AVR in the US in 2016, according to the 2019 Update on Outcomes and Quality of the Society of Thoracic Surgeons Adult Cardiac Surgery Database (**Fig. 4**).[3] Due to technical issues with anchoring a transcatheter valve in the absence of annular calcium, TAVR has only a limited role in treating patients with isolated AR.[4]

Although it has not yet been evaluated in a large-scale or randomized trial, there is an increasing experience in treating a degenerated bioprosthetic valve with a new transcatheter valve. This procedure, termed "valve-in-valve TAVR," seems to be feasible whether the original bioprosthetic was implanted using open surgical or transcatheter technique.[32,33] Because the alternative to valve-in-valve TAVR is re-operative AVR, valve-in-valve TAVR represents a potentially promising alternative for select patients with degenerated bioprosthetic aortic valves.

Before the advent of TAVR, balloon aortic valvuloplasty, which was first introduced in 1985, was the only transcatheter treatment used for AS.[34] Outside of a few specific indications this therapy has largely been abandoned due to high rates of restenosis

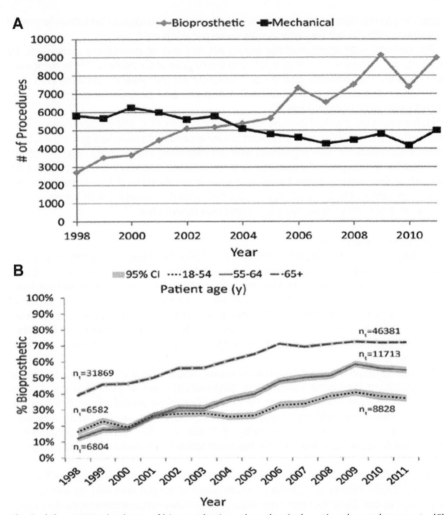

Fig. 3. (*A*), estimated volume of bioprosthetic and mechanical aortic valve replacements. (*B*), percentage of aortic valve replacements in which a bioprosthetic valve was used by age. (Reproduced from Isaacs et al.[30])

and symptom recurrence within 6 to 12 months.[4,35] Currently, balloon valvuloplasty is used as a palliative procedure or as a bridge to SAVR in patients with decompensated heart failure.[4]

Aortic valve repair is an alternative procedure to replacement used in the setting of isolated AR with or without aortic root dilation or aneurysms of the ascending aorta. A case series of patients in Germany demonstrated comparable freedom from reoperation and mortality in the appropriate setting, and European guidelines state that it is reasonable to perform repair over replacement in the appropriate clinical setting.[36]

Mitral Regurgitation

In mitral regurgitation (MR) retrograde flow across an incompetent valve can lead to symptomatic limitations, decompensated heart failure, and need for surgery. MR is classified as primary or secondary and as acute or chronic based on its etiology.[9] In

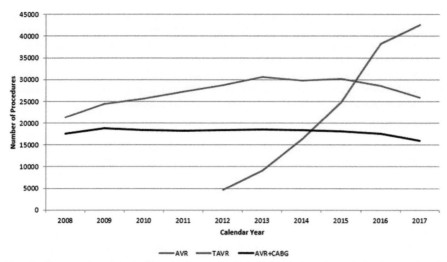

Fig. 4. Change in procedure volume over time for aortic valve replacement (AVR), AVR + Coronary Artery Bypass Grafting (CABG), and transcatheter aortic valve replacement (TAVR). (Reproduced from D'Agostino et al.[3])

this section we will discuss the overall prevalence of the disease, the prevalence of the various subcategories, the clinical significance, and relevant factors regarding treatment.

Although AS is the most significant form of VHD in terms of mortality, MR is the most common form of VHD in the US population overall.[2,37] A population-based study in the US that included 11,900 patients who underwent echocardiography gives the best estimate of the prevalence of MR in developed countries. This study demonstrated the prevalence of MR to be 1.7%, with increasing prevalence with age, ranging from 0.5% in those aged 18% to 44% to 9.3% in those ≥75. At that time the adult population in the US was roughly 200 million people, so approximately 3.4 million adults in the US had some degree of MR.[10] Similar rates were demonstrated in patients more than 65 years of age screened in the UK. In this study 4700 patients underwent echocardiography. The overall prevalence of moderate or greater MR was 3.5% in those ≥ 65. Similarly, the prevalence increased with age with rates of MR of 2.0% in patients 65% to 74%, and 7.7% for patients greater than 75 years old.[37]

Chronic MR can be subdivided into primary and secondary etiologies, which sometimes are referred to as organic and functional etiologies, respectively. In primary MR, regurgitation is due to pathology of the valve apparatus (leaflets, chordae, papillary muscle, and/or annulus) and secondary MR is due to disease of the ventricle or atria. Mitral valve prolapse (MVP) caused by myxomatous degeneration of the mitral valve is the most common etiology of chronic primary MR in high-income countries.[4] Other less common causes include infective endocarditis, RHD, cleft mitral valve, and radiation heart disease. The causes of secondary chronic MR include ischemic cardiomyopathy and idiopathic dilated cardiomyopathy as well as hypertrophic cardiomyopathy.[38] A multicenter study in 2001 in Europe including 4900 patients with known VHD from 92 centers representing both academic and nonacademic hospitals assessed the etiologies of chronic MR. In those with chronic MR, the majority had a primary etiology (>75%) with degenerative and rheumatic causes being most common at 61.3% and 14.2%, respectively. Ischemia was the next most common etiology at 7.3%.[17]

Acute severe MR is a medical emergency that may manifest as severe decompensated heart failure. Similar to chronic MR, acute MR can be subdivided into organic and functional etiologies.[39] The most common organic etiologies include perforation from infective endocarditis, chordal rupture secondary to myxomatous degeneration, papillary muscle rupture, and primarily in developing nations, acute rheumatic fever with carditis.[17,40] Acute functional MR is a relatively rare phenomenon; ischemia and cardiomyopathies are among its more common causes.[17]

Mitral Stenosis

The predominant cause of mitral stenosis (MS) worldwide is RHD. The prevalence in industrialized countries is low, affecting approximately 0.1% of the population.[9,10] In a multicenter prospective study in Europe, rheumatic disease accounted for 85% of cases of MS, followed by degenerative causes at 12.5%.[17]

Mitral Valve Disease Treatment

In 2017 14,000 mitral valve replacements (MVR) and more than 16,000 mitral valve repairs were performed in the US, according to the Society of Thoracic Surgeons 2019 report of outcomes and quality.[3] This represents a nearly 2-fold increase from the 16,000 total mitral valve interventions performed in 2005.[41]

Treatment for mitral regurgitation

In cases of acute MR, afterload reduction with medications and/or intra-aortic balloon pump counter-pulsation to improve forward flow followed by prompt surgical intervention is recommended by the ACC and AHA.[4] For chronic MR, medical treatment of left ventricular (LV) dysfunction and hypertension with renin–angiotensin system blocking medications, diuretics, and aldosterone antagonists according to available guidelines is recommended.

Mitral valve repair or replacement is indicated in patients with symptomatic severe MR or asymptomatic MR with signs of LV dysfunction.[4] When feasible repair is preferable to replacement as results seem to be superior when repair is performed.[4,37,42,43] Transcatheter edge-to-edge repair is an approved option for treating MR in those at prohibitive surgical risk, and with improvements in technique is now being offered to many patients with advanced age or high surgical risk.[4] The most established technique uses the MitraClip system (Abbott Cardiovascular, Plymouth, MN).[44] Several relatively small studies have demonstrated the safety and efficacy of this device in appropriately selected patients.[44,45]

A retrospective review of the National Inpatient Sample database found that 656,030 interventions were performed on the mitral valve for MR from 2000 to 2016 in the US.[46] An analysis of the trends overtime demonstrated that the number of replacement procedures decreased by 5.6% per year from 2000 to 2010, whereas the number of repair procedures increased by 8.4% per year from 2000 to 2006. Additionally, there was a steep increase of 84.4% per year of MitraClip procedures from 2013 to 2016.[46] These trends are graphically represented in **Fig. 5**.

Treatment for mitral stenosis

Patients with MS who also have atrial fibrillation should be anticoagulated to decrease the risk of embolic events, unless there is a contraindication to anticoagulation.[4] In those with a normal rhythm but who are tachycardic there is evidence that rate-controlling medications (beta-blockers, calcium channel blockers, and ivabradine) can improve MS symptoms. For rheumatic MS, when indications for intervention are met, percutaneous mitral balloon commissurotomy (PMBC) is the first-line procedure of choice whereby there is appropriate anatomy. The number of PMBC

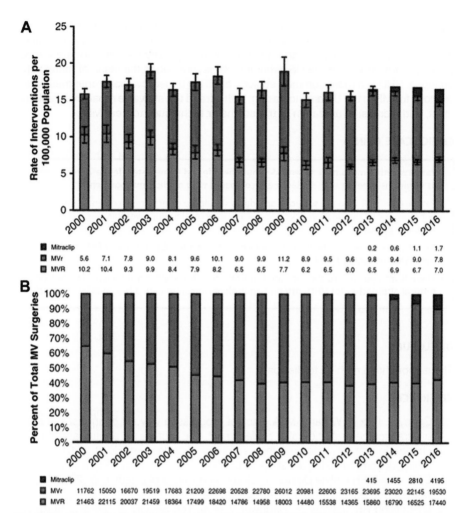

■ Mitraclip														0.2	0.6	1.1	1.7
▨ MVr	5.6	7.1	7.8	9.0	8.1	9.6	10.1	9.0	9.9	11.2	8.9	9.5	9.6	9.8	9.4	9.0	7.8
▤ MVR	10.2	10.4	9.3	9.9	8.4	7.9	8.2	6.5	6.5	7.7	6.2	6.5	6.0	6.5	6.9	6.7	7.0

■ Mitraclip														415	1455	2810	4195
▨ MVr	11762	15050	16670	19519	17683	21209	22698	20528	22780	26012	20981	22606	23165	23695	23020	22145	19530
▤ MVR	21463	22115	20037	21459	18364	17499	18420	14786	14958	18003	14480	15538	14365	15860	16790	16525	17440

Fig. 5. Trends in mitral valve interventions from 2000 to 2016. (*A*), Rate of interventions per 100,000 people in US population more than 18 years of age. (*B*), percent distribution of interventions. MVr, mitral valve repair. MVR, mitral valve replacement. (Reproduced from Zhou et al.[46])

procedures performed has decreased overtime with 22.6 procedures/10 million populations performed between 1998 and 2001 and 22.7/10 million populations from 2008 to 2010, representing a 7.5% decrease.[47] Surgical commissurotomy or MVR are acceptable alternatives if PMBC is not available, the patient is not a candidate, or if they have previously failed PMBC.[4] For patients with nonrheumatic MS, MVR is generally necessary as the calcification of the annulus and base of the leaflets is the main pathologic cause, rather than commissural fusion.[4]

SUMMARY

Although there are various pathologies of the 4 heart valves that are of clinical relevance, acquired diseases of the aortic and mitral valves are the most common cause of morbidity and mortality. AS is increasing in incidence in the US, driven largely by an aging demographic, and is the most common indication for valve intervention. Aortic valve replacement is the only effective treatment of AS, is increasingly accomplished via transcatheter techniques, and has a dramatic mortality benefit. MR is the most common form of VHD in the US, whereby MR is most often the result of mitral valve prolapse; RHD is a more common etiology of MR in underdeveloped countries. Interventions for MR in the US are increasing, with a trend toward valve repair over replacement, and increasing utilization of transcatheter techniques to treat MR.

CLINICS CARE POINTS

- Patients with symptomatic severe AS should be referred immediately for valve replacement as survival is superior with replacement compared with medical management.
- Patients with AR who are surgical candidates should be offered replacement before severe symptoms or LV dysfunction develops as early intervention improves long-term outcomes for these patients.
- Mitral valve repair is preferred over replacement when feasible for cases of MR and is being used with increasing frequency.
- There is a trend toward the increased utilization of transcatheter interventions over open surgical approaches for VHD, offering equivalent outcomes with a less invasive approach.

DISCLOSURE

The authors have nothing to disclose.

REFERENCES

1. Coffey S, Cox B, Williams MJA. Lack of progress in valvular heart disease in the pre-transcatheter aortic valve replacement era: Increasing deaths and minimal change in mortality rate over the past three decades. Am Heart J 2014;167(4). https://doi.org/10.1016/j.ahj.2013.12.030.
2. CDC WONDER Online Database. Underlying Cause of Death 1999-2019. https://wonder.cdc.gov/controller/datarequest/D76.
3. D'Agostino RS, Jacobs JP, Badhwar V, et al. The Society of Thoracic Surgeons Adult Cardiac Surgery Database: 2019 Update on Outcomes and Quality. Ann Thorac Surg 2019;107(1):24–32.
4. Otto CM, Nishimura RA, Bonow RO, et al. 2020 ACC/AHA Guideline for the Management of Patients with Valvular Heart Disease: A Report of the American College of Cardiology/American Heart Association Joint Committee on Clinical Practice Guidelines. Circulation 2021;E72–227. https://doi.org/10.1161/CIR.0000000000000923.
5. Siu SC, Silversides CK. Bicuspid Aortic Valve Disease. J Am Coll Cardiol 2010;55(25):2789–800.
6. Roberts WC, Ko JM. Frequency by decades of unicuspid, bicuspid, and tricuspid aortic valves in adults having isolated aortic valve replacement for aortic stenosis, with or without associated aortic regurgitation. Circulation 2005;111(7):920–5.
7. Lindman BR, Clavel MA, Mathieu P, et al. Calcific aortic stenosis. Nat Rev Dis Primers 2016;2. https://doi.org/10.1038/nrdp.2016.6.
8. Coffey S, Cox B, Williams MJA. The prevalence, incidence, progression, and risks of aortic valve sclerosis: A systematic review and meta-analysis. J Am Coll Cardiol 2014;63(25 PART A):2852–61.

9. D'Arcy JL, Coffey S, Loudon MA, et al. Large-scale community echocardio-graphic screening reveals a major burden of undiagnosed valvular heart disease in older people: The OxVALVE Population Cohort Study. Eur Heart J 2016;37(47): 3515–3522a.

10. Nkomo V, Gardin J, Julius M, et al. Burden of valvular heart disease: a population-based study. Lancet 2006;368:1005.

11. Coffey S, Cairns BJ, Iung B. The modern epidemiology of heart valve disease. Heart 2016;102(1):75–85.

12. Watkins DA, Johnson CO, Colquhoun SM, et al. Global, Regional, and National Burden of Rheumatic Heart Disease, 1990–2015. N Engl J Med 2017;377(8): 713–22.

13. Enriquez-Sarano M, Tajik AJ. Aortic Regurgitation. 2021. www.nejm.org.

14. Singh J, Evans J, Larson M, et al. Prevalence and clinical determinants of mitral, tricuspid, and aortic regurgitation (the Framingham Heart Study). Am J Cardiol 1999;83(6):897–902.

15. Fox E, Wilson R, Penman A, et al. Epidemiology of pure valvular regurgitation in the large middle-aged African American cohort of the Atherosclerosis Risk in Communities study. Vasc Congenit Heart Dis 2007;154(6):1229–34.

16. Lebowitz N, Bella J, Roman M, et al. Prevalence and correlates of aortic regurgi-tation in American Indians: the Strong Heart Study. J Am Coll Cardiol 2000;36(2): 461–7.

17. Iung B, Baron G, Butchart EG, et al. A prospective survey of patients with valvular heart disease in Europe: The Euro Heart Survey on valvular heart disease. Eur Heart J 2003;24(13):1231–43.

18. Carabello B. Aortic Stenosis. N Engl J Med 2002;346(9):677–82.

19. Clark MA, Arnold Sv, Duhay FG, et al. Five-year clinical and economic outcomes among patients with medically managed severe aortic stenosis: Results from a medicare claims analysis. Circ Cardiovasc Qual Outcomes 2012;5(5):697–704.

20. Ross J Jr, Braunwald E. Aortic stenosis. Circulation 1968;388(1):61–7.

21. Campo J, Tsoris A, Kruse J, et al. Prognosis of Severe Asymptomatic Aortic Ste-nosis With and Without Surgery. Ann Thorac Surg 2019;108(1):74–9.

22. Sharabiani MTA, Fiorentino F, Angelini GD, et al. Long-term survival after surgical aortic valve replacement among patients over 65 years of age. doi:10.1136/openhrt-2015

23. Viktorsson SA, Helgason D, Orrason AW, et al. Favorable Survival after Aortic Valve Replacement Compared to the General Population. J Heart Valve Dis 2016;25(1):8–13.

24. Bonow R0, Rosing DR, Mcintosh CL, et al. The natural history of asymptomatic patients with aortic regurgitation and normal left ventricular function. Circulation 1983;68(3):509–17. http://ahajournals.org. Accessed October 11, 2021.

25. Bonow R, Lakatos E, Maron B, et al. Serial Long-term Assessment of the Natural History of Asymptomatic Patients With Chronic Aortic Regurgitation and Normal Left Ventricular Systolic Function. Circulation 1991;84(4):1625–35.

26. Dujardin K, Enriquez-Sarano M, Schaff H, et al. Mortality and morbidity of aortic regurgitation in clinical practice. A long-term follow-up study. Circulation 1999; 99(14):1851–7.

27. Tornos P, Sambola A, Permanyer-Miralda G, et al. Long-term outcome of surgi-cally treated aortic regurgitation: influence of guideline adherence toward early surgery. J Am Coll Cardiol 2006;47(5):1012–7.

28. Klodas E, Enriquez-Sarano M, Tajik A, et al. Optimizing timing of surgical correction in patients with severe aortic regurgitation: role of symptoms. J Am Coll Cardiol 1997;30(3):746–52.
29. Chaliki HP, Mohty D, Avierinos J-F, et al. Outcomes After Aortic Valve Replacement in Patients With Severe Aortic Regurgitation and Markedly Reduced Left Ventricular Function. Circulation 2002;106(21):2687–93.
30. Isaacs AJ, Shuhaiber J, Salemi A, et al. National trends in utilization and in-hospital outcomes of mechanical versus bioprosthetic aortic valve replacements. J Thorac Cardiovasc Surg 2015;149(5):1262–9.e3.
31. Russo M, Taramasso M, Guidotti A, et al. The Evolution of Surgical Valves. http://emh.ch/en/services/permissions.html.
32. Cizmic A, Kuhn E, Eghbalzadeh K, et al. Valve-in-Valve TAVR versus Redo Surgical Aortic Valve Replacement: Early Outcomes. Thorac Cardiovasc Surgeon 2021. https://doi.org/10.1055/s-0041-1735476.
33. Tuzcu EM, Kapadia SR, Vemulapalli S, et al. Transcatheter Aortic Valve Replacement of Failed Surgically Implanted Bioprostheses: The STS/ACC Registry. J Am Coll Cardiol 2018;72(4):370–82.
34. Cribier A, Saoudi N, Berland J, et al. Percutaneous transluminal valvuloplasty of acquired aortic stenosis in elderly patients: an alternative to valve replacement? Lancet 1986;327(8472):63–7.
35. Ancona R, Pinto S. Mitral valve incompetence: epidemiology and causes. Eur Soc Cardiol 2018;16(11).
36. Salem R, Zierer A, Karimian-Tabrizi A, et al. Aortic Valve Repair for Aortic Insufficiency or Dilatation: Technical Evolution and Long-term Outcomes. Ann Thorac Surg 2020;110(6):1967–73.
37. Cahill TJ, Prothero A, Wilson J, et al. Community prevalence, mechanisms and outcome of mitral or tricuspid regurgitation. Heart 2021;107(12):1003–9.
38. Levine RA, Hagége AA, Judge DP, et al. Mitral valve disease-morphology and mechanisms. Nat Rev Cardiol 2015;12(12):689–710.
39. Stout KK, Verrier ED. Acute valvular regurgitation. Circulation 2009;119(25):3232–41.
40. Watanabe N. Acute mitral regurgitation. Heart 2019;105(9):671–7.
41. D'Agostino RS, Jacobs JP, Badhwar V, et al. The society of thoracic surgeons adult cardiac surgery database: 2016 update on outcomes and quality. Ann Thorac Surg 2016;101(1):24–32.
42. El-Eshmawi A, Castillo JG, Tang GHL, et al. Developing a mitral valve center of excellence. Curr Opin Cardiol 2018;33(2):155–61.
43. Bonow RO, Adams DH. The Time Has Come to Define Centers of Excellence in Mitral Valve Repair. J Am Coll Cardiol 2016;67(5):449–501.
44. Lesevic H, Karl M, Braun D, et al. Long-Term Outcomes After MitraClip Implantation According to the Presence or Absence of EVEREST Inclusion Criteria. Am J Cardiol 2017;119(8):1255–61.
45. Mauri L, Foster E, Glower DD, et al. 4-Year results of a randomized controlled trial of percutaneous repair versus surgery for mitral regurgitation. J Am Coll Cardiol 2013;62(4):317–28.
46. Zhou S, Egorova N, Moskowitz G, et al. Trends in MitraClip, mitral valve repair, and mitral valve replacement from 2000 to 2016. J Thorac Cardiovasc Surg 2021;162(2):551–62.e4.
47. Badheka AO, Shah N, Ghatak A, et al. Balloon mitral valvuloplasty in the United States: A 13-year perspective. Am J Med 2014;127(11):1126.e1–12.

Moving?

Make sure your subscription moves with you!

To notify us of your new address, find your **Clinics Account Number** (located on your mailing label above your name), and contact customer service at:

Email: journalscustomerservice-usa@elsevier.com

800-654-2452 (subscribers in the U.S. & Canada)
314-447-8871 (subscribers outside of the U.S. & Canada)

Fax number: 314-447-8029

Elsevier Health Sciences Division
Subscription Customer Service
3251 Riverport Lane
Maryland Heights, MO 63043

*To ensure uninterrupted delivery of your subscription, please notify us at least 4 weeks in advance of move.

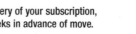

Printed and bound by CPI Group (UK) Ltd, Croydon, CR0 4YY

03/10/2024

01040476-0001